AF815660

Volker Langholf

Medical Theories in Hippocrates

Untersuchungen zur antiken Literatur und Geschichte

Herausgegeben von
Winfried Bühler, Peter Herrmann und Otto Zwierlein

Band 34

Walter de Gruyter · Berlin · New York
1990

Medical Theories in Hippocrates

Early Texts and the 'Epidemics'

by

Volker Langholf

Walter de Gruyter · Berlin · New York
1990

Als Habilitationsschrift auf Empfehlung des
Fachbereichs Geschichtswissenschaft der Universität Hamburg
gedruckt mit Unterstützung der Deutschen Forschungsgemeinschaft

Gedruckt auf säurefreiem Papier
(alterungsbeständig – pH 7, neutral)

CIP-Titelaufnahme der Deutschen Bibliothek

Langholf, Volker:
Medical theories in Hippocrates early texts and the 'Epidemics' / von Volker Langholf. – Berlin ; New York : de Gruyter, 1990
(Untersuchungen zur antiken Literatur und Geschichte ; Bd. 34)
Zugl.: Hamburg, Univ., Habil.-Schr.
ISBN 3-11-011956-0
NE: GT

© Copyright 1990 by Walter de Gruyter & Co., D-1000 Berlin 30.
Dieses Werk einschließlich aller seiner Teile ist urheberrechtlich geschützt. Jede Verwertung außerhalb der engen Grenzen des Urheberrechtsgesetzes ist ohne Zustimmung des Verlages unzulässig und strafbar. Das gilt insbesondere für Vervielfältigungen, Übersetzungen, Mikroverfilmungen und die Einspeicherung und Verarbeitung in elektronischen Systemen.
Printed in Germany
Satz und Druck: Arthur Collignon GmbH, Berlin 30
Buchbinderische Verarbeitung: Lüderitz & Bauer, Berlin 61

Contents

Introduction

This book is about the application and evolution of medical theories in the so-called Hippocratic treatises. According to *Epidemics I*, ch. 5 Li. (= ch. 11 Kw., Jones), "the art (*tékhnē*) [of medicine] has three [aspects]: the disease, the patient, and the physician."[1] The medical author understood that these three aspects were mutually complementary (or, put otherwise, each aspect was a function of the other two). The text continues: "The physician is the servant of [or, has an ancillary function in] the art: together with the physician, the patient must fight the disease."[2] The ancient physician was, of course, aware of further, more special aspects, which were comprised within the above-mentioned ones. There was, for instance, a rich tradition in pharmacology; there was prognosis; dietetics (i. e. knowledge concerning the interaction between food and bodily exercise); there was what we would today call physiology (i. e. knowledge concerning the parts and humours of the human body and how they work); yet another aspect was that the medical craft had historically evolved from simple beginnings to more sophisticated stages, that this evolution was a continuing process, and that certain developments were erroneous.[3]

Thus, considering the broad spectrum of different viewpoints from which it would be possible for the modern scholar to study Hippocratic medicine, it might appear that the aspect chosen as the subject of this book, the application and evolution of theories, offers but a limited approach. Since, however, Hippocratic theories presuppose plenty of concrete facts related to all aspects of medicine and are never so 'theoretical' and abstract as not to influence directly the daily occupation of the Hippocratic physician, it will, in the course of this study, be necessary to recall or to reconstruct many of these concrete facts.

To give a definition of the modern term 'theory' as used in this book proves a difficult undertaking. The Hippocratic Collection has numerous 'theories' and even uses the word *theōríē*, from which 'theory' is derived, but *theōríē* in the Collection has a more narrow sense than 'theory.' There

---

1 *Epid. I* 2.636.1–2 Li. = 1.190.3–4 Kw. = 1.164 Jones Ἡ τέχνη διὰ τριῶν· τὸ νόσημα καὶ ὁ νοσέων καὶ ὁ ἰητρός.

2 *Epid. I* 2.636.2–4 Li. = 1.190.4–6 Kw. = 1.164 Jones Ὁ ἰητρὸς ὑπηρέτης τῆς τέχνης· ὑπεναντιοῦσθαι τῷ νοσήματι τὸν νοσέοντα μετὰ τοῦ ἰητροῦ.

3 See here in particular the treatise *On Ancient Medicine* (Περὶ ἀρχαίης ἰητρικῆς).

is still a close semantic connection with the verb *theōreín*, 'to look at,' 'to behold,' also 'to contemplate in one's mind,' 'to consider.'[4] Studying the semantics of Greek terms cannot be a starting point for the present investigation, and particularly the meaning of the Greek word *theōríē* as indicated above does not help in defining what a Hippocratic theory is. In fact, when speaking of 'theories' in the Hippocratic Collection, one brings an unhistorical, even anachronistic element into one's research. But there seems to be no way for us to avoid that. Since we are so highly accustomed to thinking in modern terms, we cannot dismiss them, even if they are inadequate in historical contexts. Just as the Egyptian god Ammon (Amun) became Zeus for the ancient Greek historian in the *interpretatio Graeca*, so ancient Greek medical concepts and ideas for which there was no generic term during their time become 'theories' in our modern *interpretatio*.[5] Both procedures have their merits because they facilitate one's initial orientation in a strange world, as well as their limits because they may be misleading. We shall, therefore, use the modern term 'theory' as a heuristic tool rather than a descriptive label. There is no need to begin this investigation by giving a precise definition of what is to be understood by 'theory,' and we shall even avoid starting from a modern definition or concept of 'theory.' Instead, the word will be taken in its rather vague modern everyday meaning.[6] The word 'doctrine' will be used synonymously.

It is not yet possible, and perhaps it will never be so, to describe with chronological accuracy the formation of the medical theories in the Hip-

[4] Hannelore Rausch, Theoria. Von ihrer sakralen zur philosophischen Bedeutung, München, 1982 (= Humanistische Bibliothek, ser. I, vol. 29). Significant passages in the Hippocratic Collection: θεωρίη 'consideration' *Lex* 4.640.6 Li. = 2.264 Jones. θεωρέω 'to consider' *Acut.* 2.268.5 Li. = 1.119.9 Kw. = 2.78 Jones. *Acut. (Sp.)* 2.444.1 Li. = 1.159.10 Kw. *Epid. II* 5.76.11. *Coac.* 5.692.21. *Sept.* 7.448.14, 19 Li. = *Oct.* 80.6, 10 Gr. θεωρητός *Aph.* 4.476.12, 13 Li. = 4.114 Jones.

[5] The *interpretatio Graeca* may imply an adulteration of the original concepts, whereas our use of the word 'theory' and of other modern terms will, it is to be hoped, not have the effect of creating misunderstandings. Generally cf. Lloyd, Magic 1 f.; Mansfeld, Theoretical and empirical attitudes 378. For similar problems in modern historiography, see Karl Christ, "Theodor Mommsen und die römische Geschichte," in: Theodor Mommsen, Römische Geschichte, vol. 8, München, 1976, 35 f.

[6] The Hippocratic treatises distinguish between mental and manual activities: e. g. *VM* 1.572.1–2 Li. = 1.1.18–19 Kw. = 1.12 Jones οἱ δημιουργοὶ πολλὸν ἀλλήλων διαφέρουσιν κατὰ χεῖρα καὶ κατὰ γνώμην. *Morb. I* 6.150.6–20 Li. = 16.2–18 Wittern κατὰ γνώμην ... κατὰ δὲ χειρουργίην. Cf. Kudlien, Beginn 44. When translating these passages into modern languages, one might, of course, use the scheme of 'theoretical' and 'practical' activity, but it should then be kept in mind that these terms are anachronistic and imply too narrow an interpretation. In fact, either group of activities described in the *Morb. I* passage implies theoretical as well as practical elements. The whole chapter is about the daily routine of the physician.

pocratic Collection. There exists, so far, no history of early 'Hippocratic' medicine, not even a generally acknowledged chronology of the Hippocratic treatises, which have all been transmitted under the name of Hippocrates but cannot have been written by one person.

Considerable scepticism has prevailed since the middle of the twentieth century as to the possibility of solving the 'Hippocratic question,' namely the problem, which of the texts have been written by the historical Hippocrates, son of Herakleides, ca. 460—370 B.C. Few scholars have in recent decades attempted to demonstrate or ventured to assert that certain treatises are 'genuine,'[7] and since agreement is unlikely to be reached on this topic, no effort will be made in this book to distinguish between 'Hippocratic' and 'non-Hippocratic' (or 'spurious') works of the Collection.[8]

Apart from the specific problem of authorship, scholars have proposed dates for each of the treatises. However, because of the scarcity of evidence, to speak of dates is most often to tread on unsafe ground. Even the modern term 'treatise' is suspect. Many of the Hippocratic writings, although possessing well attested titles in quotations since antiquity, are compilations which are so heterogeneous in their contents and style that such normally indispensable tools of philology like the terms 'treatise,' 'author,' 'compiler,' 'redactor' are of no or little use.[9] In any such 'treatise' it is occasionally possible to date certain passages, but it is not always wise to extend automatically the date to the entire work. Apart from absolute dating of treatises, attempts to establish a relative chronology among the Hippocratic works meet with similar difficulties and objections. In this book, however, one assumption about the relative date of *On Diseases II*,

---

[7] Although Wesley D. Smith's study, The Hippocratic tradition (1979), suggests that rethinking the methodological basis for ascriptions of authorship in the Corpus Hippocraticum is not unwarranted, his assertion that a particular treatise, *On Regimen* (*De victu*) is by Hippocrates is open to the same objections hitherto raised to earlier such proposals: *(i)* contemporary information on the historical Hippocrates is scarce; *(ii)* congruences between such testimonies and extant medical treatises of the Corpus are not necessarily proofs of authorship. (Smith, Hippocratic tradition, ch. 1, gives a good account of previous research and scholarship on the subject; cf. Lloyd, Hippocratic question. For additional bibliography, see Joly, Question hippocratique.) More recently, in fact, after completing the manuscript of the present book, I have myself proposed some new arguments in favour of the authenticity of *On Breaths* (*De flatibus*), a treatise or rather speech which appears to be referred to by the early Aristotelian school (Menon, 'Anonymus Londinensis'), by Antiphanes (fourth century B.C., middle Attic comedy), and by the early Alexandrian librarian, Callimachus (see Langholf, Kallimachos). Since, however, the Hippocratic question is beyond the scope of the present book, *On Breaths* will not be discussed in the following pages except for occasional mentions.

[8] For the problems posed by these very categories of literary criticism as applied to the Hippocratic Collection, see Langholf, Kallimachos 21—30.

[9] For the terms 'treatise' etc., see Langholf, Kallimachos 21—30.

ch. 12–75, is fundamental: namely, that these chapters reflect a stage of development of Greek medicine prior to that of the *Epidemics*.[10]

This is not the place to go into details of chronology, but a word should be said about our justification for dealing with the evidence of a historical process, application and evolution of medical theories, in a field where even fundamental historical facts are as yet not known to us and may never be known. Not only is useful information lacking concerning the identities of Hippocratic authors and the dates of their 'treatises,' but also we have very little concrete evidence for their geographic provenance. In recent years much of what modern scholarship believed to be true about the organizational and social framework within which Greek medicine of the fifth and fourth centuries was practised and the treatises were written, in particular the scholarly assumptions about the 'medical schools' of Kos and Knidos, have proved to be unsubstantiated by the sources and, therefore, questionable. The attempt to assign treatises to ancient medical 'schools' resulted in Karl Deichgräber's influential book, Die Epidemien und das Corpus Hippocraticum. Voruntersuchungen zu einer Geschichte der koischen Ärzteschule (1933; 2nd ed. 1971); the discussion of the issue reached its climax with the publication of two books full of valuable observations: Hermann Grensemann, Knidische Medizin (1975), and Jacques Jouanna, Hippocrate. Pour une archéologie de l'école de Cnide (1974). These two 'Knidian' studies immediately provoked opposition[11] and were countered by arguments which were in principle those already put forward some months before publication of either book in a brilliant article by Wesley D. Smith, Galen on Coans versus Cnidians (1973). Smith demonstrated that the passages in Galen, on whose basis the Hippocratic treatises were customarily divided into 'Koan' and 'Knidian,' do not justify the belief that in these two neighbouring cities "rigid schools existed with peculiar and exclusive doctrines."[12] The view that there existed in fifth and fourth century Kos and Knidos a situation "school versus school" cannot be substantiated. Jutta Kollesch and Fridolf Kudlien concluded subsequently that between the physicians of the two towns a mutual give and take in matters of doctrine and therapeutic methods must have been necessarily usual.[13]

I follow this new interpretation, of which the principal arguments will be presented in Chapter I. It will be apparent that the historically more

---

10 For the date of the *Epidemics*, see below p. 77f.; for the relative chronology of *On Diseases II*, ch. 12–75, see below p. 25, 37, 52f., 123–126.

11 Kudlien, Bemerkungen. Kollesch, Stellung. Volker Langholf, Gymnasium 83 (1976), 475–477. Fridolf Kudlien, Gnomon 55 (1983), 360–362. Di Benedetto, Cos e Cnido.

12 Smith, Galen on Coans 572.

13 See their articles referred to above.

acceptable thesis of a free exchange of ideas and techniques between the medical centres allows for a more complete historical reconstruction of Greek medicine in the fifth and fourth centuries B. C. Evolutions of medical theories and practices, which were hitherto thought to have been more or less confined to one side respectively of the straits dividing (or rather connecting) the island of Kos and the peninsula of Knidos, can now be studied as constituents of a more widespread, perhaps general, development. In particular, the historical and systematic relationship between the *Epidemics* and the traditional nosology of *On Diseases II*, ch. 12–75 can now be more adequately understood. The view that treatises of the Hippocratic Collection can be traced to a Koan or to a Knidian medical 'school' respectively has been given up in the present study. Although there are texts in the *Epidemics* and in other treatises which appear to originate in a situation in which a medical teacher instructed pupils or apprentices,[14] nothing can be made out about any doctrinal or organizational affiliations to medical 'schools.'[15]

---

[14] See below p. 140–145.

[15] A different approach has been followed in a study by Antoine Thivel, Cnide et Cos? Essai sur les doctrines médicales dans la Collection hippocratique (1981). He begins with the assumption that *On Diseases II* and *On Internal Diseases* (*Morb. II* and *Int.*) are Knidian, and that certain other treatises of the Collection are Koan; cf. his two indices s. v. 'Coaques (médecins),' p. 400, and 'Cos,' p. 408. Then he gathers arguments in support of the view that the physicians of the two cities adhered to essentially the same medical doctrines and practices. Thivel's initial assumption is, however, not intended to be merely an auxiliary construction. He does not aim at carrying this assumption *ad absurdum*. Although he employs in a few instances quotation marks (in the sense of 'so-called') with such expressions like 'Knidian treatises,' and although he states in a footnote (p. 220) that the expressions 'Koan treatise' and 'Knidian treatise' should be taken only in the sense that the treatises are customarily assigned to these cities, Thivel yet posits certain minor doctrinal differences between the two medical centres; he does so relying on a classification of the Hippocratic treatises as Koan or Knidian (e. g., p. 211, 270). He does not go so far as to state explicitly that such a classification is unjustified, albeit the weight of his own arguments should have carried him to this inference. Instead, he cogently demonstrates with abundant evidence that it is more productive to classify the treatises according to other criteria. This demonstration is the valuable feature of his book (cf. the review by Otta Wenskus, Gnomon 55 (1983), 410–414). Subsequently, Thivel has clarified his standpoint by stating that he should rather have spoken of "so-called" Knidian and Koan treatises (Médecine hippocratique et pensée ionienne, in: Formes de pensée 211–232, in particular 217). The reader will find that Thivel's book and mine overlap with regard to the Kos and Knidos subject, but that the evidence put forward is rarely the same. This is an indication that there might be more evidence. In such instances I have quoted Thivel's work whenever I found that he provides additional details of relevance. These quotations (in my notes) are added merely as postscripts, since Thivel's book was published after the substance of my Chapter I had been formulated. I have not systematically discussed his results, since Thivel and I basically agree that the Hippocratic Collection does not betray fundamental doctrinal differences between Koan and Knidian physicians.

Caution is similarly not out of place with regard to the above-mentioned problem of modern terminology. Louis Bourgey, Observation et expérience chez les médecins de la Collection hippocratique (1953), has stimulated me more than might appear from the number of explicit references made to it. His method is different from mine. He commences by arranging the Hippocratic works in three groups according to various types of authors: theoretical physicians (special chapters on p. 47–50; 109–144), empirical physicians (p. 50–56; 145–188), and positivist or rational physicians (p. 56–66; 189–275).[16] The 'Knidian' treatises form part of his second group, the 'Koan' constitute his third group. It is obvious already from his chapter headings that Bourgey's classification depends on the use of modern terminology, which he uses as an analytical tool, first to arrange the ancient treatises in groups, and secondly to describe each group. This methodological approach is legitimate as far as its principles are concerned. I shall be following it myself in the present study. The analysis or interpretation of the Hippocratic treatises, however, will yield more insights to the historian who uses as few modern terms as possible. Albeit one cannot do completely without such terminology, and the terms 'empiricism,' 'positivism,' 'rationalism,' or 'theory' are heuristically useful at times for the historian in labelling certain tendencies or characteristics of texts of the fifth and fourth centuries, still it is doubtful whether such terms can serve as the basis for reconstructing the complex development of human activity and thought during an epoch wherein the concepts signified by the terms had not yet formed. Modern terminology should serve a more modest, peripheral function.

At the present stage of Hippocratic scholarship it is possible to formulate some historical problems more precisely and less anachronistically

---

No reference will be made to two recent studies which appeared after the manuscript of the present book had been completed: *(i)* Vincenzo Di Benedetto, Il medico e la malattia. La scienza di Ippocrate, Torino, 1986 (Einaudi Paperbacks, 172); cf. my review in Anzeiger f. d. Altertumsw. 42 (1989), 24 f. *(ii)* Hermann Grensemann, Knidische Medizin, Teil II: Versuch einer weiteren Analyse der Schicht A in den pseudohippokratischen Schriften De natura muliebri und De muliebribus I und II (Hermes Einzelschriften, 51), Wiesbaden/Stuttgart 1987. Despite its small size of 91 pages, this methodologically important study is fundamental for further research in the gynaecological treatises and, moreover, in the earliest history of Greek medicine. The book opens new and surprising perspectives in suggesting (p. 69 f.) that certain therapeutical specialties, which appear to be historically related to Knidos (see below p. 28–30), occur predominantly in Grensemann's text stratum A 2. New light is also shed on the early history of humoral pathology (p. 70–72).

[16] Bourgey uses the following short formulas (p. 66): "... trois orientations intellectuelles, ... trois grandes familles d'esprit: les médecins théoriciens, les médecins à tendance empirique, les médecins capables enfins de lier correctement l'observation à la raison, et que nous appellerons les médecins positifs."

than philologists and medical historians of previous decades could. Certain obstacles which hinder a solution to some of these problems can now be recognized more clearly. With regard to our special problem, how medical theories evolved and were applied, the historical sources will permit, I believe, tentative answers to the following questions:

(i) What are the medical theories contained in the writings of the Hippocratic Collection?
(ii) To what extent do these theories contradict each other?
(iii) To what extent are they compatible with each other?
(iv) Can these theories be grouped as stages of a general historical development of Greek medicine?
(v) If so, on what general outlines did this development take place, and what are the specific steps involved?

It should, however, be kept in mind that these questions cannot be asked simply sequentially, and that it is not wise to regard any answers given to any one question as a firm basis for further inferences. Conclusions remain proposals. I shall, therefore, not attempt to reconstruct the development of Greek medical theory in the fifth and fourth centuries with any completeness. Since the source material is fragmentary and only roughly dated, nothing more can be expected than to achieve some insight into a few features and principles of this development.

Now, let us survey briefly the contents of this book. Chapters I and II are intended to provide the background to Chapter III ("The *Epidemics* treatises"). Chapter I deals with the above-mentioned problem of medical 'schools' in Kos and Knidos. Chapter II starts by describing a development in meaning of some 'medical' substantives, tracing their unspecific and rather comprehensive usage in archaic and in colloquial texts to a narrower, almost terminological application in the Hippocratic treatises, where their signification is more directly related to sensory perception. The chapter then describes the methods of cognition applied by the authors of the oldest extant nosological[17] texts (exemplified by the chapters 12–75 of *On Diseases II*). As Grensemann and Jouanna have set forth, these texts stand nearest to a lost inferred common source for all of the nosological treatises of the Collection and reflect, therefore, a relatively ancient stage of medical thought and practice.[18] I shall demonstrate that these texts, which cannot be proved to have originated from a Knidian 'school,' are

[17] The substantive 'nosology' in its modern sense 'general description of the species of diseases' seems not to have been used in antiquity. Liddell/Scott/Jones quote only the verb from Anonymus Londin. XI 40 τὸ αἴτιον οὕτως νοσολογεῖ, words that are dubiously transmitted (cf. Diels's edition, p. 17).

[18] *Passim* in their books quoted above.

'forerunners' of the *Epidemics* in their methods of cognition and of disease description.

In Chapter III, which constitutes the central section of the book, the *Epidemics* are examined in the light of the results obtained in the preceding chapters. The perspectives are varied: What doctrine on *krísis* and critical days do the *Epidemics* set forth or presuppose (III 1)? What are the roots of this doctrine (III 2)? What research methods can be reconstructed from the extant *Epidemics* texts (III 3)? This latter section is subdivided into a series of smaller studies which are not designed to form a logical or systematic sequence. Their purpose is rather to present some more or less autonomous results. Here as in other sections of the book I have avoided as much as possible reconstructing a 'system' of medical theories out of these results, mainly for two reasons: first, our historical sources do not permit us to assess how systematic the theories underlying the *Epidemics* were, because these composite books, as many others of the Collection, are not very explicit with regard to their medical doctrines; second, the authors of the treatises are involved in speculations, and any modern attempts at reconstructing their speculations must to some degree be speculative themselves. The results thus obtained by the medical historian must not be used as building-stones for constructing a 'system' which might prove to be merely a house of cards.

Chapter IV, which deals with "Prognosis and divination," is a loosely attached appendix. This chapter could alternatively have been located between Chapters II and III; there, however, it would have been too disruptive. Although it describes, as Chapters I and II do, the 'background' of the *Epidemics*, its contents are not presupposed in Chapter III.

The notorious problem of the origins of Hippocratic doctrines in contemporary or earlier natural philosophy[19] has been touched upon where necessary, but has generally been beyond the scope of this book, which deals primarily with the *medical* aspects of Hippocratic theories and with the application and evolution of medical doctrines within the medical profession.

With regard to quotations and references, the following principles have been adopted: Except for the footnotes, quotations of Greek and Latin texts have in each instance been translated, and single Greek words have been transliterated. Quotations in Greek and Latin language have been confined to the footnotes. Variant readings are documented there whenever they modify the sense of a passage or are otherwise of interest. Critical annotations enclosed in round brackets ( ) indicate, as a rule, the readings from all the relevant Greek Hippocratic manuscripts and from extant

[19] See, for instance, *passim* in Schumacher, Antike Medizin; Lonie, Hippocratic treatises; Thivel, Cnide, and the bibliography listed in these works.

ancient commentaries on Hippocratic treatises. Since some of these commentaries have a rather rich manuscript tradition of their own, their variant readings cannot always be quoted *in toto*.

The numerous Hippocratic manuscripts are not all relevant. Many are only copies of available older ones and can, therefore, be dismissed as text sources.[20] No manuscript contains the whole Collection: each of the important ones has its own unique selection of treatises.[21] Quite often two or more codices overlap with regard to contents. The Hippocratic manuscripts are referred to by the letter symbols current in modern philological literature.[22]

The mutual relationship of these manuscripts is as follows: A, C′ and θ have equal claim to authenticity. M and V *together* (i. e., if they agree with each other) have the same claim as any one of the group A, C′, θ. The '*recentiores*' H, I, R replace lost pages of M. Apart from the Hippocratic manuscripts proper, the aforementioned ancient commentaries[23] contain the Hippocratic texts on which they comment, or parts of texts. Several of the commentaries are available in their original Greek version; others are extant only in Arabic or Latin translations made in the middle ages.

---

[20] For recent literature see the articles by A. Anastassiou and S. Byl in Hippocratica 17–31 and 73–85 respectively; also Manetti/Roselli (ed.), Ippocrate, Epidemie, Libro sesto; Grensemann, Gynäkologie 62–76.

[21] M and its copies are, of course, more uniform.

[22] The following list is complete only as far as the quotations in this book are concerned:

A = Parisinus Graecus 2253, 11th/beginning of 12th c.
C′ = Parisinus 446 suppl., 10th c.
H = Parisinus Graecus 2142, 14th c. (its more recent part)
I = Parisinus Graecus 2140, 13th/14th c.
M = Marcianus Venetus 269, 10th/11th c.
R = Vaticanus Graecus 277, 14th c.
V = Vaticanus Graecus 276, 12th c.
θ = Vindobonensis medicus 4, 10th/11th c.

For more details, see the prefaces of the modern critical editions of the respective treatises (cf. the bibliography).

[23] The abbreviations used are:

Gal. = Galen
Joh. = Johannes Alexandrinus
Pall. = Palladios (Pall. cod. U = Palladii codex Urbinas Graecus 64).

For details, see bibliography.

Other abbreviations used in the critical annotations are:

add. = addidit, addiderunt
in explic. = in explicatione [in the interpretative part of a commentary]
in lemm. = in lemmate [in the text quoted at the beginning of an interpretation in a commentary]
in marg. = in margine
om. = omisit, omiserunt
rec. = recentior(es).

The Hippocratic text of each of these commentaries has, again, the same claim to authenticity as have A or C′ or θ or the agreement of M and V.[24]

References to passages of the Hippocratic Collection are indicated by the title of the treatise,[25] the book (in Roman numerals), and the chapter (Arabic numerals); also the respective volumes and pages of modern editions are given. The basic edition still used today is Littré's, therefore it seemed necessary to refer to it.[26] But, despite two reprints, its availability in libraries is limited. The four Hippocrates volumes issued so far in Loeb's Classical Library (edited by Jones and Withington, with a useful English translation) have a wide circulation but are of limited philological value. Their chapter numbers sometimes differ from Littré's, and Littré's pages are not indicated in them. This may make it cumbersome to find a Littré reference in the Loeb text. Therefore, the Loeb volumes have been quoted in addition to Littré. But this seemed still insufficient, because neither Littré's text (which is antiquated) nor the one edited by Jones and Withington comes up to modern standards. For this reason, a third edition has been referred to whenever available, and whenever it seemed necessary to do so.[27] The texts reproduced in the quotations are taken from the best

[24] The descent can be represented simply as follows:

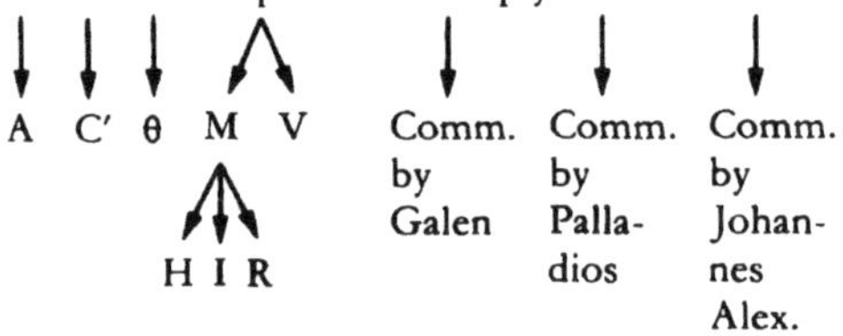

For a more nuanced description see Grensemann, Gynäkologie 39 ff.

[25] The abbreviations of ancient authors' names and works are, with occasional modifications, those of Liddell/Scott/Jones, A Greek-English dictionary.

[26] Littré did not number his lines. It is customary in modern publications to count them including the titles, but excluding the pagination and the page headlines.

[27] The abbreviations are:

Gr.	=	Grensemann
Kw.	=	Kühlewein
Li.	=	Littré
Per. ... La.	=	'Perikope' [i. e., paragraph] in Langholf, Syntaktische Untersuchungen.

Since recent editions, e. g. the one of *Prog.* by Alexanderson, and especially those published in the Corpus Medicorum Graecorum and in the Budé series (Collection des universités de France), indicate Littré's pages, it seemed unnecessary always to mention them in the quotations, although they have in every instance been consulted.

References without further indications are to Littré.

Other abbreviations:

K.	=	Kühn (editor of Galen)
CMG	=	Corpus Medicorum Graecorum.

For details, see bibliography.

editions or based on the evidence of the relevant Greek manuscripts (microfilms) and ancient commentaries. Occasionally I have changed the wording of the editions. Since the texts are often highly technical or otherwise difficult to understand, I have abridged the quotations as little as possible and provided a translation, thereby enabling the non-Hellenist to follow the main arguments throughout. In transcribing the Greek, I have marked long vowels by horizontal strokes. Accents (always acute) indicate stressed syllables. Greek proper names have been transcribed without such auxiliary signs; very common proper names occur in their best-known form.[28]

I wish to express my gratitude to those persons in Hamburg and elsewhere who have read typed versions of this book, and whose help in the fields of philology, medical history, and/or English grammar has encouraged me over the years. Among them are Patricia and Lawrence Bliquez (Seattle), Karen Faulkner (Philadelphia), Hermann Grensemann (Hamburg), Mirko D. Grmek (Paris), Jacques Jouanna (Paris), Fridolf Kudlien (Kiel), Fernand Robert (Paris), Wesley D. Smith (Philadelphia). I owe a special debt of gratitude to Winfried Bühler (Hamburg), who, in addition to his numerous critical suggestions, has helped me in various ways, and to Joanne H. Phillips (Cambridge, Mass.), who has purged my text thoroughly. There is scarcely a page that has not profited from her acumen and learning, thanks to her method of administering the *absinthia taetra* (Lucretius *I* 936, *IV* 11). William Beck (Hamburg) has not only read the manuscript in an early stage but has also shared the burden of proof-reading.

Furthermore, I am pleased to mention several institutions whose aid made my research and its publication possible. From spring 1977 to the end of 1979, I was supported by a stipend granted by the Deutsche Forschungsgemeinschaft (DFG) and by a Resident Fellowship (summer 1977 to spring 1978) at the Center for Hellenic Studies, Washington, D. C. (Trustees for Harvard University). I wish to thank both the DFG and the former Director of the Washington Center, Bernard M. W. Knox, for enabling me to concentrate on my subject for almost three years. Thanks are due to the DFG also for a publication grant. I am, last but not least, very much indebted to those colleagues who have read the manuscript *ex officio*, and to the Thesaurus Linguae Graecae (Hamburg): The typescript of the recently published Index Hippocraticus has been an indispensable tool.

---

[28] This leads to inconsequences such as "Hippo*c*rates, son of Hera*k*leides" (Latin form versus transliteration).

I. Medical Practice and 'Schools' in Pre-Alexandrian Times: Kos and Knidos

Before we begin to discuss some medical expressions and medical theories of the Hippocratic treatises, it will be useful to examine the problem of 'medical schools' as outlined above. Since the nineteenth century, philologists and historians of medicine have attempted to assign these treatises to two (or even more) 'schools' which allegedly flourished in the fifth and fourth centuries B. C. One of them is the Koan 'school,' with which Hippocrates, a native of the island of Kos, was supposed to have been associated; another one is the Knidian 'school,' situated in the city of Knidos on the Asian peninsula of the same name, some 20 miles off Kos.

After Littré[1] and Ermerins,[2] the two great nineteenth century editors of the Hippocratic Collection, it was an almost undisputed belief among Hippocratic scholars that these two 'schools' (Kos and Knidos) were opposed to each other and defended certain doctrines and approaches to medicine which were peculiar to each of them.[3] Until recently, this modern belief underlay practically all that was written about the development of Greek medicine in the pre-Alexandrian age. It was not until the 1970's that the hypothesis was more closely inspected in a short article which deservedly became influential. Its author, Wesley D. Smith,[4] examining the relevant evidence found in the works of Galen, came to the conclusion that in modern scholarship "the very material ... was ignored or used very selectively." "Questions asked in research, and data accepted, have been dictated by the construct [of the two doctrinally opposed schools of Kos and Knidos] and then results thought to support it."[5]

---

[1] Œuvres complètes d'Hippocrate, cf. the bibliography.

[2] Hippocratis et aliorum medicorum veterum reliquiae, cf. the bibliography.

[3] On the earlier history of this belief since the seventeenth century see Lonie, Cos.

[4] Smith, Galen on Coans. An earlier sceptic in the Kos/Knidos question was a young scholar whose highly original book appeared in the same year as Deichgräber's influential work on "Die Epidemien und das Corpus Hippocraticum. Voruntersuchungen zu einer Geschichte der koischen Ärzteschule": Adolf Palm, Studien zur hippokratischen Schrift Περὶ διαίτης (dissertation, Dr. phil.), Tübingen, 1933. Another sceptic before Smith was Kudlien, Beginn 35–36.

[5] Both quotations from p. 585.

Smith does not question the well-attested fact that Kos[6] and Knidos[7] were medical centres, nor does he deny the possibility that in both cities medical literature was written. In fact, we possess, among the treatises of the Hippocratic Collection, a compilation called "Koan Prognoses" (*Kōi-akaí prognṓsies*); its title would seem to indicate that the work derived from Kos — but the earliest attestation of the title is in the second century A. D., although there are good reasons to believe that the book itself dates from the fourth century B. C. Its title may be just as old.[8] Furthermore, there is reference in the Hippocratic Collection to a lost work with the title "*Knidian Signs*" (*Knídiai gnṓmai*),[9] traces of which survive partly in

---

6 For Kos cf. Sherwin-White, Ancient Cos 256—289; Fraser, Ptolemaic Alexandria, vol. 1. 338 ff., vol. 2. 495 ff.

7 Grensemann, Knidische Medizin *passim*.

8 Gal. *In Hp. Epid. III comm.* p. 59.5,8; 62.8,12; 63.8 Wenkebach; cf. Gal. *Gloss.* 19.69,81 K. The fundamental monograph on *Coac.* is Poeppel, Κῳακαὶ προγνώσεις. Ancient attestations are discussed in vol. 1, p. 34—39; as a date of *Coac.*, Poeppel proposes the end of the fourth century B. C., p. 62—67. The edition by Littré (5.588—732) has not yet been replaced.

9 The usual English translation of Κνίδιαι γνῶμαι is 'Knidian Opinions,' a rendering that reflects the vagueness of the original title. The normal Greek term for a philosophical or scientific 'opinion' (i. e. doctrine or *placitum*) is, however, not γνώμη but δόξα. The Greek substantive γνώμη has several meanings. In the case of this title, its ambiguity must have been felt already in antiquity. First, γνώμη is a distinguishing 'mark,' a 'token' (see Liddell/Scott/Jones); in the Hippocratic Corpus, διαγνώμη occurs with the same meaning in *Carn.* 8.614.2 Li. = 22.7 Deichgräber (διαγνώμην V, Deichgr.: διὰ γνώμην falso Li.), and διαγινώσκω, διάγνωσις are, of course, frequent; if one takes the *nomen simplex* γνώμη in this sense, one might translate the title as 'Knidian Signs' (or, anachronistically, but more precisely, 'Knidian Symptomatology'). Second, γνώμη is the 'decree' of an assembly or corporation, a 'resolution.' One might conjecture that the Κνίδιαι γνῶμαι was an official document of a Knidian group of physicians, a text containing the main principles of their nosology. One might, on the grounds of this hypothesis, translate Κνίδιαι γνῶμαι as 'Knidian Resolutions,' but the plural would in this case be somewhat puzzling (the singular, which one would rather expect, is nowhere attested to), and it would be hard to explain why in the extant fragments of, and testimonies about, the Κνίδιαι γνῶμαι only internal diseases are dealt with. The work obviously did not contain texts on surgery, an aspect of medicine so important in the epoch, when no barrier existed between 'medicine' and surgery, that no group of physicians would have neglected it. The first translation given, 'Knidian Signs,' seems therefore preferable; and the Κνίδιαι γνῶμαι would then have its counterpart in the above-mentioned Κῳακαὶ προγνώσιες, 'Koan Prognoses' (or 'Koan Prognostic Signs'). Other translations of Κνίδιαι γνῶμαι are 'Knidian Sentences,' French 'Sentences cnidiennes,' German 'Knidische Sentenzen.' All of these renderings seem to imply that the text so entitled was in the form of maxims or aphorisms (cf., for instance, the Γνῶμαι of Democritus in Diels/Kranz 68 B 35—115; Jones [ed.], Hippocrates, vol. 2, p. XXV f.). There is, however, no evidence for such an assumption. It is also risky to speak — as has been done occasionally in recent scholarship — of a 'single Knidian sentence' as long as there exists any doubt as to whether the plural γνῶμαι refers to nosological descriptions (= 'chapters') rather than to signs or symptoms.

quotations by later writers, partly through reports or criticisms of it. The testimony contained in the beginning of the Hippocratic treatise *On Regimen in Acute Diseases*[10] is the oldest, and because it has been of fundamental importance for the question of the relationship between the two centres, a translation follows:

"Those who have written the so-called *Knídiai gnõmai* did describe correctly what the patients are suffering from in each disease, and how some diseases end. Up to this point, even a non-physician could give a correct description if he skilfully asked the patients what they are suffering.

---

[10] *Acut.* 2.224.2–228.6 Li. = 1.109.2–110.13 Kw. = 2.62–64 Jones = frg. 10 Gr. (In this note, Gal. = Galen's commentary; Gal. Plac. = Galen *De placitis Hippocratis et Platonis*, ed. Phillip De Lacy, 3 vols, Berlin, 1978–1984 [CMG V 4.1.2], vol. 2. 574.) Οἱ συγγράψαντες τὰς Κνιδίας καλεομένας γνώμας ὁποῖα (ὁποῖα AMV: ὁκόσα Gal.) μὲν πάσχουσιν οἱ κάμνοντες ἐν ἑκάστοισι τῶν νοσημάτων ὀρθῶς ἔγραψαν καὶ ὁποίως ἔνια ἀπέβαινεν (αὐτῶν post ἀπ. add. Gal.: om. AMV)· καὶ ἄχρι μὲν τούτων καὶ (ἣν post καὶ add. A: om. MV, Gal.) μὴ ἰητρὸς δύναιτ' ἂν (δύναιτ' ἂν AV, Gal.: ἂν δύναιτο M) ὀρθῶς συγγράψαι, εἰ εὖ παρὰ τῶν καμνόντων ἑκάστου πυθοίατο (πυθοίατο M, Galeni pars codicum: πευθίατο A: πύθοιτο V, Galeni codices plerique) ὁποῖα πάσχουσιν. (The Hippocratic manuscripts are more in favour of the plural πυθοίατο, which implies a grammatical inconsistency of number. It is the *lectio difficilior.*) ὁπόσα δὲ προσκαταμαθεῖν δεῖ (δεῖ AMV: χρὴ Gal.) τὸν ἰητρὸν μὴ λέγοντος τοῦ κάμνοντος, τούτων τὰ (τὰ MV, Gal. in lemm.: om. A, Gal. in explic.) πολλὰ παρεῖται, ἄλλ' ἐν ἄλλοισι καὶ ἐπίκαιρα ἔνια ἐόντα ἐς τέκμαρσιν. ὁπόταν δὲ ἐς τέκμαρσιν λέγηται ὡς (ὡς V, Gal.: ἢ ὡς AM falso, cf. infra ἢ ὡς κεῖνοι) χρὴ ἕκαστα ἰητρεύειν, ἐν τούτοισι πολλὰ ἑτεροίως γινώσκω ἢ ὡς κεῖνοι (κ- A: ἐκ- MV, Gal.) ἐπεξῄεσαν· καὶ οὐ μοῦνον διὰ τοῦτο οὐκ ἐπαινέω, ἀλλ' ὅτι καὶ ὀλίγοισι τὸν ἀριθμὸν τοῖσιν ἄκεσιν ἐχρέοντο (ἐχρέοντο AMV, Gal.: χρέονται Gal. Plac.)· τὰ γὰρ πλεῖστα αὐτοῖσιν εἴρηται, πλὴν τῶν ὀξέων νούσων, φάρμακα ἐλατήρια διδόναι καὶ ὀρὸν καὶ γάλα (ε(ι)ς post γάλα add. A^3, Gal.: om. AMV) τὴν ὥρην πιπίσκειν. εἰ μὲν οὖν ταῦτα ἀγαθὰ (ἦν post ἀγ. add. M, post ταῦτ' V, Gal.: om. A) καὶ ἁρμόζοντα τοῖσι νοσήμασιν, ἐφ' οἷσι παρῄνεον διδόναι, πολὺ (πολὺ AV: ἔτι M, Gal.) ἂν ἀξιώτερα ἦν ἐπαίνου (ἦν ἐπ. AV: ἐπ. ἦν M, Gal.), ὅτι ὀλίγα ἐόντα αὐτάρκεά ἐστιν· νῦν δὲ οὐχ οὕτως ἔχει. οἱ μέντοι ὕστερον ἐπιδιασκευάσαντες ἰητρικώτερον δή τι ἐπῆλθον περὶ τῶν προσοιστέων ἑκάστοισιν. ἀτὰρ οὐδὲ περὶ διαίτης οἱ ἀρχαῖοι συνέγραψαν οὐδὲν ἄξιον λόγου· καίτοι μέγα τοῦτο παρῆκαν. τὰς μέντοι πολυτροπίας τὰς ἐν ἑκάστῃ (-ῃ A: -ῃσι MV, Gal., Gal. Plac.) τῶν νούσων καὶ τὴν πολυσχιδίην (-σχι- AMV, Gal., Gal. Plac.: -σχε- Gal. quattuor codd.) αὐτῶν (αὐτ. MV, Gal., Gal. Plac.: om. A) οὐκ ἠγνόεον ἔνιοι (ἔνιοι AMV, Gal. Plac., Gal. unus cod.: om. Gal. ceteri)· τοὺς δ' ἀριθμοὺς ἑκάστου τῶν νοσημάτων σάφα ἐθέλοντες φράζειν οὐκ ὀρθῶς ἔγραψαν· μὴ γὰρ (καὶ post γὰρ add. MV, Gal. Plac., Gal. pars memoriae: om. A, Gal. alia pars memoriae) οὐκ εὐαρίθμητον (-ον AM, Gal., Gal. Plac.: -ως V) ᾖ (ᾖ Gal. Plac., Gal. pars: εἴη AV, Gal. pars: ἦν M), εἰ τούτῳ τις σημαίνηται (-αίνηται A recte, cf. Kühner/Gerth II 474: -ανεῖται MV, Gal. Plac., Gal. pars) τὴν τῶν καμνόντων νοῦσον, τὸ (τὸ AMV, Gal. Plac.: τῷ Gal.) ἕτερον τοῦ ἑτέρου διαφέρειν τι, (ante μὴ add. τὸ Gal. Plac.: om. AMV, Gal.) μὴ τωὐτὸ δὲ νόσημα δοκέειν (δοκέειν AMV, Gal., Gal. Plac.: -εῖ edd.) εἶναι, ἢν μὴ τωὐτὸ ὄνομα ἔχῃ. (τὸ ἕτερον τοῦ ἑτέρου is neuter in the most general sense: "one thing from the other;" hence one need not supply νόσημα, πάθος, πάθημα, ἀρρώστημα or the like. διαφέρειν and δοκέειν are parallel to each other and depend on εἰ τούτῳ … νοῦσον.)

But what the physician must know beyond that, and without the patient telling him, has mostly been left out of account [by the *Knídiai gnõmai*]. It is different in the various cases and sometimes important for the assessment [of the cases].

When it comes to a discussion about the methods of treatment in each case, I am often of a different opinion as compared with their approach. It is not simply for this [more general] reason that I am unable to agree with them; it is also [more especially] because they applied only a small number of remedies. In most cases — except the acute[11] diseases — they prescribed giving evacuative drugs and, as drinks, whey and milk according to the season. If these remedies were indeed good and appropriate to the diseases for which they were prescribed, it would be the more laudable because they suffice although being few in number. But in fact that is not the case. It must be admitted though that those who later revised [these texts] proceeded more in keeping with the medical profession as far as concerns what has to be administered in each case.

What the ancients (*hoi arkhaíoi*) wrote on regimen is not worth mentioning either. They left it out of consideration, despite its importance.

Nevertheless, some were well acquainted with the manifold varieties of each disease and with their differentiation. They were mistaken, however, when, in their writings, they wanted to indicate exactly the numbers [of varieties and differentiations] of each disease, because it is obviously quite difficult to tell numbers if one identifies the disease of each patient only on the basis of [the observation] how one disease *differs* from the other [instead of identifying it, for instance, on the basis of an observation of elements *common* to others], and on the basis of the assumption that two diseases are not identical[12] unless they have the same name."

As the text has been interpreted by modern scholars, a member of the Koan 'school' is assumed to be here criticizing the Knidian 'school.' There is, however, little ground for that assumption.[13] First, nothing is known about the author of *On Regimen in Acute Diseases*: there is no stringent argument that he was a Koan. Second, even if we should hypothesize that

[11] The expression 'acute disease' occurs in several other Hippocratic works too. 'Acute fever,' πυρετὸς ὀξύς, is used in *On Diseases II*, ch. 12—75 (*Morb. II* 7.74.3,10 Li. = 184.17, 185.6 Jouanna), 'acute pain,' ὀδύνη ὀξέη, is frequent there. (For the relatively early date of these chapters see below p. 25, 52f.) Also in other nosological treatises ὀξύς is used with nouns denoting single symptoms. Although νοῦσος ὀξέη is attested once in a very old chapter (52; cf. Grensemann, Knidische Medizin p. 144) of *Mul. I* (8.112.5), it seems that ὀξύς originally denoted a solitary 'piercing' symptom such as pain and only secondarily came to be applied to the disease as a whole.

[12] Illustrative of this last statement is a 'questionnaire' scheme underlying five texts of the Collection, see below p. 157—163.

[13] Lonie, A structural pattern 236.

he was a Koan, we possess practically no information about what a 'medical school' might have been like in the decades around 400 B. C. There are texts which bear witness to oral medical instruction, but they cannot be geographically located (see below p. 140–145); and there must have existed a medical professional centre in Knidos and in Kos respectively, but nothing is known about their organization. Although the vocational training of medical beginners may have been among their responsibilities, the term 'school' is probably an anachronistic designation. The author of the text quoted does not mention a school but several people (in the plural): "those who have written the so-called *Knídiai gnṓmai*;" "those who later revised [these texts];" "the ancients;" "some." It cannot be ascertained to what extent they formed 'schools,' or belonged to groups separate from, or identical with, each other, or included in one another. How they were organized, or whether they were organized at all also remains unknown.

The *Knídiai gnṓmai* were perhaps not exclusively Knidian.[14] They could have been connected with the medical centre of Knidos in various ways. Conceivably, they may have originated there and subsequently been taken over by non-Knidians, or they may have been taken over by Knidians from sources unknown to us, sources which may also have been available to non-Knidian physicians of that epoch.[15] Indeed, the material contained in them may have been the common property of Greek physicians at any time in the fifth and fourth centuries B. C. The physicians referred to in the text are not known. To believe that these authors and revisors were exclusively Knidian and/or formed any teams or even 'schools' is a speculation which cannot be substantiated by the extant sources. Galen[16] tells us that "those who later revised" the *Knídiai gnṓmai* were "the physicians of Knidos," and that they made a second edition. Galen's comments, however, need not be taken as an authentic testimony: he probably puts forward a learned conjecture, nothing more.[17] It is by no means certain that the revisors were Knidians; likewise, we cannot be sure that there was an official second edition rather than a number of independent adaptations made inside or outside the medical centre of Knidos, and perhaps partly still extant today in nosological treatises of the Hip-

[14] The author of *Acut.* speaks of οἱ συγγράψαντες τὰς Κνιδίας καλεομένας γνώμας, a formulation which *might* indicate that the ascription of the text to Knidos was disputable (if καλ. refers to Κνιδίας rather than to γνώμας, lit. "the *gnṓmai* called Knidian"). However, the expression could as well mean "the work known as *Knídiai gnṓmai*" (if καλ. refers to both words) and can, therefore, as H. Grensemann pointed out to me, itself not be used for calling in question the Knidian origin of the *Knídiai gnṓmai*. On the problem of the 'title' see Schmalzriedt, ΠΕΡΙ ΦΥΣΕΩΣ 41, note 19. Nachmanson, Buchtitel 14–25.

[15] See Kudlien, Bemerkungen.

[16] Gal. *In Hp. Acut. comm.* p. 120.5–14 Helmreich = frg. 11 Grensemann.

[17] Cf. Grensemann, Knidische Medizin p. 65.

pocratic Collection.[18] Probably the treatise *On Regimen in Acute Diseases* was written in an epoch when the older texts (or even their authors and/or revisors, if they were not anonymous) were still so well-known that no specification as to their identity was needed, and in an epoch when polemics were still useful, i. e. when the professional methods of those physicians were not yet outdated.[19]

How far in fact do the polemics go? "Those who have written the so-called *Knídiai gnōmai* did describe *correctly* what the patients are suffering from in each disease, and how some diseases end," but according to the author they were not exhaustive. Beyond that, their methods of medical treatment were inadequate. "It must be admitted though that those who later revised [these texts] proceeded *more in keeping with the medical profession* as far as concerns what has to be administered:" their therapy was still inadequate, but better. "What the ancients wrote on regimen is not worth mentioning. *They left it out of consideration, despite its importance*:" their dietetics are not criticized, but the fact that they omitted it. "*Some were well acquainted* with the manifold varieties of each disease and with their differentiation:" they were mistaken in trying to number them and in relying too much on names given to the diseases.[20]

Implied in this passage of *On Regimen in Acute Diseases* is a belief that medicine was constantly manifesting progress.[21] The same conviction underlies the passage immediately following the text which we have been dealing with: "I believe that one has to be attentive to the whole [range

[18] Jouanna (ed.), Hippocrate, Maladies II, p. 25–50, maintains that the *Knídiai gnōmai* were "l'ouvrage fondamental de la médecine de Cnide," that they were compiled and later revised by "une communauté de médecins assez unie," probably the Asklepiads of Knidos (p. 29), as an "ouvrage collectif des Cnidiens" (p. 48); that these physicians "avaient un enseignement propre qui se distinguait par certaines caractéristiques" (p. 30). None of these conjectures can be verified. It is mistaken to claim that *On Regimen in Acute Diseases* "atteste formellement ... une association de médecins ayant son enseignement propre, consigné dans un ouvrage fondamental propre" (p. 31). The testimonium says much less than that. It rather appears that this particular Hippocratic author had "son enseignement propre," which he contrasted to the doctrines of other physicians, regardless of any 'school' affiliation. On the complex problem of a "second edition," see Emonds, Zweite Auflage, *passim*, in partic. 22; on the Κνίδιαι γνῶμαι 22–23, 353. B. A. van Groningen, ΕΚΔΟΣΙΣ, Mnemosyne, Ser. IV, 16 (1963), 1–17.

[19] "Writers of the fourth century used the term 'the ancients' to include generations not far removed from their own or even the generation of their own youth." (Edelstein, Idea of progress 73–75, with examples.)

[20] The concept underlying this criticism is the opposition between *nómos* and *phýsis* popular in the fifth and fourth centuries B. C. Names belong to the sphere of human social convention, not of *phýsis*. See, Felix Heinimann, Nomos und Physis. Herkunft und Bedeutung einer Antithese im griechischen Denken des 5. Jahrhunderts, Schweizerische Beiträge zur Altertumswissenschaft 1, Basel 1945 (= repr. Darmstadt, 1965), 46 ff. 156 ff.

[21] Cf. Edelstein, Idea of progress 33 f., 37–39, 71.

of medical] science and practice: ... one must perform everything so as to distinguish oneself from the other [physicians] for the better." The author's opinion seems to be that his professional predecessors were not "attentive" to the whole field of medicine, but only to parts of it.[22] In addition to excellence in cognition he requires of the physician excellence in performance. Cognition and performance are a unity for this medical author, and both together form what he calls *tékhnē*, i. e. science as well as professional performance, cognition as well as everyday practical routine. Those whom he criticizes were good, but not excellent, because their cognition was biased by preconceived notions of nosological entities, and because their methods of treatment were undeveloped or non-existent. The modern reader gets the impression that the author, in spite of his polemics, held the *Knídiai gnṓmai* in a certain esteem, and over-emphasized his criticism. That his reference to the "so-called *Knídiai gnṓmai*" ("even a non-physician could write correctly if he skilfully asked the patients what they are suffering") is somewhat biased by his polemical purposes can be verified directly by examination of the two extant fragments of the *Knídiai gnṓmai*.

One of them is a quotation by Galen and reads as follows: "The word *pémphix* is also used in the *Knídiai gnṓmai*, which people attribute to the physician Euryphon, thus: 'He urinates small amounts at a time, and a *pémphix* (bubble? scum? hue?) like olive oil stands on the surface, pale like a spider's web.'"[23] This observation could only be described and used

---

[22] *Acut.* 2.230.1–232.2 Li. = 1.110.14–20 Kw. = 2.64 Jones Ἐμοὶ δὲ ἁνδάνει μὲν ἐν πάσῃ τῇ τέχνῃ προσέχειν τὸν νοῦν· ... πάντα ... διαφερόντως τῶν πέλας ἐπὶ τὸ βέλτιον ποιεῖν χρή. Cf. Knutzen, Technologie 22, 41–45. I have followed Knutzen in translating τέχνη by '(medical) science and practice;' the word comprises indeed both aspects. Cf. Kudlien, Beginn 28, 44. But I cannot follow his statement that πᾶσα ἡ τέχνη denotes "die Einheit in der Distribution" (p. 22).

[23] Gal. *In Hp. Epid. VI comm.* p. 54.1–4 Wenkebach = frg. 13 Grensemann εἴρηταί γε μὴν ἡ πέμφιξ κἀν ταῖς Κνιδίαις γνώμαις, ἃς εἰς Εὐρυφῶντα τὸν [και] ἰατρὸν ἀναφέρουσι, τήνδε τὴν λέξιν· "οὐρέει ὀλίγον ἑκάστοτε αἰεὶ καὶ ἐφίσταται πέμφιξ οἷον ἐλαίου, χλωρή, ὥσπερ ἀράχνιον." Galen adds, "They [for the meaning of οὗτοι see below] seem to have called *pémphix* not the whole blister but only that which is around it outside and which resembles a spider's web." ἐοίκασι γοῦν οὗτοι πέμφιγα καλεῖν οὐχ ὅλην τὴν φλύκταιναν, ἀλλὰ μόνον τὸ περιγράφον αὐτὴν ἔξωθεν ἀραχνίῳ παραπλήσιον. "They" cannot be the authors of the fragment, because quite obviously the fragment of the *Knídiai gnṓmai* does not speak of blisters at all: in the Hippocratic Collection the word ἐφίσταμαι is never used for blisters or any other symptoms of the skin, whereas it is the usual word to express that something 'stands on the surface' of the urine. The whole fragment is about urine, and there are notable parallels in the Hippocratic Collection: *Prog.* 2.142.6–8 Li. = 1.90.21–91.1 Kw. = 2.26 Jones (in a passage on urine), "Greasy substances like a spider's web standing on the surface are to be disapproved of; they indicate emaciation." καὶ τὰς λιπαρότητας δὲ τὰς ἄνω ἐφισταμένας ἀραχνοειδέας μέμφεσθαι, συντήξιος γὰρ σημεῖα. Galen, commenting on this latter passage (Gal. *In Hp. Prog. comm.* p. 288.17–21 Heeg) compares it to the 'scum' (γραῦς) which appears when a greasy broth has cooled. *Aph.* 4.586.1–4 Li. = 4.198–200 Jones ὁκόσοισι δὲ ἐπὶ

successfully, if both the author and the reader very closely examined the urine themselves. A description given by the patient would certainly have been inadequate to identify the disease.

The same holds true of the other fragment of the *Knídiai gnṓmai* preserved as a quotation by Rufus of Ephesus: "If *nephrĩtis* afflicts [the patient], these are the signs: he urinates thick and purulent urine, and pain befalls him that stretches into the loins and flanks and groin and the pubic

---

τοῖσιν οὔροισιν ἐφίστανται (ἐφίστανται MV: ὑφ- C') πομφόλυγες, νεφριτικὰ σημαίνουσι ... ὁκόσοισι δὲ λιπαρὴ ἡ ἐπίστασις καὶ ἀθρόη, τουτέοισι νεφριτικὰ καὶ ὀξέα σημαίνει. *Epid. IV* 5.152.8–9 Li. = Per. 110 La. For a fuller discussion see Jouanna, Archéologie, p. 131, note 3b. If Galen misunderstood the *Knídiai gnṓmai* fragment, as Jouanna maintains, and took it to refer to blisters, this would be a strong indication, if not a proof that Galen did not read that work in its entirety when he wrote his commentary on *Epid. VI* but relied on quotations; which is certainly the case with regard to the material he cites from classical poets and from Thucydides in the same context on the six immediately preceding CMG pages: for these quotations he relied on philological works as he explicitly states p. 47.25–48.2. (A detailed discussion of the quotations in this passage of Galen's commentary on *Epid. VI* is found in Ernst Wenkebach, Dichterzitate in Galens Erklärung einer hippokratischen Fieberbezeichnung, Abhandlungen der phil. – hist. Klasse der Sächsischen Akademie der Wissenschaften, vol. 39, no. 1, Leipzig, 1928. Ernst Wenkebach, ΠΕΜΦΙΞ. Glossographische Verszitate in neuer Gestalt, Philologus, 86 (= N. F. 40) (1931), 300–331.) If the assumption is correct that Galen quoted the *Knídiai gnṓmai* fragment only at second hand, the same should hold true of the famous fragment of Euryphon cited one page later in his commentary (p. 55.11–16 = frg. 15 Grensemann), cf. shortly below. (Cf. also Jutta Kollesch's review of Grensemann's book, Deutsche Literaturzeitung 97 (1976), 408–412, in particular footnote 1.) Independently, however, of the question whether Galen quoted directly or at second hand, it is quite inconceivable that he should have misunderstood the fragment about the urine. Galen must have known the Hippocratic parallel material. Fridolf Kudlien in his review of Jouanna, Archéologie (Gnomon 55 [1983], 360–362) has attempted to vindicate Galen. The original meaning of φλύκταινα (< φλύω, φλύζω), he argues, must have been 'bubble,' as e. g. in boiling liquids; and although the meaning was narrowed down to 'skin blister,' Galen may in his comment on the fragment have retained the original meaning, 'bubble.' I do not find this plausible, because the meaning 'bubble' is nowhere attested for φλύκταινα. To postulate this meaning here would imply that Galen, quite contrary to his habit, expressed himself enigmatically in an obsolete vocabulary. The key to the problem, I believe, lies in the expression "they," οὗτοι, which does not refer specifically to the Knidians or to the authors of the *Knídiai gnṓmai*, but more generally to the ancient physicians including also the author of *Epid. VI* 1.14, where Galen is trying to explain πεμφιγώδεες (πυρετοί). As the word πέμφιξ or its derivatives do not occur in the Hippocratic Collection except for *Epid. VI* 1.14, Galen quotes a number of ancient authors and finally the *Knídiai gnṓmai*, in commenting: "They [the ancient authors] seem to call πέμφιξ not the whole blister, but only its outward part similar to a spider's web." The usage of πέμφιξ in the context of blisters (φλύκταιναι) is thus *analogous* to its usage in the context of urine, but φλύκταιναι do not form in urine. The fact that Galen quotes the *Knídiai gnṓmai* in order to explain *Epid. VI* indicates that he did not, at least in this context, differentiate between 'schools' of medicine.

region and sometimes also into the *alōpekes*."[24] Of course, it is the patient who informs the physician about the regions where he feels pain; the patient can directly point to them, or he can speak of some of them. It is unlikely that a patient who was not himself a physician knew what the muscles called *alōpekes* were, or what purulent urine looked like. As with regard to the first passage on the urine, this description is so technical that neither the author nor the user of this text could have relied on a patient's words. Both fragments furnish sufficient proof that the *Knídiai gnōmai* were much more professional than the author of *On Regimen in Acute Diseases* is willing to maintain. His criticism is too general and, therefore, exaggerated.

Two more text fragments have usually been regarded as originating in the *Knídiai gnōmai*. They have been transmitted as quotations by Galen. The first describes a feature criticized by the author of *On Regimen in Acute Diseases* as typical of some medical texts he knew, i. e. a tendency "to indicate exactly the numbers [of varieties and differentiations] of each disease" (cf. above). The author of *On Regimen in Acute Diseases* does not explicitly assign the mistake to "those who have written the so-called *Knídiai gnōmai*," but to "some," who may or may not be identical with them or with "those who later revised [these texts]" or with "the ancients." In his commentary on this passage of *On Regimen in Acute Diseases*, Galen quotes some words from a text of unknown provenance: "Seven diseases of the gall," "twelve diseases from the bladder," "four diseases of the kidneys," "from the bladder, four diseases of urine retention," "three tetani," "four jaundices," "three consumptions."[25] Since it is unknown whether this quotation is from the *Knídiai gnōmai* or any other Knidian source at all (there is a gap in Galen's text), and since it is uncertain whether the feature described in *On Regimen in Acute Diseases* is typical exclusively of the *Knídiai gnōmai*, the quotation in Galen should be used with due caution for any reconstructions of the *Knídiai gnōmai*.

---

[24] Ruf. p. 159.13–160.2 (Œuvres de Rufus d'Ephèse edd. Ch. Daremberg et Ch. E. Ruelle, Paris, 1879 [= repr. Amsterdam, 1963]) = frg. 14 Grensemann τοῦτο ἄρα ἦν καὶ τὸ ἐν ταῖς Κνιδίαις γνώμαις γεγραμμένον· ἐὰν δὲ νεφρῖτις ἔχῃ, σημεῖα τάδε· οὐρέει παχὺ πυῶδες καὶ ὀδύναι ἔχουσιν ἔς τε τὴν ὀσφῦν καὶ τοὺς κενεῶνας καὶ τοὺς βουβῶνας καὶ τὸ ἐπίσιον, τοτὲ δὲ καὶ ἐς τὰς ἀλώπεκας.

[25] Gal. *In Hp. Acut. comm.* p. 121.21–122.3 Helmreich, cf. 117.11–13; = frg. 12 Grensemann. Although there is a lacuna in p. 121.22, it seems quite possible that the quotation is (directly or indirectly) taken from the *Knídiai gnōmai* (cf. Grensemann p. 64 f.), because the expression is archaic and the dialect is Ionian (with the usual secondary influence of Attic Greek): εἶπον ὀλίγον ἔμπροσθεν κατ' ἀρχὰς ὅτι ἔγραψαν οἱ ἀπὸ τῆς Κνίδου ⟨...⟩ "χολῆς νοῦσοι ἑπτά," κατὰ δὲ τὸν αὐτὸν τρόπον πάλιν κατωτέρω "ἀπὸ τῆς κύστεως νοῦσοι δώδεκα," καὶ πάλιν ἔτι κατωτέρω "νεφρῶν νοσήματα τέσσαρα," καὶ μετὰ τοῦτο πάλιν "ἀπὸ τῆς κύστεως νοῦσοι στραγγουριῶν τέσσαρες," εἶτα πάλιν ἐφεξῆς "τέτανοι τρεῖς," καὶ μετὰ ταῦτα πάλιν "ἴκτεροι τέσσαρες," εἶτα μετὰ τοῦτο "φθίσιες τρεῖς."

The other quotation by Galen has also usually been considered to be a fragment of the *Knídiai gnō̂mai*, but the basis for this identification is again unsound. Galen, commenting on *Epidemics VI* 1. 14 ("Some [fevers] are livid"[26]), says, "Euryphon calls such fevers 'livid' writing thus: 'Livid: Fever seizes [the patient] and shivering from time to time, and the head aches, and pain seizes the intestines, and he vomits bile, and whenever he feels the pain, his vision is disturbed because he feels heavy, and the stool becomes dry, and the whole skin livid, and the lips as if he had eaten mulberries, and the white of the eyes becomes livid, and he looks as if he were being strangled – sometimes he suffers less from that –, and his complexion changes often.' But also in *On Diseases*, ascribed to Hippocrates, ... a disease is called 'livid.' (The *incipit* of the book is: 'Much urine is secreted when the head is overheated.') This is literally what he writes about the livid disease [*On Diseases II*, ch. 68]: 'Livid: Dry fever seizes [the patient] and rigor from time to time, and the head aches, and pain seizes the intestines, and he vomits bile, and whenever he feels the pain, his vision is disturbed and he feels heavy, and the stomach becomes dry, and the skin livid, and the lips and the white of the eyes livid, and he looks as if he were being strangled, and sometimes his complexion changes from livid to greenish.' "[27]

The congruence between the two texts (the one by Euryphon and the one transmitted in the Hippocratic Corpus, *On Diseases II*, ch. 68), is remarkable. From this similarity and from information which Galen gives

---

[26] *Epid. VI* 5.274.8 οἱ δὲ πελιοί.

[27] Gal. *In Hp. Epid. VI comm.* p. 55.10–56.8 Wenkebach = frg. 15 Grensemann τοὺς τοιούτους πυρετοὺς Εὐρυφῶν ὀνομάζει †πελιαστ† γράφων ὧδε· "Πελιδνός· πυρετὸς ἴσχει καὶ βρυγμὸς (βρυγμὸς Wenkebach: βρεγμὸς U: Knirschen mit den Zähnen Arab.) ἄλλοτε καὶ ἄλλοτε, καὶ τὴν κεφαλὴν ἀλγέει, καὶ τὰ σπλάγχνα ὀδύνη ἴσχει, καὶ ἐμέει χολήν, καὶ ὅταν ὀδύνη ἔχῃ, ἀνορᾶν οὐ δύναται ὅτι βαρύνεται, καὶ ἡ γαστὴρ ξηρὴ γίνεται καὶ ὁ χρὼς πελιὸς ἅπας καὶ τὰ χείλεα οἷάπερ μόρα τρώξαντι, καὶ τῶν ὀφθαλμῶν τὰ λευκὰ πελιά, καὶ ἐξορᾷ ὥσπερ ἀπαγχόμενος, ὁτὲ δὲ ἧσσον τοῦτο πάσχει, καὶ μεταβάλλει πολλάκις." ἀλλὰ κἀν τῷ Περὶ νούσων Ἱπποκράτει ⟨ἐπι⟩γεγραμμένῳ ... εἴρηταί τις νόσος πελιή. τοῦ βιβλίου δ' ἐστὶν ἡ ἀρχὴ ἥδε· "οὐρέεται πολλόν, ὅταν ὑπερθερμανθῇ ἡ κεφαλή." περὶ δὲ τῆς πελι{ν}ῆς νόσου κατὰ λέξιν οὕτω γράφει (*Morb. II* 7.104.1–7 Li. = 207.1–7 Jouanna)· "Πελιὴ ν⟨οῦσος⟩· πυρετὸς ἴσχει ξηρὸς καὶ φρὶξ ἄλλοτε καὶ ἄλλοτε, καὶ τὴν κεφαλὴν ἀλγέει, καὶ τὰ σπλάγχνα ὀδύνη ἴσχει, καὶ ἐμέει χολήν, καὶ ὅταν ἡ ὀδύνη ἔχῃ, οὐ δύναται ἐνορᾶν, ἀλλὰ βαρύνεται· καὶ ἡ γαστὴρ ξηρὰ γίνεται, καὶ ἡ χρόα πελιδνή, καὶ τὰ χείλεα καὶ τῶν ὀφθαλμῶν τὰ λευκὰ πελιδνά, καὶ ἐξορᾷ ὡς ἀγχόμενος· ἐνίοτε καὶ τὴν χρόαν μεταβάλλει καὶ ἐκ πελιδνοῦ ὑπόχλωρος γίνεται." Perhaps Πελιήν should be read for Πελιὴ ν⟨οῦσος⟩, cf. similar formations of words denoting diseases etc.: δοθιήν 'furuncle,' ἑρπήν 'shingles,' λειχήν 'kind of eczema,' ἀρυφήν 'wrinkle,' κυρτήν 'gibbus' (all Liddell/Scott/Jones). The corrupt beginning of the quotation could be corrected possibly by writing πελι⟨ῆν⟩ας instead of πελιασ, but the difficulty of the immediately following πελιδνός persists. Cf. Jouanna, Archéologie 20 f., footnotes.

about Euryphon, medical historians have argued as follows: *(i)* since, according to Galen, there was a tradition in antiquity that Euryphon, a physician from Knidos, had written the *Knídiai gnṓmai*, and since some of the features mentioned in *On Regimen in Acute Diseases* can be found in Euryphon's text on the 'livid disease,' this text is part of the *Knídiai gnṓmai*; *(ii)* since the same text is almost identical with *On Diseases II*, ch. 68, this chapter of *On Diseases II* is derived from the *Knídiai gnṓmai*; *(iii)* since the chapters 12–75 of *On Diseases II* closely resemble ch. 68 in structure, they too are derived from the *Knídiai gnṓmai*; *(iv)* since there are certain congruences between *On Diseases II*, ch. 12–75 and other treatises of the Hippocratic Collection, these latter treatises are also ultimately derived from the *Knídiai gnṓmai*.

Grensemann[28] and Jouanna[29] have based their books of the mid-seventies essentially on such arguments, which can neither be refuted nor proved correct.[30] Indeed, Galen reports (without, however, explicitly consenting) an opinion of people unnamed that Euryphon had written the *Knídiai gnṓmai*.[31] Euryphon, however, was credited with having written more than this work, namely treatises of the Corpus Hippocraticum; there are passages in Galen[32] where the opinion is expressed that Euryphon was the author of the Hippocratic treatises *On Regimen* (*Vict.*) and *On Affections* (*Aff.*). It certainly cannot be ruled out that Euryphon's text on the 'livid disease' is from the *Knídiai gnṓmai*. Euryphon might have been one of their authors or one of "those who later revised" them, but the 'livid disease' text may equally well have been quoted from some other work of Euryphon.[33]

The above-mentioned chain of arguments is expanded by Grensemann[34] and Jouanna[35] to include the following: The author of *On Regimen*

---

[28] Grensemann, Knidische Medizin.

[29] Jouanna, Archéologie.

[30] Grensemann, Knidische Medizin p. 207, tries to leave the burden of proof with those who deny the Knidian origin of certain Hippocratic treatises; but this procedure would be appropriate only if the arguments in favour of his hypothesis were more cogent. Jouanna (ed.), Hippocrate, Maladies II, p. 48 has slightly modified his argumentation: "Par suite de l'existence de rédactions parallèles entre plusieurs traités nosologiques de la *Collection hippocratique* ..., il existe un modèle commun dont ces traités dérivent ...; par suite de plusieurs analogies entre certaines caractéristiques des traités du groupe et ce que l'on sait des *Sentences cnidiennes* ou des Cnidiens en général, il y a des grandes présomptions pour que ce modèle soit cet écrit collectif des médecins de Cnide ou en dérive."

[31] Cf. above p. 18.

[32] For references, see Smith, Galen on Coans 576, 579 ff. Cf. frg. 6 a, 6 b, 6 c, 7 Grensemann.

[33] Cf. Robert Joly's comments on formulating rash conclusions in this matter, in: L'école médicale de Cnide et son évolution, Ant. Classique 47 (1978), 533 f.

[34] Knidische Medizin p. 53–56.

[35] Jouanna, Archéologie *passim*.

in Acute Diseases says about the *Knídiai gnṓmai* that they contained, *(a)* a description of "what the patients are suffering from in each of the diseases," *(b)* a description of "how some of the diseases end," *(c)* "a discussion about the methods of treatment in each case." The fact that also chapters 12–75 of *On Diseases II* usually contain these elements, and often in this order, is taken by both scholars to be an additional indication that the chapters originate from the *Knídiai gnṓmai*. To this argument, one may object that quite frequently the order is *a, c, b* (for instance in the 'livid disease' chapter). Since the content of the elements is necessitated by the subject matter and any order different from *a, b, c* or *a, c, b* would be nonsensical, the congruence between the description of the *Knídiai gnṓmai* in *On Regimen in Acute Diseases* and the structure of the chapters cannot serve by itself as a support for the modern view that *On Diseases II*, ch. 12–75 is derived from the *Knídiai gnṓmai*.[36]

Another argument is more cogent at first sight. In *On Regimen in Acute Diseases* it is stated that "they applied only a small number of remedies. In most cases ... they prescribed evacuative drugs and, as drinks, whey and milk according to the season."[37] Similar formulas, with almost the same wording, are contained in *On Diseases II*, ch. 12–75; in ch. 66 it is prescribed: "This patient must be given an evacuative drug, ... and according to the season he should be given donkey milk or whey and an evacuative drug in addition."[38] Ch. 73: "This patient should frequently be given an evacuative drug and whey and milk according to the season."[39] Also ch. 68 (the chapter corresponding to a text by Euryphon): "This patient should be given an evacuative drug ... and whey according to the season and donkey milk."[40]

A brief survey of *On Diseases II*, ch. 12–75, however, makes it clear that, although there are chapters which recommend a therapy consisting

---

[36] Georg Harig, Bemerkungen zum Verhältnis der griechischen zur altorientalischen Medizin, in: "Corpus Hippocraticum" 89–90. Fridolf Kudlien, Gnomon 55 (1983), 360–362 (in partic. 360). The elements *a, b, c* are preceded by a title often indicating the disease's name, or by a subordinate clause, "if ..."; for more details about the structure of the chapters *Morb. II* 12–75 see below p. 55–72.

[37] τὰ γὰρ πλεῖστα αὐτοῖσιν εἴρηται ... φάρμακα ἐλατήρια διδόναι καὶ ὀρὸν καὶ γάλα τὴν ὥρην πιπίσκειν. For the reference, see above p. 14, note 10.

[38] *Morb. II* 7.100.16–20 Li. = 205.4–8 Jouanna τοῦτον φάρμακα (φάρμακα θ: φάρμακον M) πιπίσκειν ... καὶ τὴν κεφαλὴν καθαίρειν ... καὶ τὴν ὥρην ὄνου γάλα ἢ ὀρὸν πιπίσκων φάρμακον προσπῖσαι.

[39] *Morb. II* 7.112.2–3 Li. = 213.7–8 Jouanna τοῦτον φάρμακον πιπίσκειν θαμὰ καὶ ὀρὸν καὶ γάλα τὴν ὥρην.

[40] *Morb. II* 7.104.7–10 Li. = 207.8–208.1 Jouanna τοῦτον φάρμακον πιπίσκειν ..., καὶ ὀρὸν τὴν ὥρην καὶ γάλα ὄνου πιπίσκειν. It is striking that the *formulation* is very similar in all of the passages. Corresponding prescriptions in different formulations can be found in ch. 12 and 13, cf. below p. 32 f., and in other passages of *Morb. II.*

of just a few prescribed remedies, there are other chapters which require of the physician a rather elaborate therapeutic programme, chapters to which the description given in *On Regimen in Acute Diseases* can by no means be applied.[41] Jouanna and Grensemann[42] try to solve the apparent puzzle by postulating that *On Diseases II*, ch. 12–75 contains material from different stages of a scientific development, namely that the chapters with the simple therapy are in content and form close to the primitive version of the *Knídiai gnōmai*, from which they are supposed to be derived; and that the more elaborate chapters are vestiges of the revision mentioned in *On Regimen in Acute Diseases*. For Jouanna in particular, the whole of *On Diseases II*, ch. 12–75 reflects a "second edition" of the *Knídiai gnōmai* in which not all passages on treatment were systematically modified, but where some (e. g. the one in chapter 68) retained their archaic character, whereas others (e. g. chapter 47 b) were revised.[43]

If there was any proof that Euryphon's text on the 'livid disease,' which has its parallel in *On Diseases II*, ch. 68, derives from the *Knídiai gnōmai*, the chain of arguments adduced in favour of the supposedly Knidian origin of *On Diseases II*, ch. 12–75 (and, accordingly, of other parts of the Hippocratic Collection) would be more cogent, and the ancillary arguments would give additional support. All we know, however, is that chapter 68 has a parallel in an unnamed work of the Knidian physician Euryphon, who was an elder contemporary of Hippocrates. Probably his period of activity was in the latter half of the fifth century B. C. His precise dates are unknown.[44]

Thus, there are good reasons to doubt that any passages or treatises within the Hippocratic Collection can be identified as having been derived from the *Knídiai gnōmai* or as being Knidian. There might be such Hippocratic texts; it cannot be ruled out that the views of Grensemann and Jouanna about the Knidian origin of several Hippocratic treatises are correct, but these views cannot be proved. Perhaps it is not just coincidence

---

41 For details, cf. below p. 68–72.

42 Jouanna, Archéologie 468 ff.; Grensemann, Knidische Medizin p. 195.

43 Archéologie 468. Another possible solution for somebody believing in the Knidian origin of *On Diseases II* would be to assume that the author of *On Regimen in Acute Diseases*, being himself primarily interested in therapy, exaggerated the alleged incompetence of the authors of the *Knídiai gnōmai* in this field; on other exaggerations of his, cf. above p. 18.

44 Grensemann, Knidische Medizin p. 197–201 suggests that Euryphon was born around 500 B. C. The testimonies, however, in Grensemann's collection of fragments are ambiguous (see his 'Sach- und Namenindex' s. v. Euryphon, p. 272; cf. also Pauly/Wissowa VI.1 (11. Halbband), 1342–1344 s. v. 'Euryphon' (M. Wellmann); it is especially uncertain whether Euryphon was earlier than Herodikos. Grensemann's frg. 4 should not be dismissed lightly in an assessment of chronology.

that none of the surviving fragments of the *Knídiai gnõmai*[45] can be found in the Hippocratic Collection.[46] Furthermore, the possibility should not be discounted that Euryphon took his 'livid disease' text over from *On Diseases II*, ch. 12–75, of which the date is uncertain, but which must be among the oldest constituents of the Hippocratic Collection, as Jouanna and Grensemann have abundantly demonstrated in their studies of its style, terminology, and, most importantly, its content.

Both scholars have proved that the text of *On Diseases II*, ch. 12–75 closely resembles a lost text which must have served as a source of several nosological treatises of the Collection. The identity of this common source with the *Knídiai gnõmai* is questionable, and so are all subsequent speculations about any 'school of Knidos;' but apart from this identity and from the problem of 'medical schools,' it is very plausible that *(i)* a common literary model directly or indirectly underlies parts of the nosological treatises, and that *(ii) On Diseases II*, ch. 12–75 comes closest to this inferred model. This conclusion is inevitable when one compares the parallel versions of each chapter of the Hippocratic nosological treatises. Such a comparison[47] permits a distinction between the common heritage and later inserted additions.[48] What Grensemann and Jouanna discovered about this internal relationship of the nosological treatises is one of the major contributions to Hippocratic scholarship in this century and is independent of the question whether these treatises are in fact of Knidian origin.

General considerations may illustrate the probable relationship between the physicians of Kos and Knidos, two cities only a few miles apart.[49] It appears that those aristocratic groups of the Koan and Knidian population from which several physicians and Hippocrates' family originated, were engaged in joint religious (and political) activities. This aristocracy, the Asklepiads of both territories, who traced their origin back to the healing

---

[45] See above p. 18–20.

[46] The Hippocratic treatise *On Internal Affections* describes — in this order — three kinds of consumption (*Int.* ch. 10–12 = 7.188.26–198.24 Li.), four diseases of the kidneys (ch. 14–17 = 7.202.1–210.6 Li.), four kinds of jaundice (ch. 35–38 = 7.252.17–260.21 Li.), and three kinds of tetanus (ch. 52–54 = 7.298.11–302.5 Li.). Jouanna, Archéologie 17, note 2 rightly calls attention to the fact that the numbers of nosological subdivisions of these diseases correspond exactly to what Galen quotes from an ancient Ionic text (perhaps the *Knídiai gnõmai*, see above p. 20), but that their order is different. Moreover, several subdivisions of the ancient text quoted are absent from the Hippocratic Collection ("seven diseases of the gall," "twelve diseases from the bladder," "from the bladder, four diseases of urine retention"). Cf. also Grensemann, Knidische Medizin p. 71 f.

[47] Apropos here is the list of parallel chapters given by Jouanna, Archéologie 519 f.

[48] For Joly's objections against this view, see below p. 52, note 84.

[49] Cf. above p. 12.

hero or god Asklepios, formed one clan and maintained far-flung relations within the Greek world, as can be inferred from an inscription found in continental Greece at Delphi and dated to around 360 B. C., i. e. from shortly after the death of Hippocrates.[50] The text reads as follows:

"It was resolved by the Association of the Asklepiads of Kos and Knidos, that any Asklepiad who comes to Delphi, whenever he needs to consult the oracle or to sacrifice, consult the oracle after he has sworn that he is an Asklepiad by descent through the male line ... [lacuna] ... And that anybody who does not follow this procedure, shall not be admitted to the oracle as the Asklepiads are, and that he not receive any other privilege that may be granted to the Asklepiads by the Delphians unless he acts in accordance with this prescript."[51]

Although this inscription is short and some lines are missing in the middle, it yields valuable information. First, the Asklepiads of Kos and Knidos formed *one* organization, the name of which was *tó koinón*, a very common term for 'association.'[52] Second, it must be concluded that the Asklepiads of Kos and Knidos used the oracle of Delphi not just occasionally but regularly, which implies that the Asklepiads must have had some economic and political influence in Kos and Knidos, and that the religious cult played a certain rôle in this organization, as has to be expected anyway. Third, in order to obtain the privileges of the Asklepiads in Delphi, one had to swear an oath: I am an Asklepiad by descent through the male line. Other sources[53] allow us to understand this latter statement

---

[50] This date was proposed by the first editor on the basis of the shape of the letters: Jean Bousquet, Inscriptions de Delphes, Bullet. de Corresp. Hellénique 80 (1956), 579—590. Bousquet emphasizes the possibility that the inscription might even be from the beginning of the fourth century. Cf. Jeanne and Louis Robert, Bulletin épigraphique, Rev. Ét. Grecques 71 (1958), 254.

[51] Translation by Lawrence J. Bliquez. The latest edition is by Georges Rougemont, Corpus des inscriptions de Delphes, I: Lois sacrées et règlements religieux, Paris, 1977, p. 122—124. Rougemont's text, which comprises a new unedited fragment, reads (for the accents in δίδοται and ποιῆι, I follow the earlier editors): Ἔδοξε Ἀσκλαπιαδᾶ|ν τῶι κοινῶι Κώιων | καὶ Κνιδίων· τὸν ἀφ|ικνεύμενον Ἀσκλα|πιάδαν ἐς Δελφούς, | αἴ κα χρήζηι τῶι μα|ντείωι χρῆσθαι ἢ θ|ύεν, ὀμόσαντα χρῆσ|θαι ἔμεν Ἀσκλαπ[ιά]|δας κατὰ ἀνδρο[γέν]|ειαν ... (Sequitur lacuna nonnullorum versuum, in qua nil nisi aliquot litterae vestigiaque sunt servata.) ὃς δ[έ κα παρβάλλ]ηι | ταῦτα, μ[ὴ ἔμεν α]ὐτῶ|ι εἴσοδον ἐ[ς τ]ὸ μαν|τεῖον καθάπε[ρ] Ἀσκλ|απιάδαις, μηδέ, [α]ἴ τ|ι ἄλλο γέρας δίδο[τ]|[α]ι Ἀσκλαπιάδα(ι)ς πα|[ρ]ὰ Δελφῶν, μὴ δίδοσ|[θ]αι αἴ κα μὴ ποιῆι κ|[ατ]ὰ τὰ γεγραμένα. Edited also by F. Sokolowski, Lois sacrées des cités grecques, Supplément, Paris, 1962, p. 86 f. Cf. H. W. Pleket, Arts en maatschappij in het oude Griekenland, Tijdschrift voor Geschiedenis 96 (1983), 325—347 (in partic. 334). Kudlien, Sozialgeschichte des frühgriechischen Arztes 133—136.

[52] Erich Ziebarth, Das griechische Vereinswesen, Stuttgart, 1896 (= repr. Wiesbaden, 1969), 136; Poland, Vereinswesen 163—167.

[53] See Grensemann, frg. 1 and his commentary on it.

as: I am a descendant of Asklepios through the male line. Obviously there were also other Asklepiads: e. g. by descent through the female line, or through adoption.[54] Irrespective of its restricted genealogical sense, the word 'Asklepiad' may already have had, even at that early period, the broader meaning of 'physician' frequently attested in subsequent periods of antiquity.

The aristocratic clan of Asklepiads, although not all of its members were physicians, must have had some influence on the medical profession in Kos as well as in Knidos. In the family of Hippocrates, e. g., which traced its origin back to Asklepios,[55] there were several medical men,[56] and the leadership (*diadokhḗ*) of the 'school' (whatever this may have been) in Kos was handed down within this family.[57]

The relationship between the Koan and Knidian Asklepiads makes probable the assumption that the two medical centres were not isolated from each other. Galen mentions that the Knidian physician Ktesias criticized Hippocrates (who was his elder contemporary) for a particular method of treatment, and adds that Ktesias was a "relative of his, because he was like him an Asklepiad by descent."[58] Another passage in Galen written in a somewhat flowery style metaphorically alluding to lyric or dramatic contests suggests the same conclusion: "In olden times there was a considerable contest. Kos and Knidos competed to outdo each other in the multitude of their discoveries and inventions. The clan of Asklepiads in Asia was then still twofold after the extinction of the one in Rhodos. They had the good competition commended by Hesiod,[59] and with them

---

[54] Cf. the so-called Hippocratic *Oath* transmitted in the Corpus Hippocraticum: "I swear by Apollo the physician and Asklepios and Hygieia and Panakeia and all gods and goddesses making them witnesses ...: I shall hold my teacher in this craft (*tékhnē*) equal to my parents, and I shall share my livelihood with him, and when he is in need I shall support him, and I shall esteem his descendants as my brothers, and I shall teach them this craft ..." (*Jusj.* 4.628.2–630.1 Li. = 4.2–8 Heiberg = 1.298 Jones.) In *Prorrh. II* 9.20.12–13, the author says that he has talked to physicians, and to their sons and pupils, παισί τε καὶ μαθητῇσιν ἐλεσχηνευσάμην.

[55] Soranus, ed. Ioannes Ilberg, Corpus Medicorum Graecorum IV, Leipzig, 1927, p. 175.3–5; cf. *Yppocratis genus, vita, dogma* in the Codex Bruxellensis nr. 1342–1350, fol. 52 v–53 v, ed. Hermann Schöne, Rhein. Mus. (N. F.) 58 (1903), 56–66, especially 56–57, 61–63. More material in Pauly/Wissowa VIII.2 (16. Halbband), 1801–1852 s. v. 'Hippokrates 16' (Gossen), and Pauly/Wissowa, Suppl. VI, 1290–1345 (Edelstein).

[56] For references, see the literature quoted in the preceding footnote.

[57] Richard Walzer, Galens Schrift 'Über die Siebenmonatskinder,' Rivista degli studi orientali 15 (1935), 323–357 (in partic. 345); 16 (1936), 227. Gal. *In Hp. Nat. Hom. comm.* ed. Mewaldt, p. 8.24–25. Hp. *Or. Thess.* 9.424.2–3. Cf. Grensemann, Arzt Polybos 4–5.

[58] Gal. *In Hp. Art. comm.* 18 A. 731 K. (on *Art.* 4.288.11–12 Li.) κατεγνώκασιν Ἱπποκράτους ἐπεμβαλεῖν τὸ κατ᾽ ἰσχίον ἄρθρον, ὡς ἂν ἐκπῖπτον αὐτίκα, πρῶτος μὲν Κτησίας ὁ Κνίδιος συγγενὴς αὐτοῦ· καὶ γὰρ αὐτὸς ἦν Ἀσκληπιάδης τὸ γένος.

[59] *Op.* 21–24.

strove the physicians from Italy, Philistion, Empedokles, Pausanias, and their colleagues. These were three admirable choirs of physicians competing with each other. The choir from Kos had, through good fortune, the most numerous and best members; the one from Knidos came nearest to it; but also the one from Italy was by no means insignificant."[60] There is nowhere any mention of different approaches to healing, of different systems of medical doctrines, or of any basic differences as to the principles of the craft. As a matter of fact, 'competition' generally presupposes a basic agreement among all of the competitors. They "competed to outdo each other in the *multitude* of their discoveries and inventions,"[61] not necessarily by initiating independent or even mutually incompatible approaches.

There are testimonies about therapeutic measures which were of Knidian origin. Yet these texts must not be taken as testifying to a Knidian 'school' with exclusive tenets. Galen reports that Knidian physicians developed a method to remove pus from the lungs by pouring a liquid into the trachea and thus provoking a cough.[62] The method is recommended and described in several passages of the Hippocratic Collection (e. g. *On Diseases II*, ch. 47),[63] and it is therefore obvious that these passages are influenced by the Knidian innovation. One should not, however, hastily conclude that the respective Hippocratic treatises are, therefore, of Knidian origin themselves, or even that they are derived from the *Knídiai gnōmai*.[64]

---

60 Gal. *De meth. med.* 10.5–6 K. = frg. 2 a Grensemann καὶ πρόσθεν μὲν ἔρις ἦν οὐ σμικρὰ νικῆσαι τῷ πλήθει τῶν εὑρημάτων ἀλλήλους ὀριγνωμένων τῶν ἐν Κῷ καὶ Κνίδῳ. διττὸν γὰρ ἔτι τοῦτο τὸ γένος ἦν τῶν ἐπὶ τῆς Ἀσίας Ἀσκληπιαδῶν, ἐπιλιπόντος τοῦ κατὰ Ῥόδον. ἤριζον δ' αὐτοῖς τὴν ἀγαθὴν ἔριν ἐκείνην, ἣν Ἡσίοδος ἐπῄνει, καὶ οἱ ἐκ τῆς Ἰταλίας ἰατροί, Φιλιστίων τε καὶ Ἐμπεδοκλῆς καὶ Παυσανίας καὶ οἱ τούτων ἑταῖροι. καὶ τρεῖς οὗτοι χοροὶ θαυμαστοὶ πρὸς ἀλλήλους ἁμιλλωμένων ἐγένοντο ἰατρῶν. πλείστους μὲν οὖν καὶ ἀρίστους χορευτὰς ὁ Κῷος εὐτυχήσας εἶχεν, ἐγγὺς δ' ἔτι τούτῳ καὶ ὁ ἀπὸ τῆς Κνίδου, λόγου δ' ἦν ἄξιος οὐ σμικροῦ καὶ ὁ ἀπὸ τῆς Ἰταλίας. Cf. also Kudlien, Beginn 35 f. An Arabic tradition mentions a chronological sequence in the development of medicine (without speaking of 'schools'): ʿAlī ibn Riḍwān, 'Über den Weg zur Glückseligkeit durch den ärztlichen Beruf,' ed. by Albert Dietrich, Göttingen, 1982 (Abh. d. Akad. d. Wiss. in Göttingen, Philol.-hist. Kl., 3. Folge, no. 129), 24 (cf. 53): "... die Medizin bestand anfangs auf der Insel Rhodos, deren Bewohner sie von den Philosophen der Ägypter übernommen hatten. Dann gelangte sie zu den Angehörigen dieser Familie [viz. of Asklepiads] auf der Halbinsel Knidos, dann nach der Insel Kos." The author lived 998–1061 (or 1068) and directly used ancient Greek sources.

61 εὑρήματα means both discoveries and inventions, cf. Liddell/Scott/Jones s. v.

62 Gal. *De opt. secta ad Thrasyb.* 1.128 f. K. = frg. 17 Grensemann.

63 *Morb. II* 7.66.16–68.19 Li. = 179.16–181.10 Jouanna; for the other Hippocratic texts see frg. 17 Grensemann, commentary.

64 It is nowhere stated that the Knidian infusion method was described in the *Knídiai gnōmai*.

Another therapeutic measure of Knidian physicians was the use of the 'Knidian berry' (*Knídios kókkos*). According to Rufus of Ephesus, the best Knidian berry grew in Karia, where Knidos was located. "That is why it has this name, and also because the Asklepiads from Knidos use it most often and on a large scale."[65] Indeed, the *Knídios kókkos* is frequently mentioned in the Collection.[66] Sometimes the berry is referred to simply as *kókkos*, and it has been suggested that these particular passages where 'Knidian' is missing were written by Knidian authors.[67] At first glance it seems reasonable that in texts intended for use within a Knidian 'school' the word *kókkos* might have been sufficient to denote the *Knídios kókkos*; however, this conclusion is too far-reaching. In Hippocratic prescriptions there occur at least half a dozen kinds of berries (*kókkos*) of various plants. Accordingly, even a Knidian reader would have had some difficulty understanding correctly without further specifications what *kókkos* was supposed to mean. Therapeutic prescriptions within the Hippocratic Collection are not always explicit as to the drugs and ingredients. There are of course some texts which are very explicit; other texts, however, presuppose a considerable knowledge of pharmacology.[68] This reduces the *kókkos* argument to an ubiquitous linguistic phenomenon without any particular significance. It will suffice here to quote a few examples: "She should drink the [preparation] containing pine."[69] Clysters are denoted the same way: "the one from wild figs;"[70] "the one with vinegar."[71] Pessaries: "the one with narcissus;"[72] "the ones with buprestis [beetle]."[73] Quite often, a 'beetle' (or 'beetles') as an ingredient in recipes is mentioned without any specification as to the species. The physician was expected to know this information.[74] Similarly one might simply write "the drug" because every informed reader was supposed to know which one was referred to: "She must not swallow the drug;"[75] "he swallowed the drug."[76]

---

[65] Ruf. ap. Oribas. *Collect. med. VII* 26.30 = vol. 1, p. 231.7–14 Raeder = frg. 25 Grensemann.

[66] Cf. Grensemann, Knidische Medizin, p. 37–39, where Eubulos (frg. 128 Kock, Edmonds; from an unknown comedy) should be added; 67–70.

[67] Grensemann, *loco laud.*

[68] For the problem whether this obscurity was intentional see below p. 139.

[69] *Nat. Mul.* 7.324.15 Li. = 76.15 Trapp πινέτω δὲ τὸ σὺν τῇ δαιδί.

[70] *Nat. Mul.* 7.336.20 Li. = 82.20 Trapp τῷ ἀπὸ τῶν ὀλόνθων.

[71] *Nat. Mul.* 7.338.16–17 Li. = 83.16–17 Trapp τῷ σὺν τῷ ὄξει.

[72] *Nat. Mul.* 7.338.14 Li. = 83.14 Trapp τὸ σὺν τῇ ναρκίσσῳ.

[73] *Nat. Mul.* 7.316.1–2 Li. = 72.1–2 Trapp τὰ σὺν βουπρήστει.

[74] κανθαρίς, κανθαρίδες e. g. *Nat. Mul.* 7.324.1 Li. = 76.1 Trapp; 338.20 Li. = 83.20 Trapp; 346.14–15 Li. = 87.14–15 Trapp; 360.2 Li. = 94.2 Trapp; "apply the pessary with the beetle" προσθεῖναι τὸ σὺν τῇ κανθαρίδι *Nat. Mul.* 7.314.3–4 Li. = 71.3–4 Trapp; 338.15 Li. = 83.15 Trapp.

[75] *Nat. Mul.* 7.316.6–7 Li. = 72.6–7 Trapp μηδὲ τὸ φάρμακον πίνειν.

[76] *Epid. V* 5.204.9 ἔπιε τὸ φάρμακον.

Likewise, "On the twelfth day he drank juice," i. e. barley gruel.[77] These examples taken from therapeutic prescriptions or descriptions could be multiplied;[78] thus, there is sufficient cause for not concluding too quickly that Hippocratic passages mentioning *kókkos* without the adjective *Knídios* are necessarily Knidian in origin.

Knidian physicians seem to have had some influence on nosological terminology according to Galen: "The kinds of *kholérē* [got their name] from the Knidian physicians, perhaps also the *leukophlegmatíās hýderos* goes back to them."[79] Grensemann has rightly emphasized that the disease name *kholérē* also appears in Hippocratic treatises which have never been regarded as Knidian by any modern scholar.[80] The *leukophlegmatíās hýderos* is not attested in the Hippocratic Collection at all.

Apart from the above innovations, the Knidian physicians were credited with having adhered to the simple therapeutic method which consisted of giving "evacuative drugs and, as drinks, whey and milk according to the season."[81] It has been mentioned above that there are passages in the Hippocratic Collection where this unsophisticated treatment is recommended, and that such passages have usually been considered Knidian, although the basis for this inference is tenuous.[82] It can be further noted here that the same simple therapy is also found in Hippocratic treatises which have never been regarded as Knidian.[83] There are various passages in the *Epidemics* where milk or whey or both are recommended as a drug or as a diet, or where its usage is attested for historical cases of illness. In some of these passages, both the therapeutic indication and the mode of application are quite simple: *Epidemics II* 5.14 "If the ear aches, he should keep using milk."[84] *II* 6.13 "When the intestines are wounded, the breath

---

[77] *Epid. VII* 5.366.8–9 δωδεκάτῃ ἐρρύφησε χυλοῦ.

[78] In other medical contexts, adjectives or genitives determining a substantive are also sometimes omitted: ὀπός (viz. σιλφίου ? Cf. Gal. *Gloss.* 19.126 K.; e. g. *Morb. II* 7.60.11,20 Li. = 174.12, 175.3 Jouanna); ῥίζα (cf. Gal., *ibid.* p. 126, 135; e. g. *Mul. II* 8.262.19); φύλλον (sed cf. Gal., *ibid.* p. 153; *Mul. II* 8.298.14); ἄνθος instead of ἄνθος χαλκοῦ (e. g. *Morb. II* 7.50.18 Li. = 167.18 Jouanna; 52.3,20,24 Li. = 168.9, 169.11, 16 Jouanna; στόμα or στόμαχος can stand instead of στόμα(χος) τῆς μήτρης or στόμα(χος) τῆς ὑστέρης (frequent in the gynecological treatises), and for στῆθος τοῦ ποδός one can say simply στῆθος (*Epid. IV* 5.144.4–5 Li. = Per. 66 La.). More examples in Lloyd, Science 126–129; Langholf, Syntaktische Untersuchungen p. 148 (on Per. 157). All this is possible in a jargon used by specialists in a well-defined field of activity.

[79] Gal. *De meth. med.* 10. 81 f. K. = frg. 18 Grensemann.

[80] Grensemann, Knidische Medizin p. 31.

[81] See above p. 15.

[82] Cf. p. 23.

[83] On treatment with milk, see Deichgräber, Milchtherapie; Thivel, Cnide 283 f.

[84] *Epid. II* 5.130.17 ἢν τὸ οὖς ἀλγέῃ, τῷ γάλακτι διαχρήσθω. According to Galen, *In Hp. Epid. II comm.* p. 393 Pfaff, milk was poured into the ear against ear pain. Whether this interpretation is correct cannot be decided.

imperceptibly descends through the wound, and the chest is emptied. Give milk or, alternatively, wine blended with the same amount of water."[85] *II* 6.23 "Against restlessness, rigor, yawning: wine blended with the same amount of water or [as an alternative to this mixture] milk."[86] *II* 6.28 "Secretion of water [in cases of dropsy?]: give 8 *kotýlai*[87] of milk to drink."[88] *VI* 6.3.[89] In an individual case, *Epidemics VII* 52, in which the stomach seemed likely to be disturbed, milk was the only food the patient accepted.[90] *VI* 2.21 "In *empyḗmata* of those [patients] whose stomachs are disturbed and going to become purulent: whey [viz. as an appropriate diet]?"[91]

The last cited text (whose interpretation is not quite certain) is probably a question of a type often found in the *Epidemics* and in kindred treatises; namely the formulation of a problem which, in the author's opinion, needs further research by himself or his readers.[92] If this interpretation is correct, treatment with whey was not obsolete for the author. Akin to this kind of question are statements about therapeutical failures due to the author or his colleagues or somebody else: *Epidemics VII* 50 "The kinswoman of Euxenos, ... having drunk a drug [for evacuation] and whey, was harmed more."[93]

Besides the simple prescriptions hitherto quoted, milk is sometimes prescribed in combination with other liquids, also together with other therapeutic measures: *Epidemics II* 5.4 "If the skull is broken, give milk

---

85 *Epid. II* 5.134.23–136.2 τρωθέντος ἐντέρου ἡ ἀναπνοὴ ἔρχεται κάτω ἀφανὴς κατὰ τὸ τρῶμα, καὶ κενοῦται τὰ στήθεα· διδόναι οὖν γάλα ἢ (ἢ add. V: om. HIR) καὶ οἶνον ἴσον ἴσῳ.

86 *Epid. II* 5.136.18–19 ἀλύκης, φρίκης, χάσμης· οἶνος ἴσος ἴσῳ ἢ γάλα.

87 1 *kotýlē* is 0.27 liter.

88 *Epid. II* 5.138.4–5 ὕδατος ἀφιεμένου, γάλακτος ὀκτὼ κοτύλας δοῦναι πιεῖν.

89 *Epid. VI* 5.324.3–6.

90 *Epid. VII* 5.420.11–422.3.

91 *Epid. VI* 5.288.10–11 ἦ (ἢ MV: om. Li.) ἐν τοῖσιν ἐμπυήμασιν ὀρός (ὀρὸς vel ὀρρὸς codices recent.: ὅρος MV), οἷσι μέλλουσιν ἐκπυεῖν αἱ κοιλίαι ἐκταράσσονται;

92 Cf. below p. 179–190, in partic. 182, n. 248; 187 f., n. 273. ἦ is used to indicate 'sentence-questions' in the Hippocratic Collection, though rarely (the more usual particle being ἆρα): a sure instance of it is *Coac.* 306 (5.650.18–19), where ἢ is transmitted (and printed by Littré); but only ἦ is meaningful here. Less convincing is *Epid. II* 5.88.11 = Per. 18 La. (ἦ ῥήιον ci. Diller: ἤρεον HIR: εἴρεον V: εἰ ῥήιον Nikitas, fortasse recte).

93 *Epid. VII* 5.418.5–11 ἡ Εὐξένου ... φάρμακον πιοῦσα καὶ ὀρὸν ἐβλάβη μᾶλλον. There are some more statements about harmful or useless milk treatment which will not be discussed here as they are of no general importance, and cannot serve as a proof that the authors of the *Epidemics* were opposed to this therapy: *Epid. III* 3.138.3–11 Li. = 1.242.12–22 Kw. = 1.278 Jones; cf. 140.4–5 Li. = 243.2–3 Kw. = 280 Jones, where it is said that sometimes the stool seemed to be milky. *Epid. IV* 5.182.10–13 Li. = Per. 246 La. *Epid. VII* 5.432.3–4.

and wine, half and half."[94] Cf. *II* 5.6.[95] *VII* 45 "Bloodletting, helleborus, drinking cow-milk after drinking donkey-milk was useful and stopped evacuation, drinking water [instead of wine] from the beginning and walks and purgations of the head."[96] *VII* 115 "He [the patient] was given boiled goat-milk and one fifth of water, 3 *kotýlai* altogether, in the morning." [In the evening he got bread and vegetables and wine, and his looseness stopped.] ... "He drank milk until the urine returned to its normal condition."[97] The following statement is particularly interesting because the physician mentioned, Pythokles, was perhaps a member of a Koan family, in which this name, according to inscriptions, was customary:[98] *V* 57 = *VII* 75 "Pythokles gave the patients water, with milk admixed into much water, and they started to recover."[99] Important to note here is that all of these passages taken from the *Epidemics* indicate that treatment with milk cannot be said to be particularly Knidian.

The author of *On Regimen in Acute Diseases*, describing the treatment recommended in the original version of the *Knídiai gnōmai*, uses the expression: "To give ..., as drinks, whey and milk according to the season."[100] This formula recurs in the nosological treatises, which, as demonstrated above, need not be necessarily of Knidian origin.[101] Not hitherto noted, there are several passages which allow us to understand more precisely what the formula means and confirm further that it would be premature to regard the therapeutic use of "whey and milk according to the season" as a specifically Knidian method.

In Greek (as in Roman) antiquity, milk was available for longer periods of time during the year than was whey. *On Diseases II*, ch. 12 "If it is the season of the year, he should then drink whey after it [after the previous treatment]."[102] Ch. 13 "If it is the season, he should also drink whey after

94 *Epid. II* 5.128.14–16 ἢν τῆς κεφαλῆς τὸ ὀστέον καταγῇ, διδόναι γάλα καὶ οἶνον ἴσον ἴσῳ.

95 *Epid. II* 5.130.2–5.

96 *Epid. VII* 5.414.7–9 φλεβοτομίη, ἐλλέβοροι, γαλακτοποσίη βοείου, πρότερον δὲ ὀνείου ξυνήνεγκε καὶ τὰς ὑποχωρήσιας ἔπαυσεν, ὑδροποσίη ἀπ' ἀρχῆς καὶ περίπατοί τε καὶ κεφαλῆς καθάρσιες.

97 *Epid. VII* 5.462.10–17 πρωῒ μὲν ἐδίδοτο γάλα αἴγειον καὶ ὕδατος πέμπτη μερὶς ἀνεζεσμένον, τὸ πᾶν κοτύλαι (-αι edd.: -ας MV) τρεῖς ... ἐγαλακτοπότησε δ' ἕως τὰ οὖρα ἀποκατέστη.

98 Sherwin-White, Ancient Cos 518 f. Herzog, Heilige Gesetze p. 27. Deichgräber, Milchtherapie 52.

99 *Epid. V* 5.238.17–18 = *VII* 5.434.1–2 Πυθοκλῆς τοῖς κάμνουσιν ὕδωρ γάλα πολλῷ τῷ ὕδατι μιγνὺς ἐδίδου, καὶ ἀνέτραφον (καὶ ἀνέτραφον [= aor. II intr.] in *Epid. VII* scripserim: καὶ ἀνέτρεφον MV in *Epid. VII*: καὶ ἀνέτρεφεν Li. in *Epid. VII*: om. *Epid. V*).

100 Cf. above p. 15.

101 Cf. above p. 24 f.

102 *Morb. II* 7.22.8 Li. = 144.18–145.1 Jouanna ἢν ὥρη ᾖ τοῦ ἔτεος, ἔπειτα ὀρὸν μεταπῖσαι.

it [after the previous treatment]."[103] Whey is a by-product in various methods of cheese-making, and the production of cheese was essentially confined to the summer months. "People make cheese from the [heliacal] rising of the Pleiades in spring until the [apparent acronychal rising of the] Pleiades in summer," says Varro,[104] and this period seems to have extended from May 19 to September 19.[105] Later ancient authors recommend producing cheese in April and May, and in summer around harvest time.[106]

In the *Epidemics*, two patients are mentioned whose treatment can best be interpreted in the light of this ancient information on the availability of whey. *VII* 3–4, "The kinsman of Eratolaos, around the autumnal equinox, was seized with *dysenteríē* ... After drinking whey and drinking hot milk, the pain and the blood in his stool became less. ... [After more than a month,] when he drank about 9 Attic *kotýlai* of boiled donkey milk during two days, his excrements became very bilious, the pain diminished, and his appetite returned. After that he drank about 4 Attic *kotýlai* of unboiled cow-milk, 2 *kýathoi*[107] a day, at first mixing it with one sixth of water and a little red, astringent wine." He had one meal a day consisting of bread, fish, and meat. "He drank milk for forty days, after the first ten days without water ... For Ktesikrates, [milk] with flour[108] was more

---

103 *Morb. II* 7.24.3–4 Li. = 146.5 Jouanna ἦν δὲ ὥρη ᾖ, καὶ ὀρὸν μεταπιέτω.

104 Varro *R. rustic. II* 11.4 Caseum facere incipiunt a vergiliis vernis exortis ad aestivas vergilias.

105 According to the first list given by Boll, 'Fixsterne,' in: Pauly/Wissowa VI.2 (12. Halbband), 2427 f., the vernal heliacal rising of the Pleiades in the year 430 B. C. (which is roughly the period when the older Hippocratic treatises were written) was on May 19 for the latitude of Athens. Varro's expression "aestivae vergiliae" is not quite clear, but it should mean September 19 since there are no observable risings or settings of this star in summer except its apparent acronychal rising (September 19 according to Boll's list). Except for a few days' difference, this applies to Varro's time as well: cf. Boll's second list for the year 45 B. C. and for the latitude of Rome, *op. cit.*, 2428 f. – On ancient astronomical time-reckoning and on general problems involved see Phillips, Hippocratic physician.

106 For references, see Pauly/Wissowa X.2 (20. Halbband), 1492 s. v. 'Käse' (Kroll). Columella *XII* 13 recommends harvest-time for making cheese for domestic use, and gives two reasons: at that season the cows yield but little milk and it is, therefore, not worth the trouble to market the small quantities obtainable. Moreover the cheese would then be liable to spoil in the heat during transport. The statement by W. D. Hooper/H. B. Ash (M. Porcius Cato and M. Terentius Varro, On Agriculture, Cambridge, Mass., 1935 [Loeb Classical Library], 414), that "Columella (*XII* 13) advises July for cheese-making," is based only on 12.2 "rising of the dog-star;" but the overall context in Columella is clearly late summer and autumn (e. g. 10.1 per aestatem circa messem vel etiam exactis iam messibus); since calves and lambs were born in spring, July was the period of maximum lactation, not of "little milk."

107 1 *kýathos* is 0.045 liter, i. e. $^1/_6$ *kotýlē* (0.27 liter).

108 Cf. *Vict. II*, ch. 42 (6.540.18–20 Li. = 166.4–5 Joly = 4.312 Jones).

useful than goat whey ..., in [the month of] *Agriánios*; but in [the month of] *Karneíos*, boiled donkey milk was useful."[109] In Littré's edition, this report is divided into two paragraphs, but in fact the reference made to Ktesikrates is but a complementary note added to the case history of Eratolaos' kinsman, who drank whey and milk around the autumnal equinox, i. e. at the end of the season during which cheese was produced according to the sources quoted, and who, more than a month later, i. e. in October, had to be content with donkey and cow milk because whey was no longer available.[110]

Until recently it was not known at which time of the year the Koan months *Agriánios* and *Karneíos* had their chronological place. New research on the calendar of Rhodos (which largely resembled the one from neighbouring Kos) has furnished the result that *Agriánios* roughly corresponded to May, and *Karneíos* to October.[111] What is reported about Ktesikrates

---

[109] *Epid. VII* 5.368.14–18, 370.23–372.3, 372.10–14 Ὁ Ἐρατολάου περὶ φθινοπωρινὴν ἰσημερίην δυσεντερικὸς ἐγένετο... ὀροποτήσαντι δὲ καὶ γάλα πεπυρωμένον πιόντι μετριώτερα ἐγένοντο (ἐγένοντο V: ἐγένετο M) τὰ ἀλγήματα καὶ τὰ ὕφαιμα... πίνοντι ἄπεφθον ὡς (ἄπεφθον ὡς codices recent.: ἀπεφρόνως MV) ἐννέα Ἀττικὰς (κοτύλας post Ἀττ. add. codices recent.: om. MV) ὄνειον (ὄνιον M: ὤνιον V) ἐπὶ δύο ἡμέρας χολώδης ἐγένετο σφόδρα ἡ (σφόδρα ἡ codices recent.: σφοδρὴ MV) κάθαρσις, καὶ ἔληξαν αἱ ὀδύναι, καὶ σιτίων ἐπιθυμίη ἐγένετο. μετὰ δὲ ταῦτα βοείου γάλακτος ὡς τέσσαρας κοτύλας Ἀττικὰς ὠμοῦ (ὠμοῦ Lind.: ὁμοῦ MV) ἔπινε κατὰ δύο κυάθους δι' ἡμέρης, τὸ πρῶτον ὕδατος τὸ ἕκτον μίσγων καὶ μέλανος οἴνου καὶ αὐστηροῦ σμικρόν... ἡ δὲ πόσις τοῦ γάλακτος ἐπὶ τεσσαράκοντα ἡμέρας ἄνευ ὕδατος μετὰ τὰς πρώτας δέκα ἡμέρας... Κτησικράτει δὲ τὸ (τὸ V: τῶι M) ἐν τῷ ἀλεύρῳ μᾶλλον τοῦ αἰγείου (αἰγείου M: αἰγεί [sic] V) ὀροῦ ξυνήνεγκεν..., καὶ Ἀγριανίῳ (Ἀγριανίῳ Herzog: ἀδριανίω MV) ταῦτα· τῷ δὲ Καρνείῳ (Καρνείῳ Herzog: καινίου V: καινείου M) τὸ ὄνειον ἑφθόν. Cf. Herzog, Heilige Gesetze p. 50. Christoph Börker, Der rhodische Kalender, Zeitschrift für Papyrologie und Epigraphik, 31 (1978), 193–218, regards the names of the two months in *Epid. VII* as later additions because elsewhere in the Collection events are dated by solstices, equinoxes, and constellations (p. 217). The two names of months are indeed unique. But this is not a sufficient argument for an athetesis; and as will be shown below, the names fit very well into the therapeutic chronology, even on the basis of Börker's results.

[110] The notice on Ktesikrates has been misunderstood by the Byzantine scribes as well as the later editors. Instead of the correct form Ἀγριανίῳ, the relevant manuscripts have a nonsensical ἀδριανίω. As Littré remarked in a footnote to the passage, this Roman name cannot be authentic here. He rightly proposed to change δ into γ, but he thought that the form was a personal name derived from the name of a Koan month. He did not draw the much simpler conclusion that the form was a temporal indication. Καρνείῳ appears in the manuscripts with ι instead of ρ (a simple majuscule blunder) and could be a rare personal name (Καινίας or Καινίης), so the editors did not notice what was hiding behind the transmitted letters.

[111] Börker in his article quoted above, which gives bibliographic information on the Koan calender. Cf. Alan E. Samuel, Greek and Roman Chronology, Handbuch der Altertumswissenschaft I, 7, München, 1972. (Several centuries after the classical time of Greece, *Agriánios* had slightly shifted forward in comparison with the Julian calender: cf. P. Oxyrh.

fits, again, perfectly with what is known about cheese production. Whey was available in May, but in October this patient had to be content with donkey milk, like the kinsman of Eratolaos.[112]

Thus, while in the Hippocratic Collection there are some direct or indirect traces of the activity of Knidian physicians (viz. infusion into the lungs; the use of the Knidian berry; the disease name *kholérē*), these traces prove insufficient for concluding that the treatises which contain them are Knidian themselves or are derived from Knidian literary models. Furthermore, the treatment with "whey and milk according to the season" appears not to have been a specifically Knidian therapeutic practice at all.[113]

Indeed, Jouanna and Grensemann have had considerable success in discovering which of the so-called nosological treatises of the Collection are more developed or more primitive. Their results about the relative chronology of these treatises remain plausible; their conclusion, however, that any of the nosological works trace their origin from Knidian sources and represent a development of medical science which took place within the medical 'school' of Knidos, cannot be verified.[114]

2771 [from A. D. 323], where June 24 is said to fall within *Agriánios*. See also Sherwin-White, Ancient Cos, p. 5, note 2. *Karneíos* in Byzantine times analogously corresponded to November (Herzog, Heilige Gesetze p. 50, cf. Pauly/Wissowa X.2 [20. Halbband] 1993 s. v. 'Karneios.') — Little is known about the calender of Knidos: Samuel quotes four months, three of which have their namesakes in the Koan and Rhodian calenders; although *Agriánios* and *Karneíos* are not among these attested ones, they might, therefore, have been Knidian too.

112 Arist. *Meteor. IV* 7 (384a 21—22) mentions οἱ ἰατροὶ ὀπίζοντες, i. e. physicians boiling milk with vegetable juice (used as rennet): "So the whey and the cheese are separated," οὕτω δὲ χωρίζεται ὁ ὀρρὸς καὶ ὁ τυρός. This proves that at his time (if not earlier) medical men had contrived means for whey therapy independent of dairy activities. More details in Rufus Ephes. (ap. Oribas. *Coll. med. VII* 26.127 = vol. 1, p. 238.1—3 Raeder = frg. 26 Grensemann) Οἶδα δὲ τοὺς περὶ Καρίαν ἰατροὺς καὶ ὀρὸν γάλακτος εἰς κάθαρσιν σκευάζοντας ἀπὸ τοῦ κνήκου.

113 Although Rufus Ephes. (see preceding note) may have observed the therapy in Karia (Knidos?), as Grensemann assumed.

114 It is easier to follow Grensemann, who does not maintain that the demonstrable development was confined only to the Knidian 'school.' Grensemann even suggests that *On Affections* (*Aff.*) and *On Diseases I* (*Morb. I*) are of Koan origin and possibly related to Dexippos of Kos, p. 205—217. Similar are his views about *On Diseases III* (*Morb. III*), which, according to him, exhibits "einen Synkretismus ..., den wir nicht als knidisch bezeichnen können". "Es liegt vielmehr nahe zu vermuten, daß hier die koische Schule eingewirkt habe," p. 146, 162. Cf. Spaet, Entwickelung, in particular 37—40 (on *Morb. I, Aff.*) and 27 (on *Morb. III*). Jouanna on the other hand is much stricter. He says about the nosological treatises in general "que les innovations insérées à l'intérieur des cadres cnidiens se sont opérées au sein de l'école de Cnide," p. 503. Thivel, Cnide 153, 172 believes that *On Diseases II* (*Morb. II*) and *On Internal Diseases* (*Int.*) are Knidian because they exhibit the excessive subdivision criticized by the author of *On Regimen in Acute Diseases* (*Acut.*). But who knows whether *only* the Knidians followed this procedure? Thivel himself recognizes that "parfois, une pratique inventée par un groupe passait dans les groupes voisins," as in the case of Kos and Knidos, p. 211.

Since such proof is not possible in light of the extant testimonia, the medical historian must confine himself to generally reconstructing the development of Greek medicine in the fifth and fourth centuries B. C. The evidence available suggests that the members of the influential Asklepiad aristocracy of Kos and Knidos, part of whom were physicians, stood in a close relationship with each other, regardless of their place of residence or citizenship. This is probably also true of the non-aristocratic inhabitants of the two cities including those medical men who possibly did not belong to the Asklepiad clan. Furthermore, some of the authors of Hippocratic treatises were itinerant doctors,[115] who quite naturally were not narrow-minded provincials faithful to peculiar or exclusive medical beliefs, but probably were quite open to any professional influences they deemed good and useful. There must have been a constant and intensive process of give and take across the narrow straits which divided the two medical centres of Kos and Knidos. Hence the effort made by modern historians to discover exclusively Knidian or Koan doctrinal elements within the Hippocratic Collection is likely to remain without positive results, or to end in speculations which cannot be considered a firm basis for further research.

In view of this situation, the historian investigating the development of Greek medicine (particularly of medical theory) in the fifth and fourth centuries B. C. is entitled and obliged to use as documents all the treatises available in the Hippocratic Collection which date from that epoch, regardless of any Knidian or Koan school affiliation. In the ensuing chapters, this method will be followed. Most of the important discoveries of modern Hippocratic scholarship concerning the allegedly intra-Knidian evolution of medicine can be accepted with the restriction that it cannot be proved that this undeniable evolution took place exclusively within any particular medical centre or school.

[115] Littré, vol. 5. 10–14; Bourgey, Observation 82, 102; Nikitas, Untersuchungen 60–75, 242–245.

II. Methods of Cognition in the Oldest Hippocratic Texts: Some Early Doctrines

In the historical development of Greek medicine during the fifth and fourth centuries B. C., several features hitherto obscured by the scholarly custom of assigning various treatises of the Corpus to Kos and Knidos are now more clearly distinguishable. In historical retrospect, it would appear that the nosological works of the Collection, particularly the oldest ones,[1] were forerunners of another type of Hippocratic treatise, namely the *Epidemics* (which will be the subject of the ensuing chapter III, p. 73 ff.). 'Forerunners' neither means that the authors of the nosological treatises were prescient of the evolution of medicine or consciously worked in that direction, nor does it even mean that the authors of the *Epidemics* necessarily used or knew the particular nosological works extant in the Collection (which are perhaps just random remnants of a once considerably larger nosological literature). Rather the term signifies that some of the nosological treatises are *representative* of an older approach to medicine which is presupposed in the *Epidemics*. The readers of the *Epidemics* had to have had a training in traditional nosology in order to fully understand the new approach.

That the nosological approach as exemplified by the oldest treatises of the Hippocratic Corpus was itself already – in a technical sense – highly developed, can be recognized when one compares these ancient medical writings to non-medical texts. An examination of some 'medical' or 'physiological' expressions in the Homeric poems (eighth century) and in the comedies of Aristophanes (a contemporary of Hippocrates) will help to elucidate the methods of cognition manifested by the oldest Hippocratic texts.

In Homeric poetry, there is not always a sharp distinction between what we today would call a passion (or an emotion) and a physiological constituent of the body. As the following examples evince, there are contexts in which *khólos*, 'gall' (the two words are etymologically related) clearly conveys just the meaning of 'wrath' or 'anger,' while in some

[1] *On Diseases II*, ch. 12–75, and the stratum A (according to Grensemann's nomenclature) of the gynaecological treatises. As to the internal chronology, one must follow Jouanna and Grensemann; cf. the preceding chapter, p. 25 and below, p. 52 f.

passages we are tempted to ask whether the poet intended to use a metaphor rather than to give a concrete physical description.[2] Asking questions of this kind is, however, fruitless since such terms as 'metaphor,' 'concrete,' etc. are modern labels alien to the time of Homeric poetry. Such labels can be used for heuristic purposes, but they cannot contribute to an answer which satisfies the historian. Sometimes the modern reader gets the impression that the authors of the Homeric texts avoided being unambiguous and preferred not to imply too clear a concept of what is happening in the body and/or the soul. *khólos* can 'possess' the *thȳmós* ('soul,' 'spirit')[3] (*Iliad IX* 675), can be 'put in' the *thȳmós* (*VI* 326), can 'fall into' the *thȳmós* (*IX* 436, *XIV* 207, 306, *XVI* 206), can 'penetrate into' somebody (*dýō* with accusative, *IX* 553 f., *XIX* 16, *XXII* 94), can 'seize' somebody (*lambánō I* 387, *VI* 166, *XVI* 30; *hairéō IV* 23, *VIII* 460, *XVIII* 322), or simply 'come' (*IX* 525, *XVII* 399). The word can even be used to express social interaction: just as the Homeric hero can put *khólos* into his own *thȳmós* (*VI* 326), he can put *khólos* into another's *thȳmós* (*XIV* 50).

Since we are dealing with 'medical theories,' it is useful to examine what Homer says, or rather, what Homeric poets made their ancient epic characters say, about *khólos* under the aspect of its being a concrete substance contained in the human body. *khólos* is mentioned as being pungent (*Iliad XVIII* 322) and hot, so it has to be quenched (*IX* 678). It swells like smoke (*XVIII* 110). It is localized in various parts or areas of the body: in the *stē̂thos* ('breast,' 'chest') (*IV* 24, *IX* 553 f., *XVIII* 110); in the *thȳmós* (cf. above and *IV* 513, *IX* 260, 565, 675); in the *phrénes* ('chest') (*II* 241);[4] in the *kradíē* ('heart') (*IX* 646). It can increase in volume: "... *khólos*, which makes even a wise man become angry and which, sweeter than dripping honey, waxes like smoke in men's chests (*stē̂thos*)" (*XVIII* 108–110); in *IV* 24 it is said that the *stē̂thos* of the goddess Hera could not hold the abundance of *khólos*; *khólos* can make organs of the body swell: "*khólos* makes my *kradíē* swell" (*IX* 646); it causes the *nóos* ('mind') to swell at *IX* 553 f.[5] The acrimonious Achilleus

[2] Cf. throughout Snell, Entdeckung 13 ff.; Smith, Physiology; Körner, Die ärztlichen Kenntnisse; Siegfried Laser, Medizin und Körperpflege, Archaeologia Homerica, Kap. S, Göttingen, 1983.

[3] *thȳmós* is translated in Liddell/Scott/Jones by "*soul, spirit*, as the *principle of life, feeling and thought.*" I am giving the translations of θυμός, στῆθος etc. only as a first orientation for the non-expert reader. In fact, these and the following Homeric words have no modern equivalents.

[4] For the meaning of *phrénes*, see shortly below.

[5] The word for 'swelling' in both passages is *oidánō*, which is closely related to the Hippocratic medical expressions *oidéō* and *oídēma* 'oedema.'

is once reproached for having been nursed on *khólos* (*XVI* 203).[6] It can be removed by a drug, *phármakon ákholon* (*Odyssey IV* 220 f.).[7] Finally, *khólos* can be 'digested' (literally, 'cooked') in the body (*Iliad I* 81, *IV* 513, *IX* 565).[8]

This collection of 'physiological' passages, however, should not mislead the modern reader into thinking that it is possible to reconstruct a *system* of Homeric 'physiology.' Such a reconstruction is not possible for two reasons. First, the information on 'physiology' contained in the Homeric epic is extremely fragmentary; this poetry presupposes, on the part of its contemporary listeners or readers, a basic, though not necessarily systematic, knowledge of what usually happens in man (e. g. what happens with his *khólos*, or in his *thȳmós*), and therefore these phenomena are not explicitly described. Second, the poems do not systematically differentiate between expressions for physical constituents, organs, passions, and metaphorical expressions, as we would describe them today. There existed no conceptual system to do so. Albeit for certain philological purposes as the production of dictionaries such modern expressions might prove useful, their application here would be anachronistic. In utilizing them we would assign falsely to Homer's world the disciplines and provinces of modern science and philosophy. It would, therefore, be unmethodical to try to reconstruct a Homeric 'physiology' by singling out those passages which we today would interpret in physiological terms, and ignoring the other passages.

As far as 'physiology' is concerned, there are some obvious parallels that can be drawn with regard to the Homeric and Hippocratic usage of substantives. The Hippocratic *kholḗ*, 'gall,' linguistically related to *khólos*, has according to several Hippocratic treatises the qualities 'bitter,' 'hot,' 'dry;'[9] it has to do with food and digestion; it can increase in volume; it can affect various parts and functions of the body; it can affect the mind. Homeric *khólos* has all these properties in common with Hippocratic *kholḗ*; but Homeric *khólos* has a much broader meaning. In the Hippocratic treatises neither is *kholḗ* ever applied 'metaphorically' in the sense of 'wrath' or 'anger' (for which *orgḗ, orgízō, orgílos* are used), nor does *kholḗ* mean a function of gall, e. g. a state of the body like 'disease caused by gall.'[10] To

[6] Smith, Physiology 552.

[7] Lexikon des frühgriechischen Epos, Fasc. 9, Göttingen, 1978, s. v. ἄχολος.

[8] 'To cook,' Greek *péssō* or *katapéssō*, is again the word used in the Hippocratic treatises; the root has survived in the words 'peptic' etc.; cf. below p. 88 f.

[9] πικρή, θερμή, ξηρή.

[10] In *Loc. Hom.*, several examples which might be explained as 'disease caused by gall' are better explained simply in the sense of 'gall,' e. g. 6.294.4 Li. = 48.23 Joly ἐπὴν δ' ἐς τὸν κίθαρον ῥυῇ ὑπὸ ψύχεος, χολὴ γίνεται. "Quand la fluxion se fait sur la poitrine par l'effet du froid, c'est un flux de bile qui se produit." (Joly) For the other passages in *Loc. Hom.*, see Joly's *Index verborum*.

be sure, *kholḗ* can be the cause of diseases when it abounds either throughout the body or in parts of it; it can cause bodily diseases and even mental affections which are similar to some of those which Homer calls *khólos*: "The brain is harmed," says the author of *On the Sacred Disease* (ch. 15),[11] "through phlegm and bile; by which of them, you can distinguish in the following way: Those who are disturbed by phlegm are quiet, not loud, not excited. Those [who are disturbed] by bile are shouting, malicious, not quiet; they are always liable to do something unexpected." In the Hippocratic treatises *kholḗ* is both the name of a body liquid (gall or bile) and the name of the organ that contains the liquid (the gall-bladder),[12] not the name of their function.

The situation is similar with other substantives: *phrḗn* (or its plural *phrénes*) in the Homeric poems indiscriminately denotes a bodily organ and a bodily function;[13] in the Hippocratic Collection (where it is used almost exclusively in the plural,[14] *phrénes*) it has practically lost its Homeric meaning of a function ('intelligence,' 'mind,' 'soul' etc.) and is most often used as an anatomical name equivalent to *diáphragma*, 'diaphragm' and occasionally for other membranes. In only two Hippocratic passages has the word *phrénes* kept its Homeric meaning of a body function: *Appendix to Regimen in Acute Diseases*, ch. 1 "derangement of the *phrénes*;"[15] similarly *Prorrhetic II*, ch. 9.[16] In four more passages, *phrénes* in the old meaning of a function is used within conventional Greek phrases, which illustrate only stylistic conservativism.[17] In the remaining 80 or more Hippocratic passages, the *phrénes* are an organ, and nothing else. In a famous passage,

---

11 *Morb. Sacr.* 6.388.12–16 Li. = 84.53–56 Gr. = 2.174–176 Jones.

12 There are only a few passages where *kholḗ* means 'gall-bladder;' e. g. *Oss.* 9.168.11–13 ἥπατος πέντε λοβοί· ἐπὶ τετάρτου λοβοῦ ἐπίκειται ἡ χολή, ἣ στόμα ἐπὶ φρένας, καρδίην, πλεύμονα φέρει. This is the text of the only relevant codex Marcianus 265 (M), according to Wilhelm Kahlenberg's unpublished edition of *Oss.*, which is kept in the Hamburg Thesaurus Linguae Graecae.

13 Böhme, Die Seele und das Ich (about φρένες, κραδίη, κῆρ, ἦτορ and other words). Bruno Snell, φρένες – φρόνησις, Glotta 55 (1977), 34–64; revised reprint in: *idem*, Der Weg zum Denken und zur Wahrheit, Hypomnemata 57, Göttingen, 1978, 53–90: "... solch körperliches Organ [hat] eine Funktion, und der Name des Organs kann seine Funktion bezeichnen. Die Alternative: hat das Wort 'körperliche' oder 'geistige' Bedeutung?, ist also falsch gestellt; ... das Abstrakte hebt sich vom Konkreten nicht als Eigenständiges ab." (p. 35 = repr. p. 54) Shirley M. Darcus, The phren of the noos in Xenophanes' god, Symb. Osl. 53 (1978), 25–39, and A person's relation to φρήν in Homer, Hesiod, and the Greek lyric poets, Glotta 57 (1979), 159–173.

14 The only passage with a singular is *Coac.* 5.716.7.

15 *Acut. (Sp.)* 2.396.1 Li. = 1.146.12 Kw. = 68.11–12 Joly παραλλάξιες φρενῶν.

16 *Prorrh. II* 9.28.18–19.

17 φρενῶν ἅπτεσθαι or ἅψις *Acut.* 2.332.6, 336.1, 360.10 Li. = 1.134.11, 135.15, 141.19 Kw. = 57.23, 58.24, 64.12 Joly = 2.104, 106, 118 Jones. *Mul. I* 8.128.22; in *Or. ad Ar.* 9.404.11 the epic phrase ἐνὶ φρεσὶ βαλόμενοι is Littré's conjecture.

again in the treatise *On the Sacred Disease* (ch. 17), it is even expressly stated that neither the *phrénes* nor the *kardíē* is the seat of intelligence: due to their anatomic structure, they exhibit only mechanical reactions to emotions, thus leading us to wrongly conclude that they themselves are directly responsible for sensual perception or intelligence.[18] It should be noted, however, that the older doctrine attacked in *On the Sacred Disease*, namely that the *phrénes* are the seat of intelligence, is yet encountered occasionally in the Hippocratic Collection. According to *On Affections*, ch. 10, *phrenī́tis* (affection[19] of the *phrénes*) with its usual picture of madness[20] results when the gall (*kholḗ*) is stirred and reaches the intestines and the *phrénes*; and in *On the Diseases of Virgins*, ch. 1, it is explained[21] how the blood, accumulating through imperfect menstruation, concentrates in the *kardíē* and the *diáphraxis* (this latter organ being equivalent to *phrénes*),[22] and how this concentration produces *paránoia* with frightening hallucinations. It is important to realize here that in passages such as these two, the *phrénes* are not *identified* with intelligence; rather it appears that intelligence is a function of the organ *phrénes*.

The Homeric word *kradíē* (seldom *kardíē* in Homer; both forms are etymologically and semantically related to our 'heart') is frequently used in the epic and evinces an ambiguity in meaning similar to that of the other Homeric substantives discussed above. There are numerous passages in Homer where *kradíē* clearly means an organ, e. g. when it is said that a spear stuck in somebody's *kradíē* (*Iliad XIII* 442), or that the *kradíē* beats in the chest (*XIII* 282). One can eat up one's own *kradíē* while rejecting food (*XXIV* 129). This organ is also the seat of certain 'psychic functions' (as we would call it) such as *nóos* (*XXI* 441); it can be filled or swelled with *khólos* (*IX* 646, *XXIV* 584); it can mourn in the chest (*X* 9–10; *Odyssey XX* 13; of a lion, *Iliad XX* 169); it can spring out of the breast (*X* 94). We might be inclined to label some of these passages as metaphors. A *kradíē* can be as hard as an axe (*III* 60) or a stone (*Odyssey XXIII* 103), but again, this anachronistic label does not explain very much. Finally, *kradíē* occurs in contexts where it seems to denote the psychic function itself, as when it is said that the *kradíē* is divided whether to do this or that (*Iliad XVI* 435), or that the *kradíē* was changed (*Odyssey IV* 260).[23]

In the Hippocratic Collection, *kardíē* (seldom the Homeric form *kradíē*) occurs about 150 times, and it never means anything else but an organ of

[18] *Morb. Sacr.* 6.392.4–394.8 Li. = 86.86–88.12 Gr. = 2.178–180 Jones.

[19] "*phrenitis* n'est pas une inflammation des *phrénes*, mais une affection non mieux précisée de ces organes" (Professor M. D. Grmek in a letter).

[20] *Aff.* 6.216.21–218.12; τοῦ νοῦ παρακοπή 216.24–25.

[21] *Virg.* 8.466.1 ff.

[22] Cf. a few lines further on, 468.6.

[23] Cf. Snell, Entdeckung 22, with note 32; 70, with note 29.

the body.[24] As to the function of this organ, it is quite often unclear to us whether the heart or the *ventriculus* or the *ostium cardiacum* is meant by *kardíē*.[25] The *kardíē* is the source of the blood and plays various other rôles in the various Hippocratic treatises. Just as in the case of the substantive *phrénes*, the *kardíē* can react to emotions: at *Epidemics VI* 5, ch. 5, "Excitement makes the *kardíē* and the lungs contract;"[26] in *Epidemics VII*, ch. 3, it is implied that the heartbeat is increased when somebody is running or is afraid.[27] There are very few passages in the Hippocratic Collection where the idea is expressed that the *kardíē* is the seat of emotions or intelligence.[28] One of these passages is found in *On the Diseases of Virgins* and has been quoted above in our discussion of *phrénes*; another is in the *Appendix to Regimen in Acute Diseases*, ch. 5 Littré (= ch. 7 Kühlewein, Joly), where we are told that when corrupted blood flows to the *kardíē* or to the liver or to the blood vessel (*vena cava*?), then the patients get fainting fits, speechlessness, seizures, and/or *paraplēgíē*.[29] In the treatise *On the Heart*, ch. 10, it is maintained that "the intelligence (*gnṓmē*) of man has its seat in the left side of the body cavity and rules over the rest of the soul (*psȳchḗ*),"[30] and the late, non-medical *Letter* no. 23 poetically calls the *kardíē* "the queen, the wet-nurse of anger."[31] One last passage which should be mentioned has already been quoted above: *On the Sacred Disease* (ch. 17), where the doctrine is refuted that either the *phrénes* or the *kardíē* is the seat of intelligence. Indeed, although *kardíē* may serve as the *seat* of functions, nowhere in the Hippocratic Collection is the word used for an emotion or any other bodily or psychic function itself.

Before proceeding further with our discussion, let us summarize briefly: In Homer several substantives indiscriminately denote (to put it in modern terms) either an organ (or, in the case of *khólos*, a substance) of the body or a function of the body or soul; sometimes in Homer the modern reader is tempted to apply the term 'metaphor;' in the Hippocratic treatises, on

[24] In *Epid. V* 5.254.1 *kardíē* is both the name for a disease and for an organ. The passage has to be explained in terms of style, not of lexicography: cf. Langholf, Syntaktische Untersuchungen p. 104.

[25] Once, *Morb. IV* 7.550.21 Li. = 89.6 Joly, even the liver is referred to as *kardíē*, but the Hippocratic author says that this expression is popular. For a detailed discussion of this passage and of the ambiguous meaning of *kardíē* elsewhere in the Collection cf. Lonie, Hippocratic treatises 286–288. More examples in Lloyd, Science 149–157.

[26] *Epid. VI* 5.316.5–7.

[27] *Epid. VII* 5.370.21–23.

[28] This was to be Aristotle's doctrine; see, e. g., Düring, Aristoteles 537–541.

[29] *Acut. (Sp.)* 2.406.4–11 Li. = 1.149.14–22 Kw. = 71.6–14 Joly.

[30] *Cord.* 9.88.7–9.

[31] *Ep.* 9.396.1. The view expressed is that of later popular philosophy. On the date of the *Letters* (early imperial epoch) see D. Th. Sakalis, Beiträge zu den pseudo-hippokratischen Briefen, in: Formes de pensée 499–514.

the other hand, the same substantives, or those linguistically closely related, denote organs (or bodily substances) only, or almost exclusively.[32]

Of course, several centuries separate the Homeric poems from the Hippocratic Collection. It might seem misleading to compare them, but in fact the Homeric usage of these substantives was not archaic for the Greek of the fifth and fourth centuries B. C. nor was it considered essentially poetic. The Homeric substantives or their collateral forms were applied in the Homeric way throughout the post-Homeric centuries, not only in texts inspired — directly or indirectly — by Homer's poetry (as, e. g., tragedies) but also in colloquial contexts. The usage was simply popular. This can clearly be recognized in Aristophanes' comedies, which are contemporary with many of the Hippocratic writings.[33] These comedies are representative of extant fifth and fourth century texts reflecting popular or everyday speech and thought.

In Aristophanes, *kholḗ* is as ambiguously used as *khólos* is in Homer. *kholḗ* is 'in' people (*Lysistrata* 464 f.); it can be 'stirred' (*Wasps* 403), can 'boil' when one hears something annoying (*Thesmophoriazusae* 466—468), or can simply 'come' (*Peace* 66).

The Aristophanic *kardíā* also has a range of usage that covers the bodily organ as well as certain psychic functions. The heart 'swells' (*Clouds* 1368), 'leaps' (*Clouds* 1391), can be 'shaken' (*Acharnians* 12) or 'struck' (*Frogs* 53—54), or can 'burn' (*Lysistrata* 9); one can 'love' somebody from the *kardíā* (*Clouds* 86) or 'bite' one's own *kardíā* (*Acharnians* 1); something can 'flatter' one's *kardíā* (*Thesmophoriazusae* 869). Some of these passages might also be described as 'metaphorical.'

The word *phrḗn* (or its plural, *phrénes*), which in Hippocrates is rarely used in the sense of a psychic function, frequently has this usage in Aristophanes. In a few passages, one might just as well understand it as an organ or as a metaphorical expression. Something wise is 'in' the *phrḗn* (*Birds* 429); also memory is 'in' the *phrénes* (*Knights* 1052). Most often, however, Aristophanes' *phrḗn* or *phrénes* is used synonymously with, and sometimes parallel to, words denoting 'mind.'

---

[32] Sometimes names of organs in the Hippocratic treatises seem to denote anatomical regions around the organs. *nephrós*, 'kidney,' is a good example. Material relating to the kidneys has been collected by Grmek/Wittern, Krankheit des Nikias 12—13. This extension of the meaning (as compared to modern usage) is due to an interpretation of the various contexts in terms of modern medical methods. For the Hippocratic writer and for the reader of the fifth and fourth centuries, *nephrós* may in all these contexts have had its strictest meaning, 'kidney.'

[33] For the present purpose, those passages in which Aristophanes mocks Greek tragedy have been disregarded, because their diction differs in many respects from ordinary speech. — For *kholḗ*, cf. J. Taillardat, Les images d'Aristophane, 2nd ed., Paris, 1965, 194.

Thus, it would appear that the Hippocratic use of *kholṓ*, *phrénes*, and *kardíē* is considerably narrower than the use of these words (or of their equivalents *khólos*, *phrḗn*, *kradíē* respectively) in Homer and in the colloquial language of the fifth and fourth centuries B. C., even though 'narrower' does not imply that these words are unambiguously defined in Hippocrates. As it has been stated above,[34] in numerous Hippocratic passages one can hardly determine whether *kardíē* means the heart or the *ventriculus* (= *gastḗr*) or the *ostium cardiacum*. Apart from this ambiguity, however, *kardíē* in Hippocrates has a very restricted meaning: it always means an organ, never a function; it is never used metaphorically.

Almost the same distinction applies to the *phrénes*. In the Hippocratic writings, *phrénes* is (with the few exceptions quoted above) a word for a body organ. In most of the Hippocratic passages it is equivalent to *diáphragma*, the diaphragm or midriff. This is in contrast to Homer, where, apart from other meanings (cf. above), *phrḗn* or *phrénes* obviously does not denote the midriff but the lungs[35] or, what seems still more plausible, the intricate texture of lungs, vessels, tubes, and nerves found in the chest.[36]

In a few Hippocratic passages *phrénes* as an organ has retained this Homeric meaning. In the fragment *On the Diseases of Virgins* (already quoted on two occasions), the words *phrénes* and *diáphraxis* (the latter word occurs only here) are used indiscriminately as synonyms. It should be noted that, although *diáphraxis* is a substantive linguistically very closely related to *diáphragma*, it manifestly does not mean 'diaphragm' in this passage; consequently, *phrénes* too means something special here. The fragment explains that the menstrual blood, when it has no issue from the body, "rushes up into the *kardíē* and into the *diáphraxis*. When these are filled, the *kardíē* gets stupefied. After the stupefaction, it is seized with numbness. After the numbness, with madness ... From the *kardíē* and from the *phrénes* the blood can withdraw only slowly because the vessels (*phlébes*) are horizontal (*epikársiai*). This body region is an important one and susceptible to derangement and madness. When these parts are filled, also rigor with fever quickly comes."[37] It is useful here to cite what Richard

---

[34] p. 42, with note 25.

[35] Onians, Origins 23 ff.

[36] Cf. David J. Furley, The early history of the concept of soul, in: University of London, Institute of Classical Studies, Bulletin no. 3, 1956, p. 2–3. S. Ireland/F. L. D. Steel, Φρένες as an anatomical organ in the works of Homer, Glotta 53 (1975), 183–195.

[37] *Virg.* 8.466.17–468.9 οὐκ ἔχον τὸ αἷμα ἔκρουν ἀναΐσσει ὑπὸ πλήθεος ἐς τὴν καρδίην καὶ ἐς τὴν διάφραξιν· ὁκόταν οὖν ταῦτα πληρωθέωσιν, ἐμωρώθη ἡ καρδίη· εἶτε ἐκ τῆς μωρώσιος νάρκη· εἶτε ἐκ τῆς νάρκης παράνοια ἔλαβεν ... ἐκ δὲ τῆς καρδίης καὶ τῶν φρενῶν βραδέως παλιρροεῖ· ἐπικάρσιαι γὰρ αἱ φλέβες καὶ ὁ τόπος ἐπίκαιρος (ἐκ δὲ ... ἐπίκαιρος M: om. V propter homoeotel.) ἔς τε παραφροσύνην καὶ μανίην (ἕτοιμος post μανίην add. M: om. V). ὁκόταν γὰρ (γὰρ M: om. V) πληρωθέωσι ταῦτα (ταῦτα M: αὐτὰ V) τὰ μέρεα, καὶ φρίκη ξὺν πυρετῷ ἀναΐσσει.

B. Onians has said about the Homeric *phrēn* or *phrénes*:[38] "No part of the body has less obvious claims to be the seat of ... the intelligence, than the midriff or diaphragm, the pink muscular sheet dividing the organs of the thorax from those of the abdomen." With reference to *Iliad I* 103 f. ("his [Agamemnon's] black *phrénes* were filled with fury all around"), he continues: "How a dome-shaped muscular sheet can be 'filled ...' ... is not explained. Nor is the similar difficulty met that Homer repeatedly speaks of *thȳmós*, etc. as moving *in*, being *in* or being placed *in*, not beneath, the *phrénes*." Onians rightly reminds us of the fact already known to the ancient Greek grammarians that a considerable proportion of the Greek vocabulary underwent semantic changes in the period between Homer and the fifth and fourth centuries B.C. Since the *phrénes* and the *diáphraxis* in the fragment *On the Diseases of Virgins* are indeed explicitly described as being 'filled' with blood, we are entitled to infer that these two words have retained the old Homeric meaning of *phrēn*/*phrénes* and can, therefore, be considered semantic 'fossils'[39] in the Hippocratic Corpus, wherein *phrénes* otherwise almost exclusively, and *diáphragma* always, denote the diaphragm or midriff.[40]

The statement made in *On the Diseases of Virgins* about *phrénes* or *diáphraxis* is in the same doctrinal context as *Aphorisms V* 40, "In women, a congestion of blood in the breasts indicates mental derangement."[41] This doctrine holds true generally, not only with women, according to *Epidemics II* 6. 32: "An indication of imminent mental derangement: congestion of blood in the breasts (nipples)."[42] The reason seems to be given in *Epidemics*

---

[38] Onians, Origins 23 f.

[39] 'Fossils' from archaic stages of Greek medicine can be found frequently in the Collection (Kudlien, Beginn 88–97, 100, and *passim*), particularly in therapy, e.g. *Epid. VII* 5.434.16–19, where it is prescribed to lie in sea-water, to drink light white wine, and to *urinate into the water*. This is clearly archaic folk-medicine, cf. generally Robert Muth, Träger der Lebenskraft. Ausscheidungen des Organismus im Volksglauben der Antike, Wien, 1954, 117–125. For 'fossils,' see also below p. 54 f., 134, 253 f. The metaphor 'fossil' does not imply that these doctrinal elements were of only antiquarian interest to the authors of the Collection.

[40] Another indication for the relatively early date of *Virg.* besides the archaic usage of *phrénes* is the use of *thȳmós* (8.468.13 ὁ θυμὸς κακὸν ἐφέλκεται), very much in the Homeric sense. All other instances of *thȳmós* in the Hippocratic Collection are either phraseological (βῆξαι θυμὸς ἐγγίνεται *Prog.* 2.132.1–2, 154.1 Li. = 1.86.10–11, 95.17–18 Kw. = 2.20, 34 Jones; *Coac.* 5.684.6–7; ἐκ θυμοῦ *Epid. VI* 5.316.5) or late (in *Ep.* and *Or. Thess.*).

[41] *Aph.* 4.544.16–17 Li. = 4.168 Jones γυναιξὶν ὁκόσῃσιν ἐς τοὺς τιτθοὺς αἷμα συστρέφεται, μανίην σημαίνει. Cf. Littré vol. 4. 423 f.

[42] *Epid. II* 5.138.19–20 τῷ μέλλοντι μαίνεσθαι τόδε προσημαίνει (post πρ. add. τὸ σημεῖον HIR: om. V)· αἷμα συλλέγεται ἐς τοὺς τιτθούς. Galen (comm. on the passage) had difficulties explaining this sentence.

II 6. 19: "There is a broad vein in each breast: This region takes part to a very high degree in intelligence."[43]

There are other Hippocratic passages where *phrénes* as an organ has retained its ancient meaning. In *On Diseases II*, ch. 12–75, which belongs to the oldest nosological texts of the Corpus,[44] chapter 72 describes a disease called *phrontís*, a name not clearly attested to elsewhere and etymologically related to *phrénes*. The word either means 'sorrow'[45] or 'affection of the *phrénes*.'[46] In this description it is stated that "the *phrénes* swell to the exterior,"[47] which would certainly be nonsensical if the author followed the later usage, 'midriff.'[48] For him, the *phrénes* must have been something more substantial than a sheet of muscular tissue. Another case is *On the Places in Man*, ch. 3: "The hollow vein ... is between the windpipe and the esophagus. It passes through the *phrénes* and through the *kardíē*[49] and between the *phrénes* and branches towards the groin." In this description, which suggests a downward direction, the *phrénes* cannot be the midriff.[50] Furthermore, *On Diseases III*, ch. 9, "[the patients] have pain in their *phrénes*"[51] can hardly be understood if one thinks of the diaphragm.

A particularly interesting 'fossil,' which was even to become one of the main pillars of the humoral theory expounded or presupposed in a number of Hippocratic treatises, is *kholḗ* in the concept of 'black bile.' Whereas other humours such as bile, phlegm (= mucus), blood, and water can easily be observed, 'black bile' does not exist as such: although the author of *On the Nature of Man* (*passim*) claims that it is regularly observed, Galen felt the need of circumstantially 'proving' its existence and demonstrating its alleged provenance from the spleen.[52] The observation of 'black bile' implied a good deal more interpretation on the part of the physician than did the observation of other humours. Any blackish dis-

---

43 *Epid. II* 5.136.11–12 φλὲψ ἔχει παχείη ἐν ἑκατέρῳ τιτθῷ· ταῦτα μέγιστον ἔχει μόριον συνέσιος. For ἔχω = 'to be' see, Liddell/Scott/Jones s. v., B II 1. The translation of the sentence is by no means certain. Galen (comm. on the passage) explained it differently.

44 Cf. above, p. 25, and below, p. 52 f.

45 Liddell/Scott/Jones translate 'hypochondria.'

46 Another instance of *phrontis* is dubiously transmitted in *Mul. I* 8.96.16, cf. Langholf, Syntaktische Untersuchungen p. 185 f.

47 *Morb. II* 7.110.2–3 Li. = 211.18–19 Jouanna αἱ φρένες οἰδέουσιν ἐκτός. For a fuller quotation and discussion, see below p. 54 f. Any modern translation like "the region around the midriff" only camouflages the problem.

48 Kudlien, Schwärzliche Organe 53.

49 *kardíē* is clearly 'heart' here, not 'stomach.'

50 *Loc. Hom.* 6.282.10–13, cf. 282.16–22 Li. = 42.6–10, 14–21 Joly ἡ δὲ κοίλη φλὲψ ... πέφυκε ... μεταξὺ τοῦ τε βρόγχου καὶ τοῦ οἰσοφάγου· φέρεται δὲ διὰ τῶν φρενῶν καὶ διὰ τῆς καρδίης καὶ μεταξὺ τῶν φρενῶν, καὶ σχίζεται ἐς τοὺς βουβῶνας ...

51 *Morb. III* 7.128.6 Li. = 76.20–21 Potter τὰς φρένας ἀλγέουσιν.

52 For instance in *De atra bile* 5.104–148 K.; cf. Kudlien, Beginn 77.

charges of the body were liable to be interpreted as containing 'black bile:' for instance, black stool, vomit, urine. 'Black urine'[53] must often have been caused by malaria ('blackwater fever'), which was spreading in Greece during the epoch of Hippocrates[54] and may have contributed to the formation of the concept of 'black bile.'[55] It is possible that the author of *On the Nature of Man*,[56] whose four humours were phlegm, blood, bile, and *black bile*, had practised in an epoch or/and area in which malaria was endemic, while another author, who wrote *On Generation, On the Nature of the Child, On Diseases IV*[57] and certain gynaecological texts,[58] and whose four humours were phlegm, blood, bile, and *water*, had not (not yet?) been influenced by observations of this disease when constructing his theory.[59]

In the Hippocratic Corpus, there occurs not only the expression 'black bile,' *mélaina kholḗ*, but in addition there are found a number of compounds consisting of the same elements, for instance *melagkholíē*.[60] At first sight it would seem that the compounds are derived from the expression *mélaina kholḗ*. This would correspond to the aetiology of diseases like *melagkholíē* as explained in the Hippocratic Corpus, namely that these diseases are caused by black bile.[61] The derivation is, however, extremely unlikely. In fact, the etymological origin must be from *melágkholos*,[62] an adjective once attested in Sophocles, *Trachiniae* 573. Since its context in the tragic passage poses problems of interpretation (see below p. 49 f., note 73), the word's possible range of meaning should be reconstructed by using an indirect method, namely by examining the meaning of other analogously formed compounds. Apart from *melágkholos*, there are 17 adjectives ending in *-kholos*. At least 7 out of them signify functions of the soul such as wrath or anger.[63] Examining the meaning of the denominative verb directly

---

[53] οὖρα μέλανα.

[54] Grmek, Les maladies *passim* (index 'paludisme'); on 'black urine' *ibid.* 409–436.

[55] Grmek, Les maladies 436.

[56] Polybos, Hippocrates' son-in-law; see, Grensemann, Arzt Polybos *passim*; Jouanna (ed.), Hippocrate, La nature de l'homme, p. 55–59.

[57] Lonie, Hippocratic treatises 43–51.

[58] Grensemann, Gynäkologie 9–32.

[59] Volker Langholf, Gymnasium 92 (1985), 217–219. On the inferable development of the quaternary theory of *Nat. Hom.* out of a system of 3 humours and 3 seasons, which were supplemented by black bile and its corresponding season (autumn), see, Müri, Melancholie 27 f. (= 174–176 of the reprint).

[60] μελαγχολάω, μελαγχολίη, μελαγχολικός, μελαγχολώδης.

[61] Kudlien, Beginn 78.

[62] See, e.g., Albert Debrunner, Griechische Wortbildungslehre, Heidelberg, 1917, §§ 183, 38, 43, 61; note in particular that μελαγχολάω cannot be a composit of μέλαν + χολάω.

[63] The adjectives ending in -χολος fall into 3 semantic categories (cf. Liddell/Scott/Jones): *(i)* Adjectives in which -χολος has an exclusively or predominantly medical meaning referring to the substance bile: ἀκρητόχολος, ἀπικρόχολος, γλισχρόχολος, διάχολος, κατάχολος, ξανθόχολος (hence -χολικός), περίχολος, πικρόχολος, ὑδατόχολος, ὑπό-

derived from *kholḗ*, viz. *kholáō*, and its compounds reveals that they all indicate functions of the soul.[64] Thus, it is not unreasonable that also the adjective *melágkholos* was in its meaning originally not confined to the humour bile but could refer to a function of the soul, just as *khólos* in the Homeric poems and *kholḗ* in Aristophanes could designate a temper. This inference is confirmed by examining a verb derived from *melágkholos*, viz. *melagkholáō*, which outside of the Hippocratic Collection is used in old comedy.[65] Without any medical connotation it signifies there a state of the soul, 'to be crazy.' No medical bodily humour such as bile or black bile can be ascertained in Aristophanes:[66] The colloquial expression *melagkholáō* is rather likely to reflect the unspecific meaning of *khólos* and *kholḗ* as found in Homer and in Aristophanes respectively.[67]

What, however, does *melag-*, 'black,' in this verbal compound mean if not a bodily humour which is black in appearence? It seems that *melagkholáō* belongs to a group of early Greek expressions found from Homer onward in which human 'organs' or constituents of the body (in the Homeric sense) are said to become or to be 'black.' These expressions are 'metaphorical' (in the sense described above). They do not refer to strictly anatomical or physiological constituents of the body, nor could any black colour in every instance have been seen. Fridolf Kudlien has collected and cogently interpreted the relevant material.[68] One of his typical examples is Aeschylus, *Eumenides* 459 "my mother with black *phrénes* killed him,"[69] where 'black' expresses the abomination of the criminal act: the *phrénes* are 'black' because the act of the *phrénes* is perverse. The bodily constituents turning 'black' or being 'black' are obviously but the special case of a

---

χολος. *(ii)* Adjectives in which -χολος has an exclusively or predominantly 'psychological' meaning referring to a function of the soul such as anger, wrath: ἀκράχολος/ἀκρόχολος (hence -χολέω, -χολία), ζάχολος, κρυψίχολος. *(iii)* Adjectives falling into categories *i* and *ii*; in these adjectives, -χολος may refer to the substance bile as well as to a function of the soul: ἄχολος, δίχολος, ἐπίχολος, ὑπέρχολος. — On the relationship between 'bile' and 'wrath,' 'anger' see also Müri, Melancholie 35 f. (= 187 f. of the reprint), who, however, restricts his linguistic observations to χολόομαι and χολωτός.

64 χολάω, ἐκχολάω, ὑπερχολάω.

65 Aristoph. *Av.* 14 (staged Dionys. 414), *Eccl.* 251 (of 392?), *Plut.* 12, 366, 903 (of 388).

66 Both Müri, Melancholie 34 (= 185 of the reprint), and Flashar, Melancholie 37–39, believe that bile as a humour is presupposed in Aristophanes. 'Bile' is, however, not used in a 'physiological' sense by this poet. Although he may have known a medical theory implying bile, he did not make his stage-figures allude to it, probably because bile had not yet been popularized as an important constituent of the body.

67 The verb μελαγχολάω may be an older formation than μελαγχολία (-ίη) because the latter has never brought forth a denominative *μελαγχολιάω: the older verb was too current. Cf. generally Jean Irigoin, Préalables linguistiques, in: Formes de pensée 175 f.

68 Kudlien, Schwärzliche Organe.

69 ἀλλά νιν κελαινόφρων ἐμὴ μήτηρ κατέκτα. An example to be added is Aristoph. *Ra.* 470, in tragic parody: Στυγὸς ... μελανοκάρδιος πέτρα.

considerably more common, perhaps even universal, phenomenon, namely the association of the colour 'black' with 'bad,' 'malignant,' 'sinister.'[70]

The adjective *melágkholos*, from which Aristophanes' popular verb *melagkholáō* is derived, may, therefore, originally have had a broad, unspecific meaning not narrowed down to any medical theory of 'black bile.' A physician of the first century A. D., Aretaios, who had philological interest and training,[71] explains *melagkholíē* linguistically: "*kholḗ* has the connotation of 'wrath' ('anger'), while 'black' connotes 'much' and 'wild'."[72] This appears to be a good and precise observation about the semantic range of *melagkholíē* and of kindred compounds. Aretaios may have taken it over from grammatical literature based on more primary evidence than we have today. Unfortunately, no relevant scholium or other ancient grammatical explanation is available for the difficult Sophoclean passage where *melágkholos* happens to be once attested.[73] [Cf. below, "Addendum," p. 267.]

---

[70] Cf., e. g., Liddell/Scott/Jones s. v. μέλας, which rich material. Snell, Entdeckung 182.

[71] He used an antiquarian scholarly dialect, the Ionian of the Hippocratic Collection, for his literary work, which betrays philological training throughout; cf. Fridolf Kudlien, Untersuchungen zu Aretaios von Kappadokien, Akad. d. Wiss. u. d. Lit., Abhandl. d. geistes- u. sozialwiss. Kl. 1963, no. 11, Mainz/Wiesbaden, 1964, p. 1156, 1174–1176 (cf. 1152 note 1).

[72] Aret. *III* 5 (39.19–27 Hude) καὶ τούσδε … μελαγχολικοὺς καλέομεν, χολῇ μὲν τῆς ὀργῆς ξυμφραζομένης, μελαίνῃ δὲ πολλῆς καὶ θηριώδεος. He then quotes Hom. *Il. I* 101–104, continuing: τοιοίδε γίγνονται οἱ μελαγχολώδεες, εὖτ᾽ ἂν ὑπὸ τοῦ κακοῦ κινέωνται. Cf. Flashar, Melancholie 76 f. – Müri, Melancholie 35 f. (= 188 of the reprint) finds Aretaios' observation amusing, but not helpful ("amüsant, wenn auch nicht förderlich"), although his own argumentation is similar. Important here is Kudlien, Beginn 83; Kudlien, Primitive medicine 327.

[73] The *hapax legomenon* μελάγχολος may have had the same connotations, as can be inferred from the difficult passage where the adjective is attested, Soph. *Trach.* 572–577. The text has been variously explained and even 'emended,' cf. Richard C. Jebb, Sophocles, The plays and fragments, vol. 5, Cambridge, 1908 (= repr. Amsterdam, 1962), *ad loc.* Emendations seem, however, unnecessary. It is possible that θρέμμα (v. 574) signifies 'coagulated substance' (not 'creature,' as Liddell/Scott/Jones translate: ὕδρας θρέμμα = ὕδρα would be rather redundant); see Flashar, Melancholie 37, with notes 35 f., where literature is quoted. For τρέφω = 'coagulate' cf. ἀμφίθρεπτον αἷμα v. 572, 'blood clotted round my wound' (Jebb), and Paul Demont, Remarques sur le sens de ΤΡΕΦΩ, Rev. Ét. Grecques 91 (1978), 358–384 (where, however, θρέμμα is not quoted in this sense). The expression μελαγχόλους ἰούς may well refer to a substance, if one supplements Sophocles' description with details from later mythography: After killing the Hydra of Lerne, Herakles had, according to a mythological tradition recorded in Apollod. *II* 5.2, dipped his arrows in the monster's bile. Subsequently, the arrows became poisonous and, according to Sophocles, rendered in turn the clotted blood around Nessos' wound poisonous. After Deianeira had prepared Herakles' robe with Nessos' blood ("black poison of blood," ἰὸς αἵματος μέλας v. 717), she observed how a tuft of wool soaked with the blood and exposed to the hot sun "shrivelled all away, and quickly crumbled to powder on the ground … And from the earth, where it was strewn, clots of foam seethed up, as when the rich juice of the blue fruit from the vine of Bacchus is poured

A semantic specialization of compounds such as *melagkholáō* occurred as soon as there was a medical humoral system. It was then possible to re-interpret them by postulating that a special humour was responsible for the action expressed. Whereas none of the Hippocratic compound terms such as *melagkholáō*[74] can plausibly be derived from the analytic expression 'black bile,' *mélaina kholḗ*, it is inversely quite likely that *mélaina kholḗ* is derived from these compounds; or, in other words, that the medical concept of 'black bile' has its origins in Greek language. This humour may have been 'discovered' not by observing physiological or pathological processes in the body, but by analyzing a traditional word family according to the new, strictly medical humoral categories of the fifth century, i. e. by 'dissecting' compound words. The two components of the compounds were thus semantically narrowed down, respectively, to a colour visible to the eye and a humour with well-defined material qualities. 'Black bile' could subsequently help to explain 'black urine' and other black discharges.[75]

We have examined with considerable detail now the Hippocratic usage of *kholḗ*, *kardíē*, and *phrénes*. It would appear that *(i)* in the medical language

---

upon the ground" (v. 693–704, transl. by Jebb). This effect of the venom is similar to that of black bile as described by Galen (*De atra bile* 5.111 K. ζυμοῖ τὴν γῆν ..., καὶ κατὰ τοῦτ' ἔοικεν ὄξει δριμυτάτῳ. *De loc. affectis III* 8.176 K. [black-bilious vomit] ξύει τὴν γῆν, ἐξαίρων τε καὶ ζυμῶν καὶ πομφόλυγας ἐγείρων, οἷαι τοῖς ζέουσι ζωμοῖς ἐφίστανται. Kudlien, Beginn 78 f.). Already in *Morb. II* 73 (7.110.14–19 Li. = 212.11–17 Jouanna) a black vomit is described which "makes the soil effervesce," τὴν γῆν αἴρει (cf. below p. 59), a passage which could be re-interpreted in terms of black bile, although this humour is nowhere mentioned in *Morb. II*, ch. 12–75, cf. Jouanna, Archéologie 108–114. The "black poison" of the "black-bilious arrow" in Sophocles has, therefore, some material affinity to the black bile of later medicine. Another such affinity consists in the effect on the skin: In [Arist.] *Probl. XXX* 1 ἡ πρὸ τῆς ἀφανίσεως (viz. of Herakles) ἐν Οἴτῃ τῶν ἑλκῶν ἔκφυσις γενομένη is interpreted as a symptom of black bile (953 a 17–19; in the same text black bile is repeatedly compared to wine, 953 a 33–955 a 40, which recalls the comparison in the Sophoclean passage). An important difference should, however, not be neglected: In Sophocles, the black substance is not a normal bodily humour but a venom with typical toxic effects. Nowhere in Greek medical literature is bile or black bile ever regarded as a venom. It is, therefore, plausible that the expression μελαγχόλους ἰούς, "black-bilious arrow," does not signify exclusively "arrow with black bile" but also "arrow covered with the Hydra's bile, black and sinister" or "arrow shot in sinister wrath." The word μελάγχολος in Sophocles may thus have a meaning comparable to the ones of other adjectives ending in -χολος, namely oscillate between 'bile' and 'wrath,' 'anger.' Nessos' words are ambiguous, and probably deliberately so, because the centaur must in this crucial context not draw Deianeira's attention too outspokenly to the fact that his blood had been poisoned by the arrow: otherwise she would not have risked to use it as a philtre. [Cf. below, "Addendum," p. 267.]

[74] Cf. above, note 60.

[75] This process of reification resembles the one which helped to form the concept of *krísis*, see below p. 127–134.

of fifth and fourth century B. C. physicians these words differ in their meaning from Homeric and contemporary colloquial usage, although vestiges of traditional usage are occasionally evidenced in the Hippocratic treatises; *(ii)* the Hippocratic meaning is narrower; *(iii)* there is no uniform medical terminology in the Corpus Hippocraticum as a whole, but a considerable amount of semantic overlapping (e. g. *kardíē/gastḗr*, or *phrénes/diáphragma*). Accordingly, it is important that one be continually aware of the possibility, when trying to understand Hippocratic texts, that one and the same word may have different meanings in different passages, and that medical concepts identical or very similar to each other may be expressed with different words.

The narrowing in the meaning of 'medical' words parallels a methodological postulate formulated in the *Epidemics* and elsewhere, namely that the senses of the physician should play a prominent rôle in his professional activities.[76] A concise note in *Epidemics IV* 43 reads (words to be supplied from the context are added in square brackets in the following translation): "[It has to be said (or: It has been said)] That we [observe] with the eyes, the ears, the noses, the hand. [There are] The crises, and the other things by which we make observation. [On the one hand, there is] The patient; [on the other hand, there is] the practitioner, who, in each case,[77] touches or smells or tastes and is informed about the rest: hair, complexion, skin, vessels, sinews [another possible translation: nerves], muscles, flesh, bones, marrow, brain, the blood and its effects, intestines, stomach, bile, the other humours, limbs, ... pulses, tremors, spasms, hiccups, respiration, faeces: these are the means by which we observe."[78] It is not possible to assign an exact date to this note,[79] but the idea expressed must have been of central importance because the same thought occurs in other Hippocratic treatises of around 400 B. C., although in shorter formulations: *Epidemics VI* 8.17 "It is necessary to use the body for observation: sight, hearing, nose, touch, tongue, intelligence."[80] Sim-

---

[76] Cf. throughout Lloyd, Magic 126–169; Mansfeld, Theoretical and empirical attitudes.

[77] The English "in each case" is implied in the aorists.

[78] *Epid. IV* 5.184.7–13 Li. = Per. 252–255 (cf. p. 48 f.) La. Ὅτι τοῖσιν ὄμμασι, τοῖσιν οὔασι, τῇσι ῥισί, τῇ χειρί· αἱ κρίσιες, καὶ τἄλλα οἷσι γινώσκομεν. ὁ ἀσθενέων. ὁ δρῶν· ἢ θιγὼν ἢ ὀσφρανθεὶς ἢ γευσάμενος, τὰ δ' ἄλλα γνούς· τρίχες, χροιή, δέρματα, φλέβες, νεῦρα, μύες, σάρκες, ὀστέα, μυελός, ἐγκέφαλος, καὶ τὰ ἀπὸ τοῦ αἵματος, σπλάγχνα, κοιλίη, χολή, οἱ ἄλλοι χυμοί, ἄρθρα, ... σφυγμοί, τρόμοι, σπασμοί, λύγγες, {αμφι} πνεῦμα, ἄφοδοι, οἷσι γινώσκομεν.

[79] On the date of the *Epidemics* treatises cf. below p. 77 f.

[80] *Epid. VI* 5.350.3–4 τὸ σῶμα ἔργον ἐς τὴν σκέψιν ἄγειν· ὄψις, ἀκοή, ῥίς, ἀφή, γλῶσσα, λογισμός. Cf. Democritus 68 B 11 Diels/Kranz ὄψις, ἀκοή, ὀδμή, γεῦσις, ψαῦσις, where likewise reasoning is said to supplement the senses; Maria Michela Sassi, Le teorie della percezione in Democrito, Firenze, 1978, 213–221.

ilarly in the first lines of the treatise *In the Surgery*,[81] it is stressed that the senses of the body play a prominent rôle in medical observation. 'Intelligence' (*logismós*) is mentioned only in the last place in *Epidemics VI* 8.17, and also in the treatise *In the Surgery* 'intelligence' (for which the synonym *gnṓmē* is used) occurs only after the enumeration of the senses. In *Epidemics IV* 43 it is not mentioned at all.

The oldest testimonium about "the so-called *Knídiai gnṓmai*"[82] leads in a similar direction. In his criticism, the author of *On Regimen in Acute Diseases* states that those who wrote these texts "did describe correctly what the patients are suffering from in each disease, and how some diseases end." Then he adds the reproach: "Up to this point, even a non-physician could give a correct description if he skilfully asked the patients what they are suffering." Albeit this statement, as has been demonstrated above, is probably too general and, therefore, exaggerated, there may have been passages in the *Knídiai gnṓmai* where the description of symptoms was restricted to features immediately perceptible by the senses. This can be inferred from another nosological text, *On Diseases II*, ch. 12–75. Even though its source relationship to the *Knídiai gnṓmai* cannot be determined,[83] there is little doubt, as Grensemann and Jouanna have cogently argued,[84] that it is among the oldest nosological texts contained in the Collection, together with certain gynaecological chapters which equal them in age. One can, therefore, use *On Diseases II*, ch. 12–75 as a witness for a

---

[81] *Off.* 3.272.2–6 Li. = 2.30.2–11 Kw. = 3.58 Withington.

[82] See above p. 14 f.

[83] See above p. 24 f.

[84] Grensemann, Knidische Medizin p. 175–202. Jouanna, Archéologie *passim*, particularly 152–160. This opinion has been attacked by Robert Joly (Sur une chronologie des traités cnidiens du Corpus hippocratique, Episteme 6 [1972], 3–11; Le système cnidien des humeurs, in: La Collection hippocratique 107–127; Indices lexicaux pour la datation ..., in: "Corpus Hippocraticum" 136–147; L'école médicale de Cnide et son évolution, Ant. Classique 47 [1978], 528–537). His criticism starts from a comparison of the two versions in *Morb. II*, ch. 1–11 and 12–75, which is an insufficient basis, because this approach takes too lightly the fact that a common doctrinal and literary nucleus underlying the several nosological and gynaecological treatises can be reconstructed by applying the philological methods of 'literarische Quellenkritik,' in particular by collecting the textual elements common to all (or most) of these texts, and that *Morb. II*, ch. 12–75, together with Grensemann's gynaecological "Schicht A," resembles most closely this inferable nucleus, while other treatises (e. g. *Morb. II*, ch. 1–11; *Morb. III; Aff.; Int.; Morb. I*) can plausibly be fit into an inferred historical development of medicine. I myself do not find Joly's linguistic arguments convincing, because there is so little firmly dated text material for a comparison, and because one has to reckon with the possibility of stylistic archaisms, provincialisms, and the like. Grensemann's "Schicht C" is so considerably more developed stylistically and 'rhetorically' that I find it hard to accept Joly's chronology, viz. that "Schicht C" is earlier than "Schicht A." Cf. Grensemann, Gynäkologie 36 f., note 36.

relatively early stage in the development of Greek medicine. These texts largely depend on sensory observation, as another, closer look at ch. 68 will reveal:[85] "Livid: Dry fever seizes [the patient] and rigor from time to time, and the head aches, and pain is in the intestines, and he vomits bile, and whenever he feels the pain, his vision is disturbed and he feels heavy, and the stomach becomes hard,[86] and the skin livid, and the lips and the white of the eyes livid, and he looks as if he were being strangled, and sometimes he changes his complexion from livid to greenish. To this [patient] you should give a drug [which evacuates] from below and from above, and you should give him an enema, and purge him from the head, and wash him with warm water as little as possible, but whenever he is washed, warm him in the sun. And he should drink whey according to the season and donkey milk, and use food which is as soft [= wet] and cold as possible, and abstain from pungent and salty food. He should rather use greasier and sweeter and fatter food. The disease usually dies together [with the patient]."[87]

The symptoms described can all be observed directly through the senses, partly by the physician who feels the body temperature, inspects the vomit, palpates the stomach, examines the skin, the lips, the eyes, and partly by the patient who feels rigor, headache, intestinal pain, heaviness and a disturbance of vision. There must have been a certain amount of questioning, and probably the physician was able to assess the patient's

---

[85] Part of this text is quoted by Galen (once under the name of Euryphon and once as belonging to the Hippocratic treatise), cf. above p. 21. The following citation is not from Galen as were the ones given above, but from the version contained in the regular Hippocratic manuscripts (which, however, differs slightly). The reader will thus be able to compare the versions conveniently.

[86] The quotation in Galen has "dry" instead of "hard;" in this case, *gastēr* has to be rendered either by "stomach" (which is considered dry because the stool is dry), or by "stool."

[87] *Morb. II* 7.104.1–13 Li. = 207.1–208.5 Jouanna. The following text is Jouanna's with some minor alterations (cf. his exhaustive *apparatus criticus*; for the present purpose, only the major variant readings are indicated below). Πελιή (πελιή θΜ: πελιὴν Gal., fortasse recte [cf. supra p. 21, n. 27]: πελιὴ νοῦσος Li. codices recent. secutus)· πυρετὸς ἴσχει ξηρὸς καὶ φρὶξ ἄλλοτε καὶ ἄλλοτε, καὶ τὴν κεφαλὴν ἀλγέει, καὶ τὰ σπλάγχνα ὀδύνη ἔχει (ἔχει θΜ: ἴσχει Gal.) καὶ ἐμέει χολήν, καὶ (καὶ ἐμέει χολὴν καὶ M: om. θ) ὅταν ἡ ὀδύνη ἔχῃ, οὐ δύναται ἀνορᾶν (ἀνορᾶν M: ἂν ὁρᾶν θ: ἐνορρᾶν Gal.), ἀλλὰ βαρύνεται. καὶ ἡ γαστὴρ σκληρὴ (σκληρὴ θΜ: ξηρὰ Gal.) γίνεται καὶ ἡ χροιὴ πελιδνὴ καὶ τὰ χείλεα, καὶ τῶν ὀφθαλμῶν τὰ λευκὰ πελιδνά (τ. λ. π. M Gal.: π. τ. λ. θ), καὶ ἐξορᾷ ὡς ἀγχόμενος· ἐνίοτε καὶ τὴν χροιὴν μεταβάλλει καὶ ἐκ πελιδνοῦ (ἐκ πελιδνοῦ M Gal.: ἐκπελιδνοῦται θ) ὑπόχλωρος γίνεται. τοῦτον φάρμακον πιπίσκειν καὶ κάτω καὶ ἄνω καὶ ὑποκλύζειν καὶ ἀπὸ τῆς κεφαλῆς ἀποκαθαίρειν καὶ θερμῷ ὡς ἥκιστα λούειν· ἀλλ' ἐπὴν λούηται, ἐλειθέρει (ελειθερει θ: ἐλιθέρει M: ἐλιθερεῖν M corr.)· καὶ ὀρὸν τὴν ὥρην καὶ γάλα ὄνου πιπίσκειν καὶ σιτίοισιν ὡς μαλθακωτάτοισι χρῆσθαι καὶ ψυχροῖσιν, ἀπεχόμενον τῶν δριμέων καὶ τῶν ἁλμυρῶν· λιπαρωτέροισι δὲ καὶ γλυκυτέροισι καὶ πιοτέροισι χρήσθω. ἡ δὲ (δὲ θ: om. M) νοῦσος ὡς τὰ πολλὰ συναποθνῄσκει.

subjective symptoms (e.g. intestinal pain) by secondary signs (e.g. reactions during the palpations). With regard to the aetiology of the 'livid disease,' there is no speculation. What is significant is the observation of a restricted number of signs.

Emphasis on observation — by the physician as well as the patient — is a prominent feature of *On Diseases II*, ch. 12—75;[88] ch. 68 ('livid disease') is typical in this respect. Only exceptionally subjective symptoms are listed which cannot be verified by the physician, ch. 72: "*phrontís*: In the intestines there seems to be something like a thorn that stings, and nausea seizes him, and he avoids the light and people and loves the darkness, and fear seizes him, and the *phrénes* swell to the exterior,[89] and he feels pain when he is being touched, and he is afraid, and he has frightening visions, and dreadful dreams, and sometimes sees the dead."[90] 'Seeing the dead' is unique among the subjective symptoms described in *On Diseases II*, ch. 12—75. Whereas pain can, in many cases, be verified by the physician through the patient's reactions,[91] and whereas fear and other behaviour, also dreadful hallucinations and dreams, can be recognized as such by people other than the patient, the precise content of visions and dreams cannot be determined unless the patient reports them, or unless an observer interprets what the patient says. Perhaps the symptom 'seeing the dead' is an erratic fossil left over in this description from a more archaic epoch of medicine when religious beliefs were still a more prominent element of the craft (cf. below, ch. IV). The symptom can, however,

---

[88] *Morb. II* 7.18.19—114.4 Li. = 142.1—214.20 Jouanna. The symptoms described in another nosological treatise, *Int.*, are analysed by Wittern, Zur Krankheitserkennung.

[89] Cf. above p. 46.

[90] *Morb. II* 7.108.25—110.4 Li. = 211.15—20 Jouanna Φροντίς (νοῦσος χαλεπή post Φρ. add. Li.: om. θM)· δοκεῖ ἐν τοῖσι σπλάγχνοισιν εἶναι οἷον ἄκανθα καὶ κεντεῖν, καὶ ἄση αὐτὸν λάζυται, καὶ τὸ φῶς φεύγει καὶ τοὺς ἀνθρώπους, καὶ τὸ σκότος φιλεῖ, καὶ φόβος λάζεται, καὶ αἱ φρένες οἰδέουσιν ἐκτός, καὶ ἀλγεῖ ψαυόμενος, καὶ φοβεῖται, καὶ δείματα ὁρᾷ καὶ ὀνείρατα φοβερὰ καὶ τοὺς τεθνηκότας ἐνίοτε. For φροντίς cf. Plat. *Resp. I* 330d—e ἐπειδάν τις ἐγγὺς ᾖ τοῦ οἴεσθαι τελευτήσειν, εἰσέρχεται αὐτῷ δέος καὶ φροντὶς περὶ ὧν ἔμπροσθεν οὐκ εἰσῄει· οἵ τε γὰρ λεγόμενοι μῦθοι περὶ τῶν ἐν Ἅιδου ... τότε δὴ στρέφουσιν αὐτοῦ τὴν ψυχὴν μὴ ἀληθεῖς ὦσιν. For 'seeing the dead' cf. also *Vict. IV* 6.658.13—22 Li. = 107.21—108.9 Joly = 4.442 Jones; Lucr. *I* 132—135 (One has to consider,) quae res nobis ... mentes terrificet morbo adfectis somnoque sepultis, cernere uti videamur eos ..., morte obita quorum tellus amplectitur ossa. Cic. *De divin. I* 63 explains why to people who are dying, ... iis occurrunt plerumque imagines mortuorum. Although the two texts are philosophical (Epicurean and Stoic respectively), the phenomenon mentioned in them was a popular issue. In *Morb. II*, not the fact that patients may see the dead is surprising, but its validity as a specific symptom. Cf. also Kudlien, Primitive medicine 330f.

[91] Cf. *Epid. II* 5.88.13—14 ὀδύνας τὰς ἰσχυροτάτας ὅτῳ τρόπῳ γνοίη (γνοίη V, erkennen Gal.: διαγνοίη HIR) ἄν τις ἰδών· ὁ φόβος (ὁ φ. VHIR: an der eigenen Angst Gal.), αἱ εὐφορίαι (εὐφ-VHIR: durch Findigkeit Gal., i.e. εὐπ-), αἱ ἐμπειρίαι καὶ αἱ δειλίαι.

in its context here, be interpreted completely rationally. (As will be demonstrated presently, there are more fossils in the treatise.)

The nosological descriptions in *On Diseases II*, ch. 12–75 are similar to each other in their structure. They usually consist of the following four parts (cf. ch. 68): *(1)* name or identification of the disease; *(2)* symptoms; *(3)* treatment; *(4)* prognosis (optional; sometimes placed before *3*, as in ch. 68).[92]

(1) The first part is usually short and consists either of the disease's name, like a title of the chapter, sometimes connected with short qualifications (e. g. "*Kynágkhē*"[93] or "Another *kynágkhē*"[94]), or it consists of an indication like "Another disease,"[95] or it has the form of a subordinate conditional or temporal clause (e. g. "When caries (*terēdṓn*) is in the bone"[96]), or it consists of a combination of several of these possible formulations.

The overwhelming majority of those symptoms which cannot be observed directly through the senses is found within this first part of the nosological description, i. e. in the 'title,' which is probably one of the most traditional elements, its function being to identify the disease. The preceding quotation is a marginal case: the translation 'caries' for *terēdṓn* is certainly correct; but the original meaning attested by several ancient writers and lexicographers[97] is 'wood-worm,' a worm that 'bores' itself into wood and eats it up.[98] Probably the disease name *terēdṓn* originally implies an archaic concept of the cause of that malady. Clearer cases of unobservable symptoms mentioned in the titles are the following: Ch. 15 "If water gets to the brain."[99] Ch. 17 "Another disease: If the little blood-vessels around the brain contain too much blood and heat the brain."[100] Ch. 18 "If the vessels in the head contain too much blood."[101] Ch. 19 "If

---

[92] Jouanna, Archéologie 85–87. Jouanna (ed.), Hippocrate, Maladies II, p. 15–23. Grensemann, Knidische Medizin p. 177–194. Cf. also above p. 21, 53.

[93] Ch. 26, *Morb. II* 7.40.9 Li. = 159.9 Jouanna, Κυνάγχη.

[94] Ch. 27, *Morb. II* 7.42.21 Li. = 161.14 Jouanna, Ἑτέρη κυνάγχη.

[95] Ch. 13, *Morb. II* 7.22.18 Li. = 145.13 Jouanna, Ἑτέρη νοῦσος.

[96] Ch. 24, *Morb. II* 7.38.11 Li. = 158.1 Jouanna, Ὅταν τερηδὼν γένηται ἐν τῷ ὀστέῳ (Τερηδών ante Ὅταν add. Li.: om. θM).

[97] Cf. Liddell/Scott/Jones; Jouanna, Archéologie 60.

[98] τερηδών is cognate to τείρω, τετραίνω 'to drill.' On diseases named after animals see Parker, Miasma 248 (note 68).

[99] *Morb. II* 7.26.24 Li. = 149.1 Jouanna Ἢν ὕδωρ ἐπὶ τῷ ἐγκεφάλῳ γένηται (Ἑτέρη νοῦσος ante ἢν add. Li.: om. θM).

[100] *Morb. II* 7.30.18–19 Li. = 151.17–19 Jouanna Ἑτέρη νοῦσος· Ἢν ὑπεραιμήσαντα (-ρεμήσ- θM) τὰ φλέβια τὰ ἔναιμα τὰ περὶ τὸν ἐγκέφαλον θερμήνῃ τὸν ἐγκέφαλον. Deichgräber, Geschichte Kritik 99–102.

[101] *Morb. II* 7.32.1–2 Li. = 152.17–18 Jouanna Ἢν ὑπεραιμήσωσιν (-ρεμήσ- θM) αἱ φλέβες ἐν τῇ κεφαλῇ (Ἑτέρη νοῦσος ante Ἢν add. Li.: om. θM).

the brain is suffering from bile."[102] Ch. 20 "If the brain is mortified."[103] Ch. 23 "Mortification of the brain: If mortification seizes [the brain]."[104] Ch. 25 "If he gets struck."[105] Ch. 40 "If a man suffers from bile."[106] Ch. 51 "Consumption of the back has its origin in the [spinal] marrow."[107] Ch. 53 "If there is a wound in the *artēríē* (wind-pipe?), cough seizes the patient, and blood is expectorated, and the *phárygx* (pharynx?) is filled with the blood unexpectedly, and he expectorates clots of blood."[108] Ch. 54 b "If both lungs suffer from spasm (or distension)."[109] Ch. 55 "If a red inflammation occurs in the lung."[110] Ch. 57 "If a growth waxes in the lung."[111] Ch. 60 "If a growth waxes in the pleura."[112] Ch. 58 "If the lung is filled."[113] Ch. 59 "If the lung prolapses against the pleura."[114] Ch. 61 "If dropsy forms in the lung."[115] Ch. 62 "If a rupture occurs in the chest and in the back."[116] Ch. 70 "Phlegmatic."[117] Ch. 71 "White phlegm."[118]

---

102 *Morb. II* 7.32.14 Li. = 153.5 Jouanna Ἢν δὲ χολᾷ ὁ ἐγκέφαλος (Ἑτέρη νοῦσος ante Ἢν add. Li.: om. θM).

103 *Morb. II* 7.34.9 Li. = 154.7 Jouanna Ἢν σφακελίσῃ ὁ ἐγκέφαλος (Ἑτέρη νοῦσος ante Ἢν add. Li.: om. θM).

104 *Morb. II* 7.38.6 Li. = 157.11 Jouanna Ἢν σφάκελος λάβῃ (Σφάκελος ἐγκεφάλου ante Ἢν add. Li.: om. θM).

105 *Morb. II* 7.38.19 Li. = 158.10 Jouanna Ἢν βλητὸς γένηται (Ἑτέρη νοῦσος ante Ἢν add. Li.: om. θM).

106 *Morb. II* 7.56.3 Li. = 171.9 Jouanna Ἢν χολᾷ ἄνθρωπος (Πυρετοὶ ἀπὸ χολῆς ante Ἢν add. Li.: om. θM; ὁ ante ἄνθρ. add. M: om. θ).

107 *Morb. II* 7.78.14 Li. = 188.8 Jouanna Νωτιὰς φθίσις ἀπὸ τοῦ μυελοῦ γίνεται (ἡ νωτιὰς φθίσις post φθίσις add. Li.: om. M: deest θ).

108 *Morb. II* 7.80.20–22 Li. = 190.3–5 Jouanna Ἢν τρωθῇ ἡ ἀρτηρίη, βὴξ ἔχει, καὶ αἷμα βήσσεται, καὶ λανθάνει ἡ φάρυγξ πιμπλαμένη τοῦ αἵματος, καὶ ἐκβάλλει θρόμβους (Ἀρτηρίη τρωθεῖσα ante Ἢν add. Li.: om. θM).

109 *Morb. II* 7.84.4 Li. = 192.5 Jouanna Ἢν δ' ἀμφότερα σπασθῶσι.

110 *Morb. II* 7.84.20–21 Li. = 193.8 Jouanna Ἢν ἐρυσίπελας ἐν πλεύμονι γένηται (Ἐρυσίπελας ἐν πλεύμονι ante Ἢν add. Li.: om. θM).

111 *Morb. II* 7.88.17 Li. = 196.6 Jouanna Ἐπὴν φῦμα φυῇ ἐν τῷ πλεύμονι (Φῦμα ἐν τῷ πλεύμονι ante Ἐπὴν add. Li.: om. θM).

112 *Morb. II* 7.92.19 Li. = 199.11 Jouanna Ἐπὴν ἐν πλευρῷ φῦμα φυῇ (Τοῦ πλευροῦ φῦμα ante Ἐπὴν add. Li.: om. θM; φυῇ θ: ἡ [= ᾗ] M).

113 *Morb. II* 7.90.10 Li. = 197.11 Jouanna Ἢν πλησθῇ ὁ πλεύμων (Πλεύμων πλησθεὶς ante Ἢν add. Li.: om. θM).

114 *Morb. II* 7.92.1–2 Li. = 198.10–11 Jouanna Ἢν ὁ πλεύμων πρὸς τὸ πλευρὸν προσπέσῃ (Ὁ πλεύμων προσπεσὼν ἐς τὸ πλευρὸν ante Ἢν add. Li.: om. θM).

115 *Morb. II* 7.94.11 Li. = 200.8 Jouanna Ἢν ὕδερος ἐν τῷ πλεύμονι γένηται (Ὕδερος πλεύμονος ante Ἢν add. Li.: om. θM).

116 *Morb. II* 7.96.9–10 Li. = 201.14 Jouanna Ἢν τὸ στῆθος καὶ (καὶ θ: ἢ M) τὸ μετάφρενον ῥαγῇ (Στῆθος ἢ μετάφρενον ῥαγὲν ante Ἢν add. Li.: om. θM). Cf. 64.1 Li. = 176.18–177.1 Jouanna ὅταν τύχῃ ῥηγματίας ὤν.

117 *Morb. II* 7.106.10 Li. = 209.9 Jouanna Φλεγματώδης (Νοῦσος ante φλ. add. Li.: om. θM).

118 *Morb. II* 7.108.4 Li. = 210.9 Jouanna Φλέγμα λευκόν.

(2) The second part of a nosological description contains the perceptible 'signs' or symptoms[119] of the disease. Almost exclusively, the signs mentioned can be observed directly by the senses. This part of the exposition presents more than just an additive series of signs (a + b + c ... + n). For example, the 'livid disease' chapter (68) mentions a simultaneous occurrence of symptoms: "Whenever he feels the pain, his vision is disturbed."[120] Some signs occur only under specific circumstances such as, when the patient performs certain movements or his body is in a certain position: Ch. 14 "Strong pain seizes the head, and if he moves only slightly, he vomits bile."[121] (Similarly ch. 16.)[122] Ch. 18 "When he stands up, vertigo seizes him."[123] Ch. 26 "When he is lying down, he suffocates."[124] Ch. 46 "When he sits up, he coughs more."[125] Ch. 54 "When he turns over, he coughs and sneezes."[126] Ch. 62 "In most cases a patient suffers this when he works with his hands or rides on a vehicle or on horseback."[127] Ch. 70 "She feels weak when she is walking, particularly uphill."[128] The symptoms may also occur in connection with food and drink: Ch. 28 "If he is forced [to drink something], it flows through his nose."[129] Ch. 40 "When he has not eaten anything, it hurts him; but when he has eaten, he suffocates."[130] Ch. 60 "He vomits warm what he has drunk."[131] Ch. 66 (cf. ch. 73) "He cannot bear being without food, and he cannot bear having eaten. When he is without food, ... [symptoms follow], but when he has eaten, ... [other symptoms follow]."[132] Ch. 71 "Whenever he has eaten, he gets respiratory troubles."[133]

---

[119] *Sýmptōma* in this sense does not occur in the Hippocratic Collection apart from one late attestation, *Decent.* 9.234.8; this treatise dates from the late Hellenistic period, cf. Fleischer, Untersuchungen 91, 108. In another passage in an older treatise, *Flat.* 6.94.3, it is *falsa lectio* (συμπτωμάτων M: συμπάντων Ermerins: πάντων A Li., Nelson).

[120] Cf. above p. 21, 53.

[121] *Morb. II* 7.24.20–21 Li. = 147.8–9 Jouanna περιωδυνίη λαμβάνει τὴν κεφαλήν, καὶ ἐπὴν κινήσῃ τις ἧσσον, ἐμεῖ χολήν.

[122] *Morb. II* 7.28.25 Li. = 150.30 Jouanna ἤν τίς μιν κινήσῃ, οὐρησείει.

[123] *Morb. II* 7.32.3–4 Li. = 152.10 Jouanna ἐπειδὰν ἀναστῇ, σκοτοδινίη μιν ἴσχει.

[124] *Morb. II* 7.40.15 Li. = 159.16 Jouanna ἢν κατακέηται, πνίγεται.

[125] *Morb. II* 7.64.12 Li. = 177.13 Jouanna ἀνακαθήμενος μᾶλλον βήσσει.

[126] *Morb. II* 7.82.17 Li. = 191.11–12 Jouanna ἢν στραφῇ, βήσσεται καὶ πτάρνυται.

[127] *Morb. II* 7.96.12–14 Li. = 201.18–19 Jouanna μάλιστα δὲ ταῦτα πάσχει, ἢν τῇσι χερσί τι πονήσῃ ἢ ἐπ' ἅμαξαν ἐπιβῇ ἢ ἐφ' ἵππον.

[128] *Morb. II* 7.106.11–12 Li. = 209.11 Jouanna ὁδοιπορέουσα δὲ ἀσθενεῖ, μάλιστα δὲ ἐπὴν πρὸς αἶπος (αἶπος Li.: ἔπος θΜ) ἴῃ.

[129] *Morb. II* 7.46.3 Li. = 163.16–17 Jouanna ἢν δ' ἀναγκασθῇ, διὰ τῶν ῥινῶν οἱ ῥεῖ (οἱ ῥεῖ θ: οἶδεῖ M).

[130] *Morb. II* 7.56.5–6 Li. = 171.11–12 Jouanna ὅταν ἄσιτος ᾖ, λυπεῖ αὐτόν· ἐπὴν δὲ καὶ (καὶ θ: om. M) φάγῃ, πνίγεται.

[131] *Morb. II* 7.92.22 Li. = 199.14 Jouanna ἀπερεύγεται τὸ πόμα θερμόν.

[132] *Morb. II* 7.100.8–16 Li. = 204.11–15 Jouanna οὐκ ἀνέχεται ἄσιτος οὐδὲ βεβρωκώς, ἀλλ' ὅταν μὲν ἄσιτος ᾖ, ...· ἐπὴν δὲ φάγῃ, ... Cf. 110.20 Li. = 212.18–213.1 Jouanna.

[133] *Morb. II* 7.108.7–8 Li. = 210.13 Jouanna ἐπὴν φάγῃ, τὸ πνεῦμα πυκινὸν ἐπιπίπτει.

Some passages testify to the significance attributed to examining the patient. Questions asked are explicitly mentioned in ch. 47: "Ask him whether his expectoration is sweeter,"[134] and ch. 51: "If you ask him, he will say that ants or the like creep down his back, starting from the head."[135] From several of the following texts, too, it can be inferred that asking the patient about his symptoms was part of the physician's task;[136] other texts refer to direct examination: Ch. 21 "If somebody calls or moves him, he moans but does not notice anything."[137] Ch. 24 "If you make an incision in it [in the pericranium], you will find the skull bloodless, rough, and reddish."[138] Ch. 26 "If you seize his tongue and examine him, the uvula is not large."[139] Ch. 41 "Another fever: Touched from outside, it is weak, but inward he is burned, and his tongue is rough, and through his nose and mouth he exhales hot breath."[140] Ch. 48 "He feels disgust at having the expectoration in his mouth."[141] Ch. 48 "If ... his expectoration, when spit on [glowing] coal, has a heavy smell, ... he will die."[142] Ch. 49 "The pus is expectorated like hailstones, and when rubbed between the fingers, it becomes hard and foul-smelling."[143] Ch. 61 "After making the incision [into the pleura], apply a tampon of raw flax and let the water flow out ... And if on the fifth or sixth day there is pus around the tampon, he generally escapes. But if there is none when you have drawn

---

134 *Morb. II* 7.66.4 Li. = 179.1–2 Jouanna εἴρεσθαι εἰ γλυκύτερον τὸ σίαλον.

135 *Morb. II* 7.78.16–18 Li. = 188.10–12 Jouanna ἢν ἐρωτᾷς αὐτόν, φήσει οἱ ἄνωθεν ἀπὸ τῆς κεφαλῆς κατὰ τὴν ῥάχιν ὁδοιπορεῖν (ὁδοιπορέειν M: κατέρχεσθαι δοκεῖν Li.: deest θ) οἷον μύρμηκας.

136 The noun *anámnēsis* does not occur in the Collection; the verb *anamimnḗskō* is once used in the sense of 'to remember (symptoms),' in *VM* 1.574.3 Li. = 1.3.4 Kw. = 1.16 Jones.

137 *Morb. II* 7.36.3–4 Li. = 155.12–13 Jouanna ἤν τις αὐτὸν καλέῃ (καλέῃ θ: -σῃ M) ἢ κινήσῃ, στενάζει, ξυνίει δ' οὐδέν.

138 *Morb. II* 7.38.13–14 Li. = 158.4–5 Jouanna καὶ ἢν τοῦτο (viz. τὸ δέρμα) ἀνατάμῃς, εὑρήσεις ἄναιμον τὸ ὀστέον καὶ τρηχὺ καὶ πυρρόν. (ἄναιμον τὸ Ermerins: ἀνατείνον θ, ἀνατεῖνον M, ἄναιμον Li.; the double καὶ requires an additional adjective qualifying ὀστέον, and the article τὸ is absolutely indispensable; ANATЄINON may have erroneously arisen out of ANAIMON with TO written *supra lineam*.)

139 *Morb. II* 7.40.12–13 Li. = 159.12–13 Jouanna ἢν καταλαβὼν τὴν γλῶσσαν σκέπτῃ, ὁ γαργαρεὼν οὐ μέγας.

140 *Morb. II* 7.58.7–9 Li. = 172.18–20 Jouanna Ἄλλος πυρετός· ἔξωθεν ἀφασσόμενός ἐστι βληχρός, ἔσωσε (ἔσωσε θ: ἔσωθεν M) δὲ καίεται, καὶ ἡ γλῶσσα τρηχείη, καὶ πνεῖ διὰ τῶν ῥινῶν καὶ διὰ τοῦ στόματος θερμόν.

141 *Morb. II* 7.72.11–12 Li. = 183.11–12 Jouanna μυσάσσεται τὸ σίαλον, ἐπὴν ἀποχρεμψάμενος ἔχῃ ἐν τῷ στόματι.

142 *Morb. II* 7.72.14–16 Li. = 184.1–2 Jouanna ἢν ... πτύοντι ἐπ' ἄνθρακας βαρὺ ὄζῃ τὸ σίαλον ...

143 *Morb. II* 7.74.23–76.1 Li. = 185.21–186.2 Jouanna ἀναβήσσεται οἷον χάλαζα τὸ πύον, καὶ διατριβόμενον ἐν τοῖσι δακτύλοισι σκληρὸν καὶ κάκοδμον γίνεται.

off the water, thirst and cough seize him, and he dies."[144] Ch. 71 "The stomach is thick when you touch it."[145] Ch. 72 "He has the impression that something like a thorn is in his intestines and stings him."[146] The following description of vomit discharged by the patient is especially remarkable for its fullness of detail: Ch. 73 "His vomit is black like lees, sometimes sanguineous, sometimes like after-wine, sometimes like sepia of a cuttle-fish, sometimes sharp like vinegar, sometimes it is saliva and mucus, sometimes yellow bile; and whenever his vomit is black and sanguineous, he has the impression that it smells like blood; then his throat and mouth are burned by the vomit, and it makes his teeth feel blunt, and the vomit makes the soil effervesce."[147]

There were methods of auscultation: Ch. 47 "Let him sit on a chair which does not move. Somebody else should hold his hands, and you should shake him at his shoulders and listen on which side of the ribs there is a noise."[148] Ch. 59 "[The chest] makes a noise like leather,"[149] and "he seems to breathe through the chest."[150] Ch. 61 "When you make an infusion [into the lungs] or fumigate or foment [them], no pus will be forthcoming. So you can recognize that there is no pus but water [in the lungs]. And if you listen for a long time, holding your ear to the ribs, there is a hissing noise inside as if from [fermenting] vinegar."[151]

---

144 *Morb. II* 7.96.3—8 Li. = 201.8—13 Jouanna ἐπὴν δὲ τάμῃς, μοτοῦν ὠμολίνῳ ... καὶ ἀφιέναι τοῦ ὕδατος (ὕδατος M: αἵματος θ) ... καὶ ἢν μέν σοι περὶ (περὶ θ: ἐν M) τῷ μοτῷ πύον περιγένηται πεμπταίῳ ἐόντι ἢ ἑκταίῳ (ἢ ἑκταίῳ θ: om. M), ὡς τὰ πολλὰ ἐκφυγγάνει· ἢν δὲ μὴ περιγένηται, ἐπὴν δ' ἐξεράσῃς (δὲ ξεράσης θ: ἐξεράσῃς M) τὸ ὕδωρ, δίψα ἐπιλαμβάνει καὶ βήξ, καὶ ἀποθνῄσκει.

145 *Morb. II* 7.108.5 Li. = 210.10 Jouanna ἡ γαστὴρ παχεῖα ψαυομένη.

146 *Morb. II* 7.108.25—110.1 Li. = 211.15—16 Jouanna δοκεῖ ἐν τοῖσι σπλάγχνοισιν εἶναι οἷον ἄκανθα καὶ κεντεῖν. Cf. above p. 54.

147 *Morb. II* 7.110.14—19 Li. = 212.11—17 Jouanna μέλαν ἐμεῖ οἷον τρύγα, τοτὲ δὲ αἱματῶδες, τοτὲ δὲ οἷον οἶνον τὸν δεύτερον, τοτὲ δὲ οἷον πολύπου θολόν, τοτὲ δὲ δριμὺ οἷον ὄξος, τοτὲ δὲ σίαλον καὶ λάπην, τοτὲ δὲ χολὴν χλωρήν· καὶ ὅταν μὲν τὸ (τὸ M: om. θ) μέλαν καὶ τὸ αἱματῶδες ἐμέῃ, δοκεῖ οἷον φόνου ὄζειν, καὶ ἡ φάρυγξ καὶ τὸ στόμα καίεται ὑπὸ τοῦ ἐμέσματος, καὶ τοὺς ὀδόντας αἱμωδιᾷ, καὶ τὸ ἔμεσμα τὴν γῆν αἴρει. On the vomit causing the soil to effervesce cf. Kudlien, Beginn 78 f.; Jouanna, Archéologie 108—114; Kudlien, Bemerkungen 100, note 26. See also above p. 49 f., note 73.

148 *Morb. II* 7.70.4—7 Li. = 181.16—20 Jouanna τοῦτον ... καθίσας ἐπὶ ἐφέδρου, ὅ τι μὴ ὑποκινήσει, ἕτερος μὲν τὰς χεῖρας ἐχέτω, σὺ δὲ τῶν ὤμων σείων ἀκοάζεσθαι ἐς ὁπότερον ἂν τῶν πλευρῶν ψοφῇ. Cf. *Morb. II* 7.96.1—2 Li. = 201.5—7 Jouanna.

149 *Morb. II* 7.92.5 Li. = 198.14—15 Jouanna τρίζει (post τρίζει add. τὸ δέρμα θ, τὸ αἷμα M: del. Li.) οἷον μάσθλης.

150 *Morb. II* 7.92.8 Li. = 198.17—18 Jouanna διαπνεῖν δοκεῖ διὰ (διὰ M: ἐκ θ) τοῦ στήθεος.

151 *Morb. II* 7.94.14—17 Li. = 200.12—15 Jouanna ἢν ἐγχέῃς ἢ θυμιᾷς ἢ πυριᾷς (ἢ θ. ἢ π. θ: ἢ π. ἢ θ. M), οὐχ ὁμαρτεῖ πύον. τούτῳ ἂν γνοίης ὅτι οὐ πύον ἀλλὰ ὕδωρ ἐστί· καὶ ἢν πολλὸν χρόνον προσέχων τὸ οὖς ἀκουάζῃ πρὸς τὰ πλευρά, σίζει (σίζει scripsi [CIZEI > OZEI]: ὄζει θM: ζέει Cornarius, Li.) ἔσωθεν οἷον ὄξος.

The nosological descriptions contained in *On Diseases II*, ch. 12–75 do not form inflexible, rigid patterns of symptoms.[152] Occasionally, a distinction is made implicitly between signs that invariably occur in every case of a certain disease, and signs that may or may not be present: Ch. 19 "With most [patients], pain seizes only half of the head, but it occurs also in the whole head."[153] Ch. 20 (after the enumeration of several signs) "Blood flows out of the nose; many, moreover, vomit [blood]."[154] Ch. 24 "With some [patients], it [the skull] is corroded down to the brain."[155] Ch. 31 "Sometimes it bursts by itself."[156] Ch. 39 "The fevers cease with some [patients]."[157] Ch. 61 "Some get oedemas in the stomach and the scrotum and the face, and some ..."[158]

Certain symptoms are more important than others since they indicate or bring it about[159] that the individual case takes a specific turn for better or worse: Ch. 40 "If he sweats after the fever, and if the sweat is cold and copious, and if the fever does not cease, the disease becomes chronic, but if he does not sweat, he [or: the disease] comes to a decision earlier."[160] Ch. 45 "His expectoration is slightly bilious and slightly sanguineous whenever he happens to suffer from a rupture [in the lungs]."[161] Ch. 48 "If he already loses hair from the head, and his head is becoming bald as from a disease, and if his expectoration, when spit on [glowing] coal, has a heavy smell, you should say that he will die within a short time, and that it is a *diárrhoia* that will kill him."[162] Ch. 57 "If pus follows the vomit:

---

152 Cf. throughout Rosanna Boncompagni, Concezione della malattia e senso dell' individualità nei testi cnidi del *Corpus hippocraticum*, Par. del Pass. 27 (1972), 209–238.

153 *Morb. II* 7.32.19–20 Li. = 153.11–12 Jouanna καὶ τοῖσι μὲν πλείστοισιν ἐς τὸ ἥμισυ τῆς κεφαλῆς ὀδύνη φοιτᾷ, γίνεται δὲ καὶ ἐν πάσῃ τῇ κεφαλῇ.

154 *Morb. II* 7.34.11–12 Li. = 154.10 Jouanna ... διὰ τῶν ῥινῶν αἷμα ῥεῖ· πολλοὶ δὲ καὶ ἐμέουσιν.

155 *Morb. II* 7.38.14–15 Li. = 158.5–6 Jouanna ἐνίοισι δὲ (καὶ post δὲ add. M: om. θ) διαβεβρωμένον πρὸς τὸν ἐγκέφαλον.

156 *Morb. II* 7.48.17–18 Li. = 166.7–8 Jouanna ἐνίοτε δὲ αὐτόματον ῥήγνυται (ῥήγνυται θ: ἐκρήγ- M).

157 *Morb. II* 7.54.20 Li. = 170.21–171.1 Jouanna οἱ πυρετοὶ ἐπαύσαντο οὖν ἐνίοισιν.

158 *Morb. II* 7.94.20–24 Li. = 200.19–201.1 Jouanna ἔνιοι δὲ καὶ οἰδίσκονται τὴν γαστέρα καὶ τὴν ὄσχην καὶ τὸ πρόσωπον· καὶ ἔνιοι ...

159 These two functions were in the case of symptoms not distinguished systematically, cf. below p. 168; 169, note 189; 224, note 450.

160 *Morb. II* 7.56.8–10 Li. = 171.15–17 Jouanna τοῦτον ἢν μὲν μετὰ τὸ πῦρ ἐξιδρῷ, καί οἱ ψυχρὸς καὶ πουλὺς ᾖ, καὶ τοῦ πυρετοῦ μὴ ἀπαλλάσσηται, ἡ νοῦσος χρονίη γίνεται· ἢν δὲ μὴ ἱδρῷ, θᾶσσον κρίνεται. For the syntactic construction of τοῦτον see Jouanna (ed.), Hippocrate, Maladies II, p. 241.

161 *Morb. II* 7.62.23–64.1 Li. = 176.18–177.1 Jouanna τὸ σίαλον πτύει ὑπόχολον, καὶ ὕφαιμον ὅταν τύχῃ ῥηγματίας ὤν.

162 *Morb. II* 7.72.14–17 Li. = 183.15–184.3 Jouanna τούτῳ ἢν μὲν αἱ τρίχες ἤδη ἐκ τῆς κεφαλῆς ῥέωσι καὶ ψιλῶται ἤδη ἡ κεφαλὴ ὡς ἐκ νούσου, καὶ πτύοντι ἐπ' ἄνθρακας βαρὺ ὄζῃ τὸ σίαλον, φάναι αὐτὸν ἀποθανεῖσθαι ἐντὸς ὀλίγου χρόνου, τὸ δὲ κτεῖνον ἔσεσθαι διάρροιαν.

if the pus is white and contains slightly sanguineous fibres, he escapes, but if it is livid and greenish and foul-smelling, he dies."[163] Ch. 63 "Often it [the disease] changes into a *peripleumoniē* (pneumonia), and he hallucinates: this is how you recognize that it becomes a *peripleumoniē*."[164]

In several passages it is said that the prognostic value of certain signs is not an absolute one, but that they are valid for prognosis only "generally" or "with most [patients]," or that they indicate a future event with a certain likelihood only: Ch. 27 "But if the disease, after the throat is healthy again and the oedemas have disappeared, turns into the lungs, fever and pain of the ribs seize [the patient], and he generally dies if this happens."[165] Ch. 29 "If the jaws are inflamed on both sides, he suffocates, but if only it [the uvula] is inflamed and not the other parts, he is less likely to die."[166] Ch. 47 "The sign whether he shall escape: if the pus is white and pure and contains fibres of blood, he generally recovers, but if it runs like egg-yolk on the first day, or if on the second it runs thick and greenish and smelling, they die after the flow of pus."[167] Ch. 57 "He suffers until the fourteenth day, because with most [patients] it is during this number of days that the *phȳma* is most enflamed... They are cleansed within fourteen days after the eruption; with many [patients] the disease will last one year."[168]

An important element still in the second part of the nosological descriptions of *On Diseases II*, ch. 12–75 is the indication as to the time it takes for a disease to develop. There are two ways of giving this indication: In terms of periods of time and points of time. The difference

---

[163] *Morb. II* 7.90.2–5 Li. = 197.2–5 Jouanna ἢν ἅμα τῷ ἐμέσματι πύον ἕπηται, ἢν μέντοι (μέντοι θ: μὲν M) τὸ πύον ᾖ λευκὸν καὶ ἶνες ἐν αὐτῷ ὕφαιμοι ἔωσιν, ἐκφυγγάνει· ἢν δὲ πελιδνὸν καὶ χλωρὸν καὶ κάκοδμον, ἀποθνῄσκει.

[164] *Morb. II* 7.96.20–22 Li. = 202.7–9 Jouanna πολλάκις δὲ καὶ μεθίσταται ἐς (ἐς θ: ὡς M) περιπλευμονίην, καὶ παρακόπτει· τούτῳ ἂν γνοίης ὅτι περιπλευμονίη γίνεται.

[165] *Morb. II* 7.44.9–12 Li. = 162.9–12 Jouanna ἢν δὲ τῆς φάρυγγος καθεστηκοίης καὶ τῶν οἰδημάτων τρεφθῇ ἐς τὸν πλεύμονα ἡ νοῦσος, πυρετὸς ἐπ' οὖν ἔλαβε καὶ ὀδύνη τοῦ πλευροῦ, καὶ ὡς ἐπὶ τὸ πολὺ ἀπ' οὖν ἔθανεν (ἀπουνέθανεν θ: ἀπέθανεν M), ἐπὴν τοῦτο γένηται.

[166] *Morb. II* 7.46.18–20 Li. = 164.18–165.2 Jouanna ἢν φλεγμήνῃ τὰ σιηγόνια ἔνθεν καὶ ἔνθεν, ἀποπνίγεται· ἢν δὲ αὐτὸς (αὐτὸς θ: αὐτὸ M) ἐφ' ἑωυτοῦ γένηται (viz. στρογγύλος τὸ ἄκρον καὶ διαφανὴς ὁ γαργαρεών), τούτων μὴ φλεγμαινόντων (φλεγμαινόντων θ: -νάντων M), ἧσσον ἀποθνῄσκει.

[167] *Morb. II* 7.72.1–5 Li. = 182.19–183.4 Jouanna σημήϊον δὲ ἢν μέλλῃ ἐκφεύξεσθαι, ἢν μὲν (ᾖ add. θ: om. M) τὸ πύον ᾖ λευκὸν (καὶ καθαρὸν add. M: om. θ) καὶ ἶνες αἵματος ἐνέωσιν, ὡς τὰ πολλὰ ὑγιὴς γίνεται. ἢν δὲ οἷον λεκιθοειδὲς ἀπορρυῇ τῇ πρώτῃ, ἢ τῇ ὑστεραίῃ ἀπορρυῇ παχύ, ὑπόχλωρον, ὄζον, ἀποθνῄσκουσιν, ἐπειδὰν ἐκρυῇ τὸ πύον.

[168] *Morb. II* 7.88.19–90.6 Li. = 196.8–197.7 Jouanna ἔστε μὲν τεσσερεσκαίδεκα ἡμέρας πάσχει (ἔστε ... πάσχει M: ἔσται ἡμέρας θ)· τοῖσι γὰρ πλείστοισι τοσαύτας ἡμέρας μάλιστα φλεγμαίνει τὸ φῦμα ... καθαίρονται δ' ἐν τεσσεράκοντα ἡμέρῃσιν ἀφ' ἧς ἂν ῥαγῇ, πολλοῖσι δὲ καὶ ἐνιαυσίη γίνεται ἡ νοῦσος.

appears to be largely a formal one. It is, therefore, neither desirable nor possible to discuss the two expressions separately. These indications about time 'foreshadow' the well-known doctrine about *krísis* (crisis of a disease) and critical days, which is fundamental in theoretically more developed treatises such as *Prognostics* and *Epidemics* (see next chapter, p. 73 ff.), and which was to become influential from antiquity onward until the nineteenth century. The *krísis* doctrine, it appears, has one of its historical roots in rudimentary theories about time such as the ones in *On Diseases II*, ch. 12–75.

With regard to periods of time, it is a common idea in *On Diseases II*, ch. 12–75 that a disease manifests itself according to a certain time scheme, the most common unit of measure being days (cf., for instance, the preceding quotation, or ch. 53: "For fifteen days he suffers this way. But after that ..."[169]).

A formula, which repeatedly occurs, is: "He dies within so and so many days; if he survives them, he recovers." Ch. 46 "This [patient] dies within twenty days; but if he survives them, he recovers."[170] Ch. 65 "This [patient] dies within seven days; but if he survives them, he recovers."[171] Ch. 27 "He generally dies if this happens; but if he survives five days, he becomes purulent inside. [I. e., the dangerous acute disease becomes chronic and less dangerous.] ... If he has survived the five days and the fever has remitted, ... [prescription follows]."[172] Ch. 45 "If he survives fourteen days, he recovers."[173]

In the statements quoted here, it is not a precise point of time at which a 'decision' occurs (the word *krísis*, 'decision,' 'crisis,' is not used at all in these chapters, the related verb *krī́nō* only exceptionally, cf. below[174]). In fact, it would be misleading to speak of a crisis here. If the patient is to die, he does so within a certain space of time, a 'decisive period' as one might say; and if he has survived this period, he has escaped the peril.

The length of the period depends not only on the disease itself (characterized by its name or by the title given at the beginning of each

---

[169] *Morb. II* 7.82.2 Li. = 190.9–10 Jouanna ἔστε (ἔστε M: ἔσται θ) μὲν πεντεκαίδεκα ἡμέρας τοιαῦτα πάσχει. μετὰ δὲ ...

[170] *Morb. II* 7.64.13–14 Li. = 177.15–16 Jouanna οὗτος ἐν εἴκοσιν ἡμέρῃσιν ἀποθνήσκει· ἢν δὲ ταύτας ἐκφύγῃ, ὑγιὴς γίνεται.

[171] *Morb. II* 7.100.6–7 Li. = 204.9–10 Jouanna οὗτος ἐν ἑπτὰ ἡμέρῃσιν ἀποθνήσκει· ἢν δὲ ταύτας ὑπεκφύγῃ (ὑπεκ- θ: ὑπερ- M), ὑγιὴς γίνεται.

[172] *Morb. II* 7.44.11–16 Li. = 162.12–163.5 Jouanna ὡς ἐπὶ τὸ πολὺ ἀπ' οὖν (οὖν θ: om. M) ἔθανεν ἐπὴν τοῦτο γένηται· ἢν δ' ὑπεκφύγῃ (ὑπεκ- θ: ὑπερ- M) ἡμέρας πέντε, ἔμπυος γίνεται ... ἢν δ' ὑπεκφύγῃ (δὲ ὑπεκφύγοι θ: δ' ὑπερφύγῃ M) τὰς πέντε ἡμέρας καὶ ὁ πυρετὸς ἀνῇ ...

[173] *Morb. II* 7.64.6–7 Li. = 177.6–7 Jouanna ἢν ὑπερφύγῃ (τὰς post ὑπ. add. codices recent., Li.: om. θM) τεσσερεσκαίδεκα ἡμέρας, ὑγιὴς γίνεται.

[174] p. 67.

chapter or description), but also on the course an individual case may take: Ch. 63 "If this [patient] is not seized with *peripleumoníē*, he recovers if he survives fourteen days; but if he is so, [he dies or recovers] within eighteen days unless he becomes purulent inside due to a lack of evacuation."[175]

The following passages, like the preceding ones, indicate 'decisive periods' consisting of several days each, but, in addition to periods of days expressed by cardinal numbers, they contain ordinal numbers[176] denoting single days on which certain events are to be expected. With regard to several of these passages it appears that the two methods of indicating days — either by cardinal or by ordinal numbers — are to some extent interchangeable: that "on the *n*th day" is synonymous to "within *n* days." Ch. 44 "If the fever ceases [or: has ceased] on the seventh day, he recovers; if it does not cease [or: has not ceased], the disease continues through eleven or fourteen days. Most [patients] die within these days; but if he survives the fourteenth day, he escapes."[177] Ch. 47 "Fever seizes him for at least fourteen days, and for at most eighteen days. During these days he coughs violently, and at first, on the seventh and eighth day, expectorates thick and pure matter, but on the ninth or tenth day after the fever has seized him he expectorates slightly sweet and purulent matter until the fourteen days are over. And if on the fifteenth day the lung is dried up and he has coughed out [what was in it], he recovers; otherwise you should wait out eighteen days. If he stops coughing during these days, he escapes ... [Follow a certain diet] until the eighteen days are over and the fever has gone. He is in greatest danger during the seven or fourteen days, but if he has survived the eighteen days, he will not die."[178]

---

175 *Morb. II* 7.96.22—98.2 Li. = 202.9—12 Jouanna οὗτος ἢν μὲν ⟨μὴ⟩ (μὴ Jouanna: om. θM) γένηται περιπλευμονικός, ἢν (ἢν θ: καὶ M) τεσσερασκαίδεκα ἡμέρας ὑπερφύγῃ, ὑγιὴς γίνεται· ἢν δὲ γένηται, ἐν ὀκτωκαίδεκα ἡμέρῃσιν, ἢν μὴ (μὴ M: μὲν θ) ἀκάθαρτος γενόμενος ἔμπυος γένηται.

176 On the numeral adjectives derived from ordinal numbers cf. the following footnote.

177 *Morb. II* 7.62.4—8 Li. = 175.13—17 Jouanna ἢν μὲν τὸ πῦρ ἀνῇ ἑβδομαῖον ἐόντα, ὑγιὴς γίνεται· ἢν δὲ μὴ ἀνῇ, ἀφικνεῖται ἡ νοῦσος ἐς τὰς ἕνδεκα ἡμέρας ἢ τὰς τεσσερεσκαίδεκα· οἱ μὲν οὖν πολλοὶ ἐν ταύτῃσιν ἀπόλλυνται· ἢν δ' ὑπερβάλῃ τὴν τεσσερεσκαιδεκάτην, ἐκφυγγάνει. — Adjectives like ἑβδομαῖος, 'being on the seventh day' are, for the present purpose, regarded as synonymous with ordinal numbers like ἑβδόμῃ, 'on the seventh day,' from which they are derived.

178 *Morb. II* 7.64.23—66.11 Li. = 178.8—179.10 Jouanna πυρετὸς ἴσχει ἡμέρας τεσσερεσκαίδεκα τὸ ἐλάχιστον, τὸ δὲ μακρότατον δυῶν δεούσας εἴκοσι· καὶ βήσσει ταύτας τὰς ἡμέρας ἰσχυρῶς, καὶ ἀποχρέμπτεται τὸ μὲν πρῶτον σίαλον παχὺ καὶ καθαρὸν ἑβδόμῃ καὶ ὀγδόῃ· ἐπὴν δὲ ὁ πυρετὸς λάβῃ ἐνάτῃ καὶ δεκάτῃ ὑπόγλυκυ καὶ πυῶδες, ἔστ' ἂν αἱ τεσσερεσκαίδεκα ἡμέραι παρέλθωσιν. καὶ ἢν μὲν ἐν τῇ πεντεκαιδεκάτῃ ἡμέρῃ ξηρανθῇ ὁ πλεύμων καὶ ἐκβήξῃ, ὑγιάζεται· εἰ (εἰ θ: ἢν M) δὲ μή, δυῶν δεούσαις εἴκοσι προσέχειν· καὶ ἢν μὲν ἐν ταύτῃσι παύσηται τοῦ βήγματος, ἐκφεύγει ... [Follow a certain diet] ἔστ' ἂν αἱ ὀκτωκαίδεκα ἡμέραι παρέλθωσι καὶ ὁ πυρετὸς παύσηται. κινδυνεύει δὲ μάλιστα

Ch. 56 "On the third or fourth day he discharges urine containing blood, and he dies on the seventh day; if he survives fourteen days, he recovers. But he is not likely to escape ... But when the fourteen days are over, [prescription follows]."[179] Ch. 64 "He dies on the seventh day, but if he survives ten days, he feels relief. On the twentieth day he becomes purulent inside, and during the first days he coughs out a little pus, later larger quantities. He is cleansed within forty days ... When the ten days are over and the fever has gone and the expectoration is clean, [prescription follows]. And when, on the twentieth day, he expectorates pus, [prescription follows]."[180]

Particularly significant for the interchangeability of cardinal and ordinal numbers is a passage in ch. 12: "He suffers this for nine days ... He discharges much white urine without trouble for twenty days ... This [patient] recovers completely on the fortieth day."[181] Does the author intend to say that the patient regains his health exactly on the fortieth day? It seems plausible that he rather means "on the fortieth day or earlier" or "around the fortieth day;" this interpretation is supported by the therapeutic prescription which follows in the same chapter: "If the forty days are over — because generally the disease ends *within* this period of time — [prescription follows]."[182] Another example is found in ch. 67, where "or earlier" is explicitly added: "This [patient] dies on the seventh day or earlier; if he survives *them*, he generally escapes. The disease is, however, deadly ... You should not give him solid food or gruel for seven days ... But when the seven days are over and the fever has remitted, he should take an electuary of millet."[183] This translation reflects a slight

---

ἐν τῇσιν ἑπτὰ ἢ ἐν τῇσι τεσσερεσκαίδεκα· ἐπὴν δὲ τὰς ὀκτωκαίδεκα ἡμέρας ὑπερβάλῃ, οὐκέτι ἀποθνήσκει. On the presumable corruptions in this passage, see Jouanna, Archéologie 596.

179 *Morb. II* 7.88.6–13 Li. = 195.16–196.2 Jouanna καὶ ἡμέρῃ τρίτῃ ἢ τετάρτῃ οὐρεῖ αἱματῶδες, καὶ ἀποθνήσκει ἑβδομαῖος. ἐπὴν δὲ τεσσερεσκαίδεκα ὑπερφύγῃ, ὑγιὴς γίνεται· ἐκφυγγάνει δ' οὐ μάλα ... ἐπὴν δ' αἱ τεσσερεσκαίδεκα ἡμέραι παρέλθωσιν ...

180 *Morb. II* 7.98.9–17 Li. = 203.1–11 Jouanna ἑβδομαῖος ἀποθνήσκει· ἢν δὲ (δὲ M: om. θ) δέκα ἡμέρας ὑπερφύγῃ, ῥᾴων γίνεται· εἰκοστῇ δ' ἡμέρῃ ἐμπυΐσκεται, καὶ βήσσει τὰς πρώτας ἡμέρας πύον ὀλίγον, ἔπειτα ἐπὶ πλέον· καθαίρεται δ' ἐν τεσσεράκοντα ἡμέρῃσι ... ἐπὴν δὲ αἱ (αἱ θ: om. M, sed v. supra, lin. 9) δέκα ἡμέραι παρέλθωσιν, ... ἢν δ' εἰκοσταῖος τὸ πύον πτύσῃ, ...

181 *Morb. II* 7.18.22–20.6 Li. = 142.3–143.4 Jouanna οὗτος ἡμέρας ἐννέα ταῦτα πάσχει ... οὐρεῖ δὲ ἀπόνως (καὶ add. M: om. θ) πολὺ καὶ λευκὸν ἐς τὰς εἴκοσιν ἡμέρας ... οὗτος τεσσαρακοσταῖος παντάπασιν ὑγιὴς γίνεται.

182 *Morb. II* 7.22.5–7 Li. = 144.15–17 Jouanna ἐπὴν δὲ αἱ (αἱ θ: om. M; sed cf. p. 20.5) τεσσεράκοντα ἡμέραι ἐξέλθωσι — καθίσταται γὰρ μάλιστα ἡ νοῦσος ἐν τοσούτῳ χρόνῳ — ...

183 *Morb. II* 7.102.8–17 Li. = 205.22–206.10 Jouanna οὗτος ἑβδομαῖος ἢ πρότερον ἀποθνήσκει· ἢν δὲ ταύτας ὑπερφύγῃ, τὰ πολλὰ ὑπεκφυγγάνει (ὑπεκ- θ: ἐκ- M)· ἡ δὲ νοῦσος θανατώδης ... σιτίον δὲ μὴ προσφέρειν μηδὲ ῥύφημα ἑπτὰ ἡμερέων (ἄχρις post ἡμ. add. codices recent., Li.: om. θM) ... ἐπὴν δὲ αἱ ἑπτὰ ἡμέραι παρέλθωσιν καὶ τὸ πῦρ μεθῇ, κέγχρον λείχειν.

grammatical inconsistency in the Greek original, where reference is made to the phrase "on the seventh day or earlier" by using the plural "them." The plural (instead of the singular, "it") would be more logical if the preceding formulation contained cardinal numbers, "within seven days." A further clear example of the oscillation between cardinal and ordinal numbers denoting days is transmitted in two parallel passages (ch. 54 and 58), whose twofold transmission guarantees that the wording is ancient and not due to faults of later copyists: "This [patient] is most likely to die on the fourth day; if he survives *them*, there is not much hope [this is the reading of ch. 54; instead of 'not much hope,' ch. 58 has 'hope generally']. Also during the seven days he is in danger; if he survives them, too, he recovers."[184] Here, as in the preceding quotation, "them" is used to refer to a phrase which literally denotes a point of time ("on the *n*th day"), but actually means a period of time ("within *n* days" or similar).

There is yet another formula: "He recovers if this or that happens; otherwise he dies within *n* days (or, less frequently, on the *n*th day)." Here, too, there are no single 'critical days' but rather 'decisive periods' of several days indicated by cardinal or ordinal numbers, within which a favourable event may or may not take place, an event that saves the patient or inaugurates his recovery. Ch. 21 "If this [patient] does not catch a fever, he dies within seven days, but if he does catch a fever, he generally recovers."[185] Ch. 22 "He generally dies within five days if he does not fall asleep."[186]

The occurrence which signifies recovery for the patient may consist of a discharge of (harmful?) matter: Ch. 16 "If this [patient] has an eruption through the nose or ears, there flows slightly purulent water, and he recovers; otherwise he generally dies within seven days."[187] Similar are the following passages: Ch. 12 "This [patient] suffers this for nine days, and if there is an eruption of water and mucus through his nose or ears,

---

[184] *Morb. II* 7.84.8–11 Li. = 192.10–12 Jouanna οὗτος τεταρταῖος μάλιστα ἀποθνήσκει· ἢν δὲ ταύτας ὑπερφύγῃ, ἐλπίδες μὲν οὐ πολλαί· κινδυνεύει δὲ καὶ ἐν τῇσιν ἑπτά· ἢν δὲ καὶ ταύτας διαφύγῃ, ὑγιάζεται. *Morb. II* 7.90.14–17 Li. = 197.16–198.1 Jouanna οὗτος τεταρταῖος μάλιστα ἀποθνήσκει· ἢν δὲ ταύτας (ταύτας θ: αὐτὰς M) ὑπερφύγῃ, ἐλπίδες ὡς τὰ πολλά· κινδυνεύει δὲ καὶ ἐν τῇσιν ἑπτά· ἢν δὲ καὶ ταύτας ὑπερφύγῃ, ὑγιάζεται.

[185] *Morb. II* 7.36.4–6 Li. = 155.14–16 Jouanna οὗτος, ἢν μιν μὴ πυρετὸς λάβῃ, ἐν τῇσιν ἑπτὰ ἡμέρῃσιν ἀποθνήσκει· ἢν δὲ λάβῃ, ὡς τὰ πολλὰ ὑγιὴς γίνεται.

[186] *Morb. II* 7.36.22–23 Li. = 156.19–20 Jouanna ἀποθνήσκει μάλιστα ἐν πέντε ἡμέρῃσιν, ἢν μὴ κατακοιμηθῇ.

[187] *Morb. II* 7.30.3–6 Li. = 150.16–151.1 Jouanna τούτῳ ἢν μὲν κατὰ τὰς ῥῖνας ἢ κατὰ τὰ ὦτα ῥαγῇ, ὕδρωψ ῥεῖ ὑπόπυος, καὶ ὑγιὴς γίνεται· εἰ (εἰ θ: ἢν M) δὲ μή, ἀποθνήσκει ἐν ἑπτὰ ἡμέρῃσιν ὡς τὰ πολλά. Cf. below p. 125f.

he is freed from the disease."[188] Ch. 14 "When he gets to the seventh day, he might die; if he survives this day, [he might die] if he has no eruption from the nose or ears ... They also die if strong pain seizes the ear, and if there is no eruption within the seven days."[189] Ch. 20 "This [patient] dies within three days; if he survives the seven days, ... if he vomits the blood and if it flows from his nose [prescription follows]."[190] A beneficial discharge can be provoked by an appropriate treatment: Ch. 17 "This [patient] dies on the fifth or sixth day ... You should warm his head, because if there is an eruption of water through his ears or nose, he escapes. If he survives the six days, [prescription follows]."[191] Ch. 25 "You should make an incision in his scalp, and when the blood has flown out, ... bandage it. If you do not make the incision, he generally dies on the eighteenth or twentieth day."[192] — A favourable or relieving discharge of (harmful?) substances is sometimes mentioned without any relation to 'decisive periods:' Ch. 55 "When he has vomited, he seems to be better, but when he has not vomited, [a description of bad symptoms follows]."[193] Ch. 66 "When he has vomited, he feels easier for a short time."[194] Ch. 69 "When he has vomited, he seems to be better. Often he vomits a little bile, about a mouthful, and pain seizes him that extends from the intestines into the lower stomach and the flanks, and whenever this happens, he feels easier."[195] Ch. 73 "When he has vomited, he seems to be better for a short time."[196]

---

[188] *Morb. II* 7.18.22–20.2 Li. = 142.3–5 Jouanna οὗτος ἡμέρας ἐννέα ταῦτα πάσχει, καὶ ἢν μὲν ῥαγῇ κατὰ τὰς ῥῖνας ἢ κατὰ τὰ ὦτα ὕδωρ καὶ πλέννα, ἀπαλλάσσεται τῆς νούσου. Cf. below p. 126.

[189] *Morb. II* 7.24.22–26.19 Li. = 147.10–148.14 Jouanna ἐπὴν δ' ἑβδομαῖος γένηται, ἐνίοτε καὶ (καὶ θ: om. M) ἀποθνῄσκει· ἢν δὲ ταύτην ἐκφύγῃ, ἐναταῖος ἢ ἑνδεκαταῖος, ἢν μή οἱ ῥαγῇ κατὰ τὰς ῥῖνας ἢ κατὰ τὰ ὦτα ... ἀποθνῄσκουσι δὲ καὶ ἢν ἐς τὸ οὖς περιωδυνίη γενομένη μὴ ῥαγῇ ἐν τῇσιν ἑπτὰ ἡμέρῃσιν.

[190] *Morb. II* 7.34.12–14 Li. = 154.10–13 Jouanna οὗτος ἐν τρισὶν ἡμέρῃσιν ἀποθνῄσκει· ἢν δὲ τὰς ἑπτὰ ἡμέρας ὑπερφύγῃ ... ἢν μὲν τὸ αἷμα ἐμῇ ἢ ἐκ τῶν ῥινῶν ῥέῃ ...

[191] *Morb. II* 7.30.23–25 Li. = 152.3–6 Jouanna οὗτος ἀποθνῄσκει πεμπταῖος ἢ ἑκταῖος ... θερμαίνειν αὐτοῦ τὴν κεφαλήν· ἢν γὰρ ῥαγῇ διὰ τῶν ὤτων ἢ διὰ τῶν ῥινῶν ὕδωρ, οὕτως ἐκφυγγάνει· ἢν δ' ἐκφύγῃ τὰς ἡμέρας τὰς ἕξ, ...

[192] *Morb. II* 7.40.6–8 Li. = 159.5–8 Jouanna σχίσαι αὐτοῦ τὸ βρέγμα, καὶ ἢν (ην θ: ἐπὴν M) ἀπορρυῇ τὸ αἷμα, ... καταδῆσαι. ἢν δὲ μὴ σχίσῃς, ἀποθνῄσκει ὀκτωκαιδεκαταῖος ἢ εἰκοσταῖος ὡς ἐπὶ (ἐπὶ θ: om. M) τὰ πολλά.

[193] *Morb. II* 7.86.3–5 Li. = 193.15–16 Jouanna ὅταν ἐμέσῃ, δοκεῖ ῥᾴων εἶναι· ὅταν δὲ μὴ ἐμέσῃ, ...

[194] *Morb. II* 7.100.11 Li. = 204.14–15 Jouanna ἐπὴν ἐμέσῃ, ῥᾴων δοκεῖ εἶναι ἐπ' ὀλίγον.

[195] *Morb. II* 7.104.16–19 Li. = 208.8–12 Jouanna ἐπὴν (ἐπὴν θ: ἐὰν M) ἀπερύγῃ, δοκεῖ ῥᾴων εἶναι. πολλάκις δὲ καὶ χολὴν ἀπεμεῖ ὀλίγην ὅσον βρόχθον· καὶ ὀδύνη λαμβάνει ἀπὸ τῶν σπλάγχνων ἐς τὴν νείαιραν (νειερὰν scripto αι supra secundum ε M: ἱερᾶν θ) γαστέρα καὶ τὴν λαπάρην, καὶ ἐπὴν τοῦτο γένηται, ῥᾴων δοκεῖ εἶναι.

[196] *Morb. II* 7.110.19–20 Li. = 212.17–18 Jouanna ἐπὴν ἀπεμέσῃ, δοκεῖ ῥᾴων εἶναι ἐπ' ὀλίγον.

It rarely occurs that the favourable event is described as happening at a certain point of time: Ch. 22 "If after inebriety he becomes speechless: if fever seizes him *immediately*, he recovers; if it does not seize him, he dies on the third day."[197]

In two descriptions the doctrine concerning days and discharges remarkably resembles the doctrines on 'critical days' contained in other treatises of the Hippocratic Collection. The two passages, to which others could be added, are mentioned here only in passing, because a detailed interpretation could be given only after a discussion of the later theories on 'critical days' (cf. below p. 126). Ch. 41 "When he reaches the fifth day, the *hypokhóndria* get hard and painful ... If rigor and strong fever seize him on the seventh day, and if he sweats, [he recovers]; otherwise he dies on the seventh or ninth day."[198] Ch. 40 "If he sweats after the fever and the sweat is cold and abundant, and if he is not [completely] freed from the fever, the disease becomes long-lasting; but if he does not sweat, it [or: the patient] is decided upon quicker ... If he sweats on the seventh day, and if the fever leaves him, [he recovers]; otherwise he generally dies on the fourteenth day."[199] This is the only passage in *On Diseases II*, ch. 12–75 where the verb *krī́nō* is used ('to judge;' translated above as 'to decide'). In another passage (end of ch. 71) the compound verb *diakrī́nō* is found with the same meaning: "The disease abides undecided in most cases."[200] The deverbative substantive *krísis*, 'crisis' (derived from *krī́nō*), does not occur in *On Diseases II*, ch. 12–75. Although these passages can, to a certain extent, be interpreted in terms of the later *krísis* doctrines, they are not exceptional within *On Diseases II*, ch. 12–75, because the same (though equally unhistoric) re-interpretation is possible for many of the passages on 'decisive periods' and on beneficial events quoted above (especially on bodily discharges which improve the patient's condition). One gets thus the impression that the later *krísis* doctrine is 'foreshadowed' in *On Diseases II*, ch. 12–75 and in similar nosological texts of the Hippocratic Collection, or, to use more strictly historical terms,

---

197 *Morb. II* 7.36.14–16 Li. = 156.10–12 Jouanna ἢν δ' ἐκ θωρήξιος ἄφωνος γένηται, ἢν μὲν αὐτίκα καὶ παραχρῆμα λάβῃ μιν πυρετός, ὑγιὴς γίνεται· ἢν δὲ μὴ λάβῃ, τριταῖος ἀποθνῄσκει.

198 *Morb. II* 7.58.9–13 Li. = 172.20–173.5 Jouanna ὅταν δὲ πεμπταῖος γένηται, τὰ ὑποχόνδρια σκληρά, καὶ ὀδύνη ἔνεστι ... τοῦτον ἢν μὲν ἑβδομαῖον ἐόντα ῥῖγος λάβῃ καὶ πυρετὸς ἰσχυρὸς καὶ ἐξιδρώσῃ· εἰ δὲ μή, ἀποθνῄσκει ἑβδομαῖος ἢ ἐναταῖος.

199 *Morb. II* 7.56.8–10 Li. = 171.15–17 Jouanna (quoted above p. 60, note 160); 58.5–6 Li. = 172.15–17 Jouanna οὗτος ἢν μὲν ἑβδομαῖος ἐξιδρώσῃ καὶ τὸ πῦρ αὐτὸν μεθῇ· εἰ (εἰ θ: ἢν M) δὲ μή, τεσσερεσκαιδεκαταῖος ἀποθνῄσκει ὡς τὰ πολλά.

200 *Morb. II* 7.108.23–24 Li. = 211.13–14 Jouanna ἡ δὲ νοῦσος μάλιστα διακρίνεται ἐν οὐδενί. Cf. Jouanna, Archéologie 432 (with note 1).

that the later doctrine has one of its roots in doctrines like those of *On Diseases II*.

(3) After examining the second part of the nosological descriptions of *On Diseases II*, ch. 12–75 including the indications about time, let us now consider the third major part, namely treatment. Considerable differences in structure are found in the various chapters. In some of them, the recommended therapeutic measures form a simple linear sequence of prescriptions; in other chapters, alternatives are offered as to whether certain measures should be taken or not, the physician's choice being made dependent on the circumstances of the individual case, for example on the presence of certain symptoms or the outcome of previous therapeutic attempts.

A typical example of the simple type is found in the now familiar chapter on the 'livid disease' (ch. 68).[201] The prescriptions made after the enumeration of the symptoms form an additive series of instructions. (In the two extracts which follow, the capital letters A, B, C ... J indicate 'disease signs,' i.e. symptoms. The minuscule letters a, b, c ... n indicate actions, mostly therapeutic measures to be taken. Round brackets ( ) enclose explanations of the letter symbols. Square brackets [ ] enclose completions of the thought necessitated by the medical subject-matter and other supplements.)

> "There is A (fever), and B (rigor), and C (headache), and D (intestinal pain), and E (vomit of bile), and F (disturbance of vision) during (C and ?) D, and G (hardening, or drying, of the stomach), and H (skin, lips, and eyes getting livid), and I (he looks as though he is being strangled), and J (his complexion changes sometimes):
>
> > To this patient do k (giving an evacuating drug), and do l (giving an enema), and do m (purging the head), and avoid n (bathing), and do o (warming in the sun), and do p (giving whey and milk according to the season), and do q (giving certain foodstuffs), and avoid r (giving certain foodstuffs)."

The more complex type is represented by ch. 14:[202]

[201] p. 53.

[202] *Morb. II* 7.24.20–26.23 Li. = 147.8–148.18 Jouanna.

"If A (headache), and if B when a (nausea during passive movements), and if C (sometimes urinary trouble and mental disorder), [remarks on prognosis follow],

then [within the initial seven days]
during A (pain), and before D (eruption from the nose and ears),

do b (warming the head with sponges).[203]
If b proves ineffective,[204]

do c (warming the head with a wine-skin), and do d (giving honey-wine).
If d proves ineffective,

do e (giving barley-water), and do f (giving porridge of peeled barley), and do g (giving diluted white wine).

After D and A

do h (giving laxative food), and do i (giving warm showers over the head), and do j (rinsing the ears), and do k (inserting sponges soaked with honey into the ears).[205] If j and k prove ineffective,[206] and if there is E (chronic flux of the ears),

do j, and do l (application of a medicine in the ears).

If F (ears being dry),

do j, and do m (fumigation of the ears).

If during A there is absence of D within the initial seven days,

do n (bathing with much warm water), and do b, [and do d, e, f, g].[203]
If [n and] b prove ineffective,

do m (fumigation of the ears), and do d, and do e, and do f, and do g."[203]

The difference between the two types of therapeutic prescriptions is striking and *might* possibly reflect a historical evolution.[207] If one takes them in their abstract structures, the simple type recalls how sequences of actions are portrayed in early Greek texts, for instance in epic poetry. Although such actions may be more complex in reality than just an addition of single elements (a + b + c ... + n), their descriptions in early literature tend to omit the logical interrelations that exist between the elements, and prefer simply to add them up. Therapeutic instructions such as those contained in ch. 68 were probably harder to execute than the more detailed ones

203 In order to provoke D, which is the principal purpose of the 'algorithmic' programme.
204 For provoking D.
205 In order to dry the ears after D.
206 For drying the ears after D.
207 Jouanna, Archéologie 454 ff.

because they required the physician to complete mentally the scarcely explicit hints. Texts of this kind are especially characteristic of an epoch when the art of healing was predominantly a craft that had to be learned through practice, and whose doctrines were to a large extent transmitted orally.[208]

Accordingly it is not unreasonable to assume that the therapeutic texts of the more complicated type are slightly more recent. The inference is, however, problematic: since it is an undeniable historical fact that considerable portions of the nosological treatises including complicated instructions trace their origin, directly or indirectly, to a common source,[209] and since this source is older than *On Diseases II*, ch. 12–75, which belongs to the oldest treatises of the Collection and is itself dependent on that source, it seems certain that even the more complicated therapeutic texts are among the most ancient constituents of the Corpus Hippocraticum. Jouanna[210] suggested that the therapeutic texts of the more complex type possibly reflect the work of physicians who, according to *On Regimen in Acute Diseases*, "later revised [the *Knídiai gnȭmai*]," and who "proceeded more in keeping with the medical profession as far as concerns what has to be administered in each case,"[211] but it has been demonstrated above[212] that there is no proof for or against the derivation of the nosological treatises from the *Knídiai gnȭmai*.

Indeed, attempts to determine the precise dates of the nosological treatises or of more or less developed passages contained therein are not likely to succeed, given the lack of other testimony and comparable textual material of unambiguous date; even studies on language and style do not yield satisfactory results. One might compare the structure of therapeutic texts to that of dated ancient Greek laws, because both kinds of texts prescribe what has to be done (or not to be done), if (or when) this or that is the condition, and both supply general cases which may have a more or less complex form. Unfortunately, however, such a comparison (which, so far as I am aware, has not been hitherto made) fails to yield results as to the dates of the therapeutic texts and illustrates only that it is quite unsafe to draw any conclusions as to chronological relations from structural simplicity or complexity of therapeutic prescriptions.[213]

An example of a law with a simple structure is exhibited by a text from the city of Teos, dated after 479 B.C. (As in the two preceding extracts, capital letters denote evidence of facts, and minuscule ones the measures to be taken.)

---

208 Lonie, Literacy.

209 Jouanna, Archéologie *passim*, particularly 501 ff.; Grensemann, Knidische Medizin *passim*.

210 Jouanna, Archéologie 468 ff.

211 For this testimonium, see above p. 14 f.

212 p. 24 f.; for the chronology see also 52.

213 The same applies to chronological conclusions drawn from the structure of prognostic aphorisms, cf. below p. 252 f.

"If A (attempt on the life of one or all of the citizens of Teos through poison or magic),
then b (death of the guilty person and of his family).
If B (cutting Teos off from supply of food),
then b.
....
....
If C (disobedience (?) towards the rulers),
then b.
....
....
If D (destruction or damage of this law inscription),
then b."[214]

A much more complex structure, however, is evinced by the text of a law considerably older, namely, the Athenian law on unintentional homicide codified by Drakon in the seventh century B. C.:

"If A (unintentional homicide),
then a (exile of the guilty person).
If B (indictment by the *basileís* that the homicide was unintentional),
then b (jurisdiction by the *ephétai*).
If C (availability of the victim's father or brother or sons),
then c (forgiveness granted by them),
unless D (veto of one of them).
If not C, and if E (availability of certain other relatives),
then c,
unless D.
If not C, and if not E, and if A, and if b, and if d (judgement that the homicide was unintentional),
then e (election by the *ephétai* of 10 members of the *phrātríā* of the victim),
then c."[215]

---

[214] For the text, see Wilhelm Dittenberger, Sylloge inscriptionum Graecarum, vol. 1, Leipzig, 1915, nr. 37 and 38 (p. 41 f.). To this and other early laws applies what the author of *On Regimen in Acute Diseases* states about the original version of the *Knídiai gnō̃mai*, namely that "only a small number of remedies" was used in them (cf. above p. 15).

[215] For the text and its interpretation see Ronald S. Stroud, Drakon's law on homicide (Univ. of Calif. Publications: Class. Studies, vol. 3), Berkeley and Los Angeles, 1968. The text is available also in Dittenberger, *op. cit.* (preced. note), nr. 111 (p. 147–150). See also, Douglas M. MacDowell, Athenian homicide law in the age of the orators, Manchester, 1963, in partic. p. 110–129. Justus Hermann Lipsius, Das attische Recht und Rechtsverfahren, Leipzig, 1915, p. 15 ff., 600 ff.

The inference that both the simple and the more complex type of therapeutic instructions in *On Diseases II*, ch. 12–75 are likely to be old as compared to other medical treatises such as the *Epidemics* exemplifies again that even the oldest texts of the Hippocratic Collection do not represent the primitive roots of the craft but an already highly developed stage.

(4) The fourth part of the single chapters of *On Diseases II*, ch. 12–75, which deals with prognosis, is optional and usually consists just of a short remark added after the third part (treatment) or inserted between the second part (symptoms) and the third. It will be left out of account here, since Jouanna[216] and Grensemann[217] have dealt with the details.

The purpose of this chapter has been to describe some of the features which characterize the stage of development of Greek medicine represented by *On Diseases II*, ch. 12–75. These features, all more or less directly related to cognition, are: the semantic change in technical vocabulary as compared to traditional and colloquial word usage (narrowing in meaning); the importance attributed to observation through the senses; the idea that diseases do not consist of inflexible, rigid patterns of symptoms; the idea that certain signs may or may not be present, may be more or less important in the individual case of a specific disease; the idea that time plays a significant part, as do certain discharges of the body. All these features are prominent in the *Epidemics* and can serve to exemplify how the nosology represented by *On Diseases II*, ch. 12–75 was presupposed by the more recent type of medical treatise to which the *Epidemics* belong.[218]

---

216 Jouanna, Archéologie 86 f.; Jouanna (ed.), Hippocrate, Maladies II, 21–23.

217 Grensemann, Knidische Medizin p. 187 f.

218 Georg Harig, Bemerkungen zum Verhältnis der griechischen zur altorientalischen Medizin, in: "Corpus Hippocraticum" 77–94, in particular 91.

III. The *Epidemics* Treatises

Although it is impossible to establish absolute dates for *On Diseases II*, ch. 12–75, it is evident, from the research of Grensemann and Jouanna, that these texts are among the most ancient in the Hippocratic Collection.[1] As has been repeatedly pointed out in the preceding chapter, one of the main features of *On Diseases II*, ch. 12–75 is a strong tendency towards considering and describing only those signs of the diseases ('symptoms,' to use the post-Hippocratic expression[2]) which can be observed – directly or indirectly – through the senses. The large majority of inferred pathological features that cannot be observed through the senses are confined to the beginnings of the descriptions, to their 'titles,' or to the 'names' of the diseases – i. e. to the most traditional and conventional part of the descriptions.

It is tempting for the medical historian to speculate that this reflects a development in Greek medicine; that the 'titles' are 'fossils' from a more ancient stage in which the causes of the various ailments were ascribed, for example, to a wood-worm in the skull-bone or to water in the brain or to mortification of the brain or to a consumption of the spinal marrow or to dropsy in the lung;[3] that the ensuing descriptions of disease signs testify to a later stage at which the aetiological 'myths' survived only for the sake of identification and classification of the diseases. The Homeric and fifth century B. C. popular usage of certain 'physiological' words[4] would, accordingly, reflect the archaic stage, while their Hippocratic use testifies to the later stage.

Such a conclusion might be correct to a certain extent, namely insofar as trends and tendencies are considered. It seems plausible that there was some kind of development from traditional speculation and traditional word usage towards sensory observation and towards a restriction in the meaning of inherited words. Efforts, however, to reduce this probable evolution to a schematic formula would be hazardous. One has to be aware of the fact that we are working with texts of fragmentary nature. If any such evolution as suggested above has indeed taken place, it was

[1] Cf. above p. 25, 52 f.
[2] Cf. above p. 57, note 119.
[3] Cf. above p. 56 f.
[4] Cf. above p. 37–51.

certainly not confined to surviving texts. It must have been a more general evolution in the mode of thinking. The medical texts which we possess represent surely less than the tip of the iceberg.[5]

The situation becomes more complicated because there must have been concurring evolutions not necessarily opposing or retrogressive, but presupposing the earlier achievements and for the most part compatible with them, although no longer leading in the same direction. It is not unreasonable that speculation about pathology, and in particular about aetiology, was revived in conjunction with careful observation and detailed description. A nosology such as that of *On Diseases II*, ch. 12–75 does not consist of static tableaux manifesting merely additions of symptoms, rather it presents flexibly applicable general cases based on observation and taking account of what happens 'generally' and also of what might happen in rarer cases. Indeed, such a nosology is an open doctrinal system with an inherent tendency towards *amplification*. Since the aim of the nosological system was its applicability to as many real cases as possible, the physician's observation of real cases necessarily resulted in a (written or non-written) amplification. An example is mentioned in the testimonium of *On Regimen in Acute Diseases*: "Some" people (related to the revisors of the *Knídiai gnṓmai*?) were "well acquainted with the manifold varieties of each disease and with their differentiation."[6]

Furthermore, there was a stimulus in this nosology towards *modifying* its system. Because the oldest stage of Greek nosology available to the historian in a representative text, *On Diseases II*, ch. 12–75, was not only to a large extent based on observation, but also encouraged it, and because there were few theoretical presuppositions[7] in this early nosology, it served as a basis, or a starting-point, for the subsequent development still traceable in the Hippocratic Collection. As Jouanna and Grensemann have demonstrated, the various versions in which nosological material has been transmitted in the Collection originated in a lost common source.[8] *On Diseases II*, ch. 12–75 gives some idea of what the source must have been like and makes it possible to trace in the Hippocratic Corpus how new theoretical concepts were added to, and amalgamated with, the inferable original nosological nucleus. These new concepts formed a cluster of theories on body humours (in particular phlegm/bile) and, closely related to it, on elementary qualities (hot/cold and moist/dry) and on the influence

---

[5] According to Xenophon there were, around 400 B.C., "many treatises by physicians" (*Mem. IV* 2.10).

[6] Cf. above p. 15.

[7] Generally on this problem Lloyd, Magic 128 f.; Mansfeld, Theoretical and empirical attitudes 384 f.

[8] Whether this source was Knidian or not, is a moot and unimportant question, as has been discussed above. Cf. p. 24 f.

of the weather and the seasons on the body. These theories enabled physicians to formulate new opinions about the causes of diseases. Unlike the traditional explanations of disease as due to a "wood-worm in the bone" or "water in the brain" or a "mortification of the brain,"[9] the new aetiologies were, to some degree, based on facts which could be observed through the senses. The ancient physician could *see* and *touch* phlegm and bile. (Today we would say: He observed whitish and grey[10] excretions like mucus of all kinds, which he interpreted as phlegm; and he observed yellowish and brownish excretions which he interpreted as bile; correspondingly with other humours such as black bile[11] and blood.) He could *feel* the warm, the cold, the moist, the dry, and the combinations thereof. The seasons as well as the weather with its changes were, of course, part of everyone's daily experiences. Several passages from a non-nosological treatise, *On the Nature of Man*, are particularly illustrative of the way in which the physicians proceeded by combining observation and theoretical speculation; ch. 5: "[The four humours] have distinct features. Phlegm has no similarity whatsoever to blood, nor blood to bile, nor bile to phlegm. For how could they be like one another, since their colours do not look the same, nor do they feel the same when you touch them with your hand — they are neither equally hot nor equally cold nor equally dry nor equally moist ... And this is how you can realize that they are not just one [substance], but that each has its own property and nature: If you give somebody a drug which brings forth phlegm, he will vomit phlegm; if you give him a drug which brings forth bile, he will vomit bile; the same way black bile will be excreted if you give him a drug which brings forth black bile; and if you make a cut in his body so that there is a wound, blood will flow." Ch. 7: "A proof that phlegm is the coldest [of the four humours]: if you touch phlegm and bile and blood, you will find that phlegm is the coldest. This is the case although it is the most viscous and is excreted with much force [i. e. pressure], almost like black bile; now, what is excreted with force, gets warmer while it is pressed with force. But even in spite of all this, phlegm appears to be the coldest because of its nature."[12] There are further examples in the same chapter, which also discusses the qualities of the seasons.

The new aetiologies were, however, only seemingly based on the observation of the principal elements. In fact there was implied a good deal of non-observational, interpretative mental operation by which the

---

9 Cf. above p. 55 f.

10 On the colour of phlegm, cf. below p. 148, note 68.

11 For black bile, see above p. 46–50.

12 *Nat. Hom.* 6.42.1–15, 46.11–17 Li. = 176.3–178.2, 182.6–11 Jouanna = 4.12–14, 18 Jones.

observable features (one might say data) were conceived of as being in a functional relationship to each other. "All diseases in people," says the compiler of the nosological treatise *On Affections* (ch. 1), "come into existence through bile and phlegm. Bile and phlegm cause the diseases when they are overdried or overmoistened or overheated or overcooled. This occurs to phlegm and bile from food and beverages, and from exercises and wounds, and from odour and noise and sight and sexual intercourse, and from the hot and the cold [as such]; it occurs, when any of the aforesaid items acts on the body either improperly, or contrary to what it is accustomed to, or more and stronger, or less and weaker. The diseases occur to people from this without exception."[13] The author of *On Diseases I*, ch. 2 states: "All diseases occur to us from internals, namely bile and phlegm, and from externals, namely exercises and wounds and from the hot, when it overheats, and the cold, when it overcools [the body]. The bile and the phlegm come into existence when the body is formed, and they are always in the body either more or less; and they produce the diseases, the ones from food and beverages as well as the ones from the hot which overheats and the cold which overcools."[14] The same concept (or similar ones) underlies other nosological treatises (with the exception of *On Diseases II*, ch. 12–75), and since this fact is well-known and has been studied in detail by Jouanna,[15] Grensemann,[16] and earlier modern historians,[17] there is no need to dwell upon it here.

---

13 *Aff.* 6.208.8–17 Li. = p. 292 Jouanna, Archéologie Νοσήματα τοῖσιν ἀνθρώποις ἅπαντα γίνεται ὑπὸ χολῆς καὶ φλέγματος· ἡ δὲ χολὴ καὶ τὸ φλέγμα τὰς νούσους παρέχει ὅταν ἐν τῷ σώματι ὑπερυγραίνηται ἢ ὑπερξηραίνηται (ὑπερυγρ. ἢ ὑπερξ. θ: ἢ ὑπερξ. ἢ ὑπερυγρ. M) ἢ ὑπερθερμαίνηται ἢ ὑπερψύχηται. πάσχει δὲ ταῦτα τὸ φλέγμα καὶ ἡ χολὴ καὶ ἀπὸ σίτων (σίτων θ: σιτίων M) καὶ ποτῶν καὶ ἀπὸ πόνων καὶ τρωμάτων καὶ ἀπὸ (ἀπὸ θ: om. M) ὀσμῆς καὶ ἀκοῆς καὶ ὄψιος καὶ λαγνείης καὶ ἀπὸ τοῦ θερμοῦ τε καὶ ψυχροῦ· πάσχει δὲ ὅταν τούτων ἕκαστα τῶν εἰρημένων ἢ (ἢ M: ἐι θ) μὴ ἐν τῷ δέοντι προσφέρηται τῷ σώματι ἢ μὴ τὰ εἰωθότα ἢ πλείω τε καὶ ἰσχυρότερα ἢ ἐλάσσω τε καὶ ἀσθενέστερα. τὰ μὲν οὖν νοσήματα γίνεται τοῖσιν ἀνθρώποισιν ἅπαντα ἀπὸ τούτων.

14 *Morb. I* 6.142.13–20 Li. = 6.5–12 Wittern = p. 310 Jouanna, Archéologie (partly) Αἱ μὲν οὖν νοῦσοι γίνονται ἡμῖν (ἡ. θ: om. M) ἅπασαι, τῶν μὲν ἐν τῷ σώματι ἐνεόντων ἀπό τε χολῆς καὶ φλέγματος, τῶν δ' ἔξωθεν ἀπὸ πόνων καὶ τρωμάτων, καὶ ὑπὸ (κ. ὑ. θ: ἀλλὰ καὶ M) τοῦ θερμοῦ ὑπερθερμαίνοντος καὶ τοῦ ψυχροῦ ὑπερψύχοντος (post ὑπερψ. add. καὶ τοῦ ξηροῦ ὑπερξηραίνοντος M; post ὑπερξ. add. καὶ τοῦ ὑγροῦ ὑπερυγραίνοντος M^3 in mg.). καὶ ἡ μὲν χολὴ καὶ τὸ φλέγμα γινομένοισί τε συγγίνεται καὶ ἔνι αἰεὶ (ἔ. αἰ. θ: ἔστιν M) ἐν τῷ σώματι ἢ πλέον ἢ ἔλασσον· τὰς δὲ νούσους παρέχει (-έχει θ: -έχεται M) τὰς μὲν ἀπὸ σιτίων καὶ ποτῶν, τὰς δὲ ἀπὸ τοῦ θερμοῦ ὑπερθερμαίνοντος καὶ ἀπὸ τοῦ ψυχροῦ ὑπερψύχοντος.

15 Jouanna, Archéologie *passim*.

16 Grensemann, Knidische Medizin *passim* (in particular as concerns parts of the gynaecological texts of the Hippocratic Collection).

17 For literature, see the two aforementioned recent monographs.

The present section of this book will be devoted to a study of certain central pathological (including aetiological) concepts underlying some Hippocratic treatises *other* than the nosological ones, and more recent than *On Diseases II*, ch. 12–75,[18] especially concepts underlying *Epidemics I* and *III* and *Epidemics II, IV*, and *VI*. (Since *Epidemics V* and *VII* contain for the most part individual case-histories and have only very little explicit theorizing, they will not be considered here.)

As in the case of other Hippocratic treatises, it is impossible to determine the authorship of the *Epidemics*.[19] Moreover there are difficulties about the chronology. Books *I* and *III* can be dated with some confidence to around 410 B.C. on the basis of inscriptions excavated in the city of Thasos.[20] The dates proposed for books *II, IV, VI* vary between 427/426 and 373/372 B.C., and in spite of the scholarly energy spent on this problem in recent years, no decisive argument seems to have been put forward in favour of more precise dates.[21] Since books *II, IV, VI* are not homogeneous works but consist of disparate materials by (probably) several authors and/or redactors, and since the identity of the *names* of patients in the *Epidemics* with the *names* of dated historical personages mentioned in other sources is not by itself a sufficient argument for an identity of *persons*,[22] I prefer to adopt a rather sceptical attitude with regard to the possibilities of narrowing down the chronological range.[23] Apart from absolute dates, attempts have been made to establish a relative chronological sequence between *Epidemics I* and *III* and *Epidemics II, IV, VI*,[24] but the evidence is equally meagre, and scepticism is not out of place. For the time being, therefore, it seems best to leave the question

---

[18] On the chronological relationship, see p. 25, 37, 52 f.

[19] Books *I* and *III* and books *II, IV*, and *VI* form two distinct groups: cf. Deichgräber, Die Epidemien 9 ff., 24 ff.; Nikitas, Untersuchungen *passim*.

[20] Deichgräber, Die Epidemien 16. J.-E. Dugand, Hippocrate à Thasos et en Grèce du nord, in: "Corpus Hippocraticum" 233–245 (this article is useful because it presents the evidence in detail; the conclusions are, however, too speculative).

[21] Littré, vol. 5.16–18; Deichgräber, Die Epidemien 74–75; Grensemann, Krankheit der Tochter 71–83; Langholf, Syntaktische Untersuchungen 15; Vincenzo Di Benedetto, Principi metodici di Ep. II. IV. VI, in: "Corpus Hippocraticum" 246–263; Grmek, Les maladies 448–452.

[22] Arguments based on the identity of names have frequently been put forward for the purpose of dating, see Deichgräber, Patienten. Critical remarks about the method are found in Wesley E. Thompson, Tot Atheniensibus idem nomen erat, in: ΦΟΡΟΣ. Tribute to B. D. Meritt, New York, 1974, 144–149. Some of the personal names of the *Epidemics* may even be place-names, cf. Langholf, *loco cit.*

[23] In Langholf, Syntaktische Untersuchungen 15, a certain date (373/372) of *Epid. IV* has been qualified as "sehr wahrscheinlich;" I now believe that other possibilities are equally probable, because the expression ἄστρον οὐ σμικρόν in *Epid. IV* 21 (5.160.13 Li. = Per. 152 La.) may refer to astronomical phenomena other than a comet.

[24] Di Benedetto, *loco cit.*; Grmek, Les maladies 452–455.

open and to date provisionally *Epidemics II, IV, VI* to around 400 B. C., plus or minus several decades, i. e. somewhere between the possible extreme dates which cover a span of 55 years.[25]

Although the title *epidēmíai* is not likely to be original,[26] it might be old. Perhaps it was given by the earliest collectors of these texts (already in the fourth century B. C.?).[27] Its meaning is not quite clear. Since the substantive as well as the adjectives *epídēmos/epidḗmios* and the verb *epidēméo* can denote the 'arrival' or 'sojourn' of persons[28] as well as of diseases,[29] the title could refer to the itinerant physicians or the oncoming diseases or both. It is, therefore, by no means certain that the title *epidēmíai* signifies unequivocally 'epidemic diseases': there are obviously more topics in the *Epidemics* treatises.[30]

The identical title of an Ionic prose work by Ion of Khios presents a similar problem of authenticity and interpretation. Although his *epidēmíai* are lost except for a few quotations by other ancient authors,[31] the extant remains seem[32] to permit the conjecture that this work described both Ion's visits abroad and the visits of guests from abroad to the author in Khios. The title, whether authentic or not, may, therefore, have been intended to be of ambiguous meaning.[33]

Ion's interest was apparently not in history or historiography as such, but in noteworthy individuals of his own time whom he had met himself. This is, apart from the title, an additional parallel to the medical *Epidemics*

---

25 One should even allow for the possibility that the books contain passages of older and/or more recent times.

26 Schmalzriedt, ΠΕΡΙ ΦΥΣΕΩΣ 44, 47. Nachmanson, Buchtitel 14–25.

27 Schmalzriedt, ΠΕΡΙ ΦΥΣΕΩΣ 73–82.

28 This is the usual meaning, cf. Liddell/Scott/Jones. It must be coincidental that this very common usage (with a personal agent) is not found in the Hippocratic Collection except for late Hellenistic pseudepigrapha.

29 ἐπίδημος *Epid. I* 2.640.10 Li. = 1.191.12 Kw. = 1.166 Jones; ἐπιδήμιος *Epid. VII* 5.424.13; *Int.* 7.214.19; 216.16; 218.9; 258.18; *Vid. Ac.* 9.158.19; ἐπιδημέω *Aer.* 2.20.4 Li. = 1.37.7 Kw. = 1.76 Jones; *Prog.* 2.188.13 Li. = 1.107.21 Kw. = 2.54 Jones; *Acut.* 2.232.10 Li. = 1.111.8 Kw. = 2.66 Jones; *Epid. I* 2.644.11 Li. = 1.192.15 Kw. = 1.168 Jones; *Epid. III* 3.70.10 Li. = 1.225.6 Kw. = 1.240 Jones; 3.92.5 Li. = 1.229.19 Kw. = 1.250 Jones; *Epid. II* 5.100.6; *Epid. IV* 5.178.1 Li. = Per. 226 La.; *Epid. VI* 5.336.11; 342.5; 348.20; *Epid. VII* 5.456.10; ἐπιδημίη is found in the titles of the seven books and in *Nat. Hom.* 6.54.18 Li. = 4.26 Jones = 190.13 Jouanna.

30 Galen, however (Gal. *In Hp. Epid. VI comm.* p. 5.16–18 Wenkebach), maintains that the title does *not* refer to the travels of the physician; unfortunately, he gives no evidence for this view.

31 Collected by Felix Jacoby, Die Fragmente der griechischen Historiker, Berlin/Leiden, 1923 ff., no. 392. Cf. Pauly/Wissowa IX.2 (18. Halbband), 1863 f. s. v. 'Ion 11' (Diehl).

32 On the condition that Jacoby's fragments 9–22 at least partly belong to the Ἐπιδημίαι, as Jacoby suggests.

33 'Encounters' would be a free, similarly ambiguous rendering of the title of Ion's and the physicians' works. Dover translates 'visits.'

treatises, whose authors show less interest in the systematic aspects of medicine than in individuals whom they had treated or examined themselves. Furthermore, Ion's *epidēmíai* may have shared with the medical *epidēmíai* books an unsystematic arrangement of the contents.[34] It is possible that Ion inaugurated a new literary form (*genus*), which was then adopted by the physicians who wrote the *Epidemics*.[35] The titles may reflect this affinity, quite independently from the problem of their authenticity.

1. krísis *and Critical Days*

The central concepts underlying the *Epidemics* are: *krísis* ('crisis' of the disease), *pépsis* ('cooking' or 'ripening' of the substances that are involved in the disease, and/or 'digestion' of food), and *apóstasis* ('segregation' or 'evacuation' of harmful substances either through excretion or through isolation, e. g. in the form of an 'abscess').[1] The comments on the matter in *Epidemics I*, ch. 5 Li. = ch. 11 Kw., Jones are apropos here: "As to what is dangerous: You should direct your attention to timely coctions (*pepasmós*, related to *pépsis*) of all substances excreted through all ways of excretion, or to good and critical (*krísimos*, related to *krísis*) segregations (*apóstasis*). Coctions indicate quickness of the *krísis*, safety, and health, but substances raw and uncooked and turning into bad segregations (*apóstasis*) indicate an absence of the *krísis* or [indicate] pain or delay or death or a return of the same [that is, a relapse]. Which out of these [possibilities] is most likely to be the case, has to be inferred from other [signs]. You must say what has happened, recognize what is happening, foretell what will happen. Address yourself to these things. You should devote yourself to two things concerning the diseases: to be of use, or not to harm."[2] These

---

[34] On the disposition of Ion's work see Dover 33 f.

[35] Jacoby *loco cit.*, "Kommentar," p. 192–194, 197. Dover 34 f.

[1] For each of these Greek words, synonyms were used, but the aforesaid words are the most common ones. Cf. Thivel, Cnide 211–216. For a brief survey of the fundamental concepts see López Férez, Historia 626–629.

[2] *Epid. I* 2.632.12–636.1 Li. = 1.189.18–190.3 Kw. = 1.162–164 Jones Ὅσα διὰ κινδύνων (διὰ κινδύνων A, Gal. interpret. Arab.: δὲ διὰ κινδύνους VIR: δ' ἀκινδύνως Gal.), πεπασμοὺς τῶν ἀπιόντων πάντας πάντοθεν ἐπικαίρους ἢ (ἢ AVIR: καὶ Gal.) καλὰς καὶ κρισίμους ἀποστάσιας σκοπεῖσθαι. πεπασμοὶ ταχυτῆτα κρίσιος, ἀσφάλειαν, ὑγιείην (ταχυτῆτα κρίσιος, ἀσφάλειαν, ὑγιεῖν, mut. in ὑγιείης (A^3) A: τ. καὶ κρ. ἀσφ. ὑγείην VI: τ. κρ. καὶ ἀσφ. ὑγιείης R, Gal. interpret. Arab.: τ. κρ. καὶ ἀσφάλειαν ὑγιεινὴν Gal.) σημαίνουσιν, ὠμὰ δὲ καὶ ἄπεπτα καὶ (καὶ AVIR: om. Gal.) ἐς κακὰς ἀποστάσιας τρεπόμενα ἀκρισίας ἢ πόνους ἢ χρόνους ἢ θανάτους ἢ τῶν αὐτῶν ὑποστροφάς. ὅ τι δὲ τούτων ἔσται μάλιστα, σκεπτέον ἐξ ἄλλων. λέγειν τὰ προγενόμενα (-γε- AVIR: -γι- Gal.), γινώσκειν τὰ παρεόντα, προλέγειν τὰ ἐσόμενα· μελετᾶν ταῦτα. ἀσκεῖν περὶ τὰ νοσήματα δύο (τὰ ν. δύο AVIR: τοῦ τὰ ν. Gal.), ὠφελεῖν ἢ μὴ βλάπτειν.

remarks are immediately followed by the equally famous sentence about three mutually complementary aspects of medicine: the disease, the patient, and the physician (cf. above, p. 1). The interrelation between *krísis, pépsis,* and *apóstasis* is not so direct. A fourth word is missing here – and it is missing in all of the relevant passages –, a word for the harmful substance that causes the disease (for instance a superabundant humour disturbing the balance of humours, or a corrupted humour). It is a rather striking fact that there is no generic word for this *materia peccans* in the whole Hippocratic Collection although the concept is clearly present.[3] This situation indicates that the idea of the 'harmful matter' is not a theoretical achievement of the authors in whose texts it is ubiquitously implicit, but a popular notion taken over into scientific medicine. In fact, 'harmful matter' can be found in several primitive and archaic systems of medicine, including that of the Egyptians. In the Collection, the substance can be overcome by the body through 'cooking' or 'coction,' whereby it becomes less harmful, and through subsequent excretion or isolation. There are several possible ways of excretion. In *Epidemics II* 1.7 it is stated: "Segregations [*apóstasis*] occur either through the vessels [*phléps*] or the sinews [*tónos*] or the bones or the tendons [*neúron*][4] or the skin or other outlets. Good are the segregations beneath the disease [beneath the diseased region], [segregations] such as varicose veins or heaviness of the loin; the best ones are the ones that go downward from above and the ones lowest in the stomach and most distant from the disease,[5] and the ones through outflow, such as blood out of the nose, pus out of the ear, urine – through outflow. Those [patients] to whom this does not occur have segregations wrought in the teeth, eyes, nose, sweat; but also swellings formed under the skin which turn outward, e. g. scrofulas and suppurations, or a wound, and eruptions of this kind, or peeling, loss of hair, white scaliness [*alphós*], leprosy [?, *léprē*], or the like, which are segregations if they occur massively and if they are not confined to one half[6] – this applies also to the other [signs] mentioned – and if they are not inadequate to the size [*peribolḗ*, lit. 'circumference'] of the disease: For example, with the niece of Timenes, there occurred a segregation [*apestḗrixen*] into a

[3] It is circumscribed as νοῦσος, 'disease,' in *Epid. II* 5.78.10, see shortly below. Lonie, Hippocratic treatises 315, 327.

[4] Both *tónos* and *neúron* could just as well refer to the nerves, which were not systematically distinguished from tendons or sinews even by Herophilos. Paul Potter, Herophilus of Chalcedon: An assessment of his place in the history of anatomy, Bull. of the Hist. of Medicine 50 (1976), 45–60; generally Fraser, Ptolemaic Alexandria I 352, II 512–514.

[5] I. e., most distant from the place where the disease manifests itself, and where the harmful substance is concentrated.

[6] Of the body, i. e. its left or right side.

finger which was unable to receive the disease [*noúsos*]; it flowed back [into the body], and she died."[7]

Krísis, pépsis, and *apóstasis* are closely interrelated with each other because all of them would appear to be functions of the harmful substance; more precisely, because its 'coction' and 'segregation' are the prerequisites of a successful *krísis*. The basic meaning of the substantive *krísis* or the verb *krī́nō* is 'judgement,' 'decision' or 'to judge,' 'to decide.'[8] Thus, the medical usage of *krísis* or *krī́nō* implies alternatives: the patient either dies or survives; if he survives, he either recovers immediately, or the disease continues; if the disease continues, it either does so being the same or having changed its appearance. Nowhere in the *Epidemics*, or to be sure in the whole Hippocratic Collection is this or a similar set of alternatives propounded systematically. It is a modern construct which can be established from abundant evidence. For example, in *Epidemics I*, ch. 12 Li. (= ch. 26 Kw., Jones), it is stated that at the critical days "the crises [*krísis*] occur towards survival or death, or tendencies [occur] towards the better or the worse."[9] The ability of the Greek physician to foretell which of these alternatives would be the outcome was necessarily a requirement of the profession. For this purpose he possessed a multitude of general and specific prognostic rules, many of which have been transmitted to us in the prognostic treatises of the Corpus (for instance *On Airs, Waters, Places;*

---

[7] *Epid. II* 5.76.17–78.10 Ἀποστάσιες ἢ διὰ φλεβῶν ἢ τόνων ἢ δι' ὀστέων ἢ νεύρων ἢ δέρματος ἢ ἐκτροπῶν ἑτέρων. χρησταὶ δὲ αἱ κάτω τῆς νούσου, οἷον κιρσοί, ὀσφύος βάρεα, ἄρισται δὲ μάλιστα αἱ (αἱ HIR: om. V) κάτω ἐκ τῶν ἄνω (sic fortasse Arabs: ἐκ τῶν ἄνω ante ἄρισται VHIR) καὶ αἱ κατωτάτω κοιλίης καὶ προσωτάτω ἀπὸ τῆς νούσου, καὶ αἱ κατ' ἔκρουν (κατ' ἔκρουν HIR: κατέκρουνοι V), οἷον αἷμα ἐκ ῥινῶν, πύον ἐξ ὠτός, πτύαλον, οὖρον – κατ' ἔκρουν. οἷσι μὴ ταῦτα, ἀποστάσιες οἷον ὀδόντες, ὀφθαλμοί, ῥίς, ἱδρώς (ἱδρώς VHIR: om. Arabs), ἀτὰρ καὶ τὰ (τὰ VH: τὸ IR) ὑπὸ δέρμα ἐς τὸ ἔξω ἀφιστάμενα (ἐς τὸ ἔ. ἀ. V: ἀ. ἐς τὸ ἔ. HIR) φύματα, οἷον (φύματα οἷον VHIR: οἷον φύματα Arabs?) ταγγαὶ (ταγγαὶ HIR: γαγγαὶ V) καὶ τὰ ἐκπυοῦντα ἢ ἕλκος καὶ τὰ τοιαῦτα ἐξανθήματα ἢ λόποι (λόποι V: λοποὶ HIR) ἢ μάδησις τριχῶν, ἀλφοί, λέπραι, ἢ τὰ τοιαῦτα ὅσα ἀποστάσιες μέν ἐστιν (ἐστιν V: εἰσιν HIR) ἀθρόως ῥέψασαι (ῥέψασαι V: ῥεύσασαι HIR) καὶ μὴ ἡμιρρόπως (ἡμιρρόπως edd.: ἡμίρροπος VHIR), καὶ ὅσα ἄλλα εἴρηται ('so ist sie doch schädlich' add. Arabs: om. VHIR), καὶ ἢν μὴ ἀναξίως τῆς περιβολῆς τῆς νούσου, οἷον τῇ Τιμένεω (τι- V: τη- HIR) ἀδελφιδῇ ἐκ νούσου ἰσχυρῆς ('wiederholt befiel, weil der Überschuß' add. Arabs: om. VHIR) ἐς δάκτυλον ἀπεστήριξεν οὐχ ἱκανὸν δέξασθαι τὴν νοῦσον· ἐπαλινδρόμησεν· ἀπέθανεν. In Thucyd. *II* 49 an *apóstasis* (this term is, however, not used) is said to have announced survival during the plague. Particularly mentioned are the genitals, hands, feet, and eyes.

[8] The word's root originally denoted 'to put asunder,' 'to divide,' and this connotation was still felt in the fifth and fourth centuries B. C., cf. Liddell/Scott/Jones s. v.

[9] *Epid. I* 2.680.6–9 Li. = 1.202.5–8 Kw. = 1.184 Jones δεῖ … εἰδέναι … κρίσιας ἐσομένας ἐπὶ σωτηρίην ἢ τὸ ὀλέθριον (ἢ τὸ ὀ. VIR: ἢ ὄλεθρον Gal.: εἴτε ὀλέθριον A) ἢ ῥοπὰς ἐπὶ τὸ ἄμεινον ἢ τὸ (τὸ AVIR: om. Gal.) χεῖρον.

Prognostics; Prorrhetics I and *II; Koan Prognoses*; parts of the *Aphorisms*,[10] and some other treatises, among them ancient works excerpting material contained in other books). Even granted, however, that the Greek doctor was able to prognosticate the development of a disease (an ability on which his professional and social standing depended[11]), the question remains: how did he manage to recognize whether a particular state in the course of a disease case was a *krísis* or not? More precisely: how did he recognize this while the pathological process was still going on, not after the supposedly 'critical' state was over, *ex eventu*?

There are two constitutive features which together make up a *krísis*. This doctrine, too, is expressed nowhere in the Hippocratic Collection in general terms but can be inferred from how it is applied: (*i*) the first and foremost feature is temporal: a *krísis* occurs only and exclusively on certain days of the disease (days numbered from its beginning); events outside of these 'critical days' are never 'critical' in the strict technical sense of the word; (*ii*) the second feature is that a *krísis* always has characteristic concomitant symptoms; a day as such, i. e. *qua* day a, b, c ... n, is never a *krísis* but a point of time at which the *krísis* may occur. Only if certain symptoms come to pass on a 'critical day,' is this a *krísis*. Just as the days are called 'critical,' the specific symptoms occurring on these days are named 'critical' (*krísimos*).

Signs of a *krísis*

Before dealing with the numerical system of 'critical days,'[12] it is useful to discuss the 'critical' symptoms. They can be divided into two classes (this division is also a modern construct and used here only for the sake of clarity in describing the *krísis* doctrine): the first class consists of the symptoms fever and rigor; the second class consists of what the Hippocratic physicians called an *apóstasis*, or 'segregation' of harmful matter.[13]

As to the first class, it was a very common phenomenon in Hippocratic medicine that during the *krísis* the fever diminished, or ceased completely. The sudden remission of fever is a well-known observation of daily life. Within a few hours, a patient may feel healthy again. Such a quick fall in body temperature is still today called 'critical,' an expression inherited

---

[10] Περὶ ἀέρων ὑδάτων τόπων, *Aer.*; Προγνωστικόν, *Prog.*; Προρρητικὸς α′, β′, *Prorrh. I, II*; Κῳακαὶ προγνώσιες, *Coac.*; Ἀφορισμοί, *Aph.*

[11] Edelstein, Περὶ ἀέρων 82–88.

[12] See below p. 93 ff., 102 ff.

[13] Cf. above p. 79–81. — Senfelder, Die hippokratische Lehre, has a good collection of textual material, although its interpretation is superficial and antiquated.

from the Hippocratics and nowadays used without any background of a general crisis-theory (i. e. the modern medical expression 'crisis' is another 'fossil').

Typical courses of fever in relation to the *krísis* are described in *Epidemics I*, ch. 11 Li. (= ch. 25 Kw., Jones). Although the Hippocratic physicians had no method of measuring the fever except by feeling the skin or the exhaled breath[14] of the patient, the following descriptions contain an almost graphical representation of the course of fever: "For instance, with some the continuous fever is strong and vigorous from the beginning and turns towards the worst, but around the *krísis* and during the *krísis* it diminishes ... With some, it begins mildly, then increases and reaches its acute stage; so it stays for some time, then it diminishes again until the *krísis* and around the *krísis*."[15]

It is equally possible that the fever rises at the *krísis*, for in the same chapter of *Epidemics I* we find: "With some, it starts slightly and almost unnoticeably, but increases and gets more acute every day, and bursts forth violently around the *krísis*."[16] In the same context it is stated that "in all cases of fever and disease" these are possibilities of development.[17]

Rigor is another symptom connected with *krísis*. Frequent shivering during convalescence, particularly after serious diseases, is a phenomenon easily observed. The Hippocratics took it as a 'critical' sign of recovery. Although rigor is once mentioned together with several forms of *apóstasis*,[18] one should not conclude that rigor was regarded as an *apóstasis*; an aphorism contained in *Epidemics VI* 1.8 even implies that there was a

---

[14] *Prog.* 2.122.13–14 Li. = 1.83.2–3 Kw. = 2.14 Jones ψυχρὸν δὲ ἐκπνεόμενον ἐκ τῶν ῥινῶν καὶ τοῦ στόματος (scil. πνεῦμα) ... Cf. *Aff.* 6.218.14–16 Li. = p. 274 Jouanna ἡ γλῶσσα τρηχέα καὶ μέλαινα γίνεται ὑπὸ θερμότητος τοῦ πνεύματος ... καὶ τὰ μὲν ἔξω ψυχρὸς γίνεται, τὰ δ' ἔσω θερμός. Cf. above p. 58, note 140.

[15] *Epid. I* 2.676.1–10 Li. = 1.200.23–201.9 Kw. = 1.182 Jones αὐτίκα γὰρ συνεχὴς ἔστιν οἷσιν ἀρχόμενος (ἀρχ. AVIR, Gal. interpret. Arab.: om. Gal.) ἀνθεῖ καὶ ἀκμάζει μάλιστα καὶ ἀνάγει ἐπὶ τὸ χαλεπώτατον (-ατον AIR, Gal. interpret. Arab.: -ερον V, Gal.), περὶ δὲ κρίσιν καὶ ἅμα κρίσει λεπτύνεται (λεπτ- A: ἀπολεπτ- VIR, Gal.) ... ἔστι δ' οἷσιν ἀρχόμενος πρηέως ἐπιδιδοῖ καὶ παροξύνεται καὶ μέχρι τινὸς ἀκμάσας πάλιν ὑφίησι μέχρι κρίσιος καὶ περὶ κρίσιν.

[16] ἔστι δ' οἷσιν ἄρχεται μαλακῶς καὶ ὑποβρύχια, ἐπαναδιδοῖ δὲ (δὲ AVIR: om. Gal.) καὶ παροξύνεται (καὶ add. A: om. VIR, Gal.) καθ' ἡμέρην ἑκάστην (ἑκ. AVIR: om. Gal.), περὶ δὲ κρίσιν (post κρ. add. καὶ ἅμα κρίσει VIR: om. A, Gal.) ἅλις ἐξέλαμψεν. (*Loco laud.*)

[17] συμπίπτει δὲ ταῦτα γίνεσθαι ἐπὶ παντὸς πυρετοῦ καὶ παντὸς (παντὸς VIR: ἐπὶ παντὸς Gal.: om. A) νοσήματος. (*Loco laud.*)

[18] *Epid. I* 2.670.11–15 Li. = 1.199.20–200.2 Kw. = 1.180 Jones ἀποστάσιες ἐπὶ τὸ ὀλέθριον καὶ κρίσιμον, ἱδρώς, ῥῖγος, ψύξις, βήξ, πταρμοί, λυγμοί, πνεύματα, ἐρεύξιες, φῦσαι ..., αἱμορραγίαι, αἱμορροΐδες. ψύξις is no *apóstasis* either, the list is not logical or systematic.

'generic' difference[19] between rigor and 'segregations' (which seems plausible in any case): "Those who have rigor do not have any segregations."[20]

The second class of symptoms present in a *krísis* consists of various forms of *apóstasis*. Some kinds of 'segregation' are more frequent than others. Excretions of sweat, urine, faeces, and blood are the most prominent.

In the Hippocratic Corpus, no explicit doctrine is found about the details of the process underlying the alleged excretion of the substance(s) causing a disease. Of course, neither sweat nor urine nor faeces nor blood were considered harmful in themselves. The modern historian trying to systematize what the ancient Hippocratic texts say about *apóstasis* may be induced to believe that the *materia peccans* was thought to be transported out of the body by means of these excretions, i. e. that these excretions served as a vehicle.

To comprehend more fully the nature of the critical symptoms that make up a *krísis*, it is instructive to analyze the 42 case-histories contained in *Epidemics I* and *III*. Of the 42 individual patients, 25 are reported to have died, and 17 to have survived.

In 5 of the 17 cases of survival, it is simply stated that the patients experienced a (successful) final *krísis*, but we do not learn what the symptoms of the final *krísis* were (absence of fever is mentioned once).[21] The fact that a detailed description of some historical cases of *krísis* was deemed dispensable by the author(s) of *Epidemics I* and *III* (and of other books, too, particularly of *Epidemics IV*) allows the conclusion that a *krísis* was something very well defined — something about which a

---

19 'Generic' difference is, again, an anachronistic description.

20 *Epid. VI* 5.270.4–5 ἀποστάσιες οὐ μάλα οἷσι ῥίγεα. This aphorism contradicts some passages where rigor plus perspiration is described: in addition to the two cases that will be quoted shortly below (p. 85, note 23; 86, note 31), cf. *Epid. III* 3.48.7–8 Li. = 1.219.16–17 Kw. = 1.228 Jones; 48.14–15 Li. = 219.23–24 Kw. = 228 Jones. There are, however, passages emphasizing that rigor is connected with urine retention, perhaps also with constipation, i. e. with a blockage of two possible means by which an *apóstasis* can be effected: *Epid. IV* 5.166.11–12 Li. = Per. 176 La.; *Epid. VI* 5.270.2–3, on which *Epid. IV* 5.168.4–7 Li. = Per. 179–181 La. seems to be dependent; cf. *Prorrh. I* 5.528.12–530.1; 544.6–8; 548.4–7 ≈ *Coac.* 5.722.19–20; 592.6–7. (On the difference between ῥῖγος and φρίκη see *Morb. I* 6.190.6 Li. = 72.10–11 Wittern.) The doctrine is fully compatible with the pathophysiological model displayed in *Flat.* 6.100.1–12 Li. = 95.7–18 Heiberg = 2.234–236 Jones. Once it is recorded that there was no rigor after an *apóstasis* had occurred, *Epid. II* 5.108.1–4 Li. = Per. 48–49 La. The aphorism quoted above may thus be a premature generalization.

21 *Epid. I* 2.690.9 Li. = 1.205.12–13 Kw. = 1.192 Jones ἐκρίθη περὶ ἑπτακαιδεκάτην. 698.5 Li. = 208.3–4 Kw. = 196 Jones ἐκρίθη τελέως ἄπυρος ὀγδοηκοστῇ. 716.14 Li. = 214.15–16 Kw. = 210 Jones ἐκρίθη τελέως ἑνδεκάτῃ. *Epid. III* 3.48.20 Li. = 1.220.5 Kw. = 1.228 Jones τελέως ἐκρίθη εἰκοστῇ. 130.1 Li. = 240.8 Kw. = 272 Jones ἐν ἑκατοστῇ εἰκοστῇ τελέως ἐκρίθη.

fundamental discussion among these authors and their colleagues must have been unnecessary. A *krísis* was probably something that had to be experienced by the physician during his medical apprenticeship through immediate 'clinical' (i. e. bedside) observation and could not be learned from books. Hence the situation that there is nowhere in the Hippocratic Collection a full general description of a *krísis*.

In 3 of the 17 cases of survival, the final *krísis* is described but proceeds in a rather complicated way. Accordingly, these cases deserve to be studied further below.[22] The remaining 9 case descriptions of final *krísis* with favourable event exhibit the following features: *Epidemics I*, case 6: "On the 80th day, there was a shivering fit, and he was seized with acute fever. He perspired abundantly. The urine had a red, smooth sediment. Complete *krísis*."[23] Case 13: "Around the 14th day, she vomited moderate amounts of bilious, yellow matters. She perspired. No fever. It was the *krísis*."[24] *Epidemics III*, 1st series, case 3: "On the 40th day, there were moderate amounts of phlegmatic, white faeces. He perspired abundantly all over. Complete *krísis*."[25] *Epidemics III*, 2nd series, case 6: "On the 4th day, around noon, he perspired abundantly with warm sweat all over. No fever. *krísis*, and no relapse."[26] Case 7: "On the 27th day, she perspired abundantly. No fever, the deafness ceased, the pain in the feet remained; but as to the rest the *krísis* was complete."[27] Case 8: "On the 34th day, he perspired all over, no fever, complete *krísis*."[28] Case 10: "On the 24th day, he discharged much white urine with much sediment. He perspired abundantly with warm sweat all over. No fever. *krísis*."[29] Case 11: "On the 3rd day ... ; towards the night of this day, she perspired abundantly with warm sweat all over. No fever, she slept, understood everything, *krísis* ... Around

---

[22] *Epid. I* 2.700.11–702.8 Li. = 1.209.4–15 Kw. = 1.198–200 Jones; 704.15–708.5 Li. = 210.15–211.14 Kw. = 202–204 Jones; *Epid. III* 3.24.3–28.6 Li. = 1.215.2–13 Kw. = 218 Jones. Cf. below p. 93, notes 65 f.; 111, note 127.

[23] *Epid. I* 2.700.8–10 Li. = 1.209.1–3 Kw. = 1.198 Jones ὀγδοηκοστῇ ἐρρίγωσε, πυρετὸς ὀξὺς ἔλαβεν· ἵδρωσεν πολλῷ· οὔροισιν ὑπόστασις ἐρυθρή, λείη. τελέως ἐκρίθη.

[24] *Epid. I* 2.716.2–3 Li. = 1.214.4–5 Kw. = 1.210 Jones περὶ δὲ τεσσαρεσκαιδεκάτην ἤμεσε χολώδεα ξανθὰ ὑπόσυχνα, ἵδρωσεν· ἄπυρος· ἐκρίθη. The adjective ἄπυρος has throughout to be understood as: "the fever *ceased.*"

[25] *Epid. III* 3.44.6–7 Li. = 1.218.20–22 Kw. = 1.226 Jones τεσσαρακοστῇ διεχώρησε φλεγματώδεα, λευκά, ὑπόσυχνα, ἵδρωσε πολλῷ δι' ὅλου, τελέως ἐκρίθη.

[26] *Epid. III* 3.120.10–11 Li. = 1.237.14–16 Kw. = 1.266–268 Jones τετάρτῃ περὶ μέσον ἡμέρης ἵδρωσε πολλῷ θερμῷ δι' ὅλου, ἄπυρος, ἐκρίθη, οὐθ' ὑπέστρεψεν.

[27] *Epid. III* 3.122.16–18 Li. = 1.238.6–8 Kw. = 1.268 Jones εἰκοστῇ ἑβδόμῃ ἵδρωσε πολλῷ, ἄπυρος, ἡ κώφωσις ἐξέλιπεν, ἡ τῶν ποδῶν ὑπέμενεν ὀδύνη, τὰ δ' ἄλλα τελέως ἐκρίθη.

[28] *Epid. III* 3.126.5–6 Li. = 1.239.4–5 Kw. = 1.270 Jones τριηκοστῇ τετάρτῃ ἵδρωσε δι' ὅλου, ἄπυρος, ἐκρίθη πάντα.

[29] *Epid. III* 3.132.9–10 Li. = 1.241.1–3 Kw. = 1.274 Jones εἰκοστῇ τετάρτῃ οὔρησε πολὺ λευκὸν πολλὴν ὑπόστασιν ἔχον· ἵδρωσε πολλῷ θερμῷ δι' ὅλου, ἄπυρος, ἐκρίθη.

the *krísis* she discharged much menstrual blood."[30] Case 12: "On the 6th day, she had a violent, abundant nose-bleeding. She shivered, and then perspired abundantly with warm sweat all over. No fever. *krísis*."[31]

In 7 out of these 9 historical cases of final *krísis* it is stated that the patient was without fever, in 2 rigor is mentioned.[32] With regard to the 'segregations,' in all 9 cases perspiration is an element of the *krísis*. Other forms of *apóstasis* are: sediment in the urine (2 cases),[33] faeces containing phlegm (1 case), vomit containing bile (1 case),[34] outflow of blood through nose-bleeding (1 case) or menstruation (1 case).

At the *krísis* there occurred also other kinds of *apóstasis* according to other books of the *Epidemics*. Urine with other qualities is mentioned in *VI* 2.19: "Such semen-like [urine] brings the *krísis*, and the excretions of urine help in such affections of the lower abdomen."[35] Faeces different from the ones described above are referred to in another individual case description which contains general reflections, *IV* 45: "In the beginning he had slightly viscous faeces; of this type the thick one brings the *krísis*. After that, suffering from insomnia, he had slightly viscous, slightly bilious, cooked faeces. When faeces which are bilious and not thin really begin to get more solid, the crises (*krísis*) are quick."[36] In addition, the following forms of *apóstasis* are reported to occur, or have occurred, in the *krísis*: cough (*VI* 7.1, in a general description of an epidemic);[37] pus (*VI* 3.4);[38]

---

[30] *Epid. III* 3.134.9–15 Li. = 1.241.12–19 Kw. = 1.276 Jones τρίτῃ ...· ἐς νύκτα δὲ ταύτην ἵδρωσε πολλῷ θερμῷ δι' ὅλου· ἄπυρος, ὕπνωσε, πάντα κατενόει, ἐκρίθη ... περὶ δὲ κρίσιν γυναικεῖα πολλὰ κατέβη.

[31] *Epid. III* 3.136.8–9 Li. = 1.242.1–3 Kw. = 1.278 Jones ἕκτῃ διὰ ῥινῶν λάβρον ἐρρύη πολύ· φρίξασα ἵδρωσε πολλῷ θερμῷ δι' ὅλου· ἄπυρος· ἐκρίθη.

[32] ἐρρίγωσε and φρίξασα respectively; the verb φρίσσω seems to denote a less intensive kind of rigor, cf. above p. 84, note 20.

[33] Cf. *Epid. IV* 5.146.20 Li. = Per. 84 La. οὔροισιν ἡ κάθαρσις καὶ ἡ κρίσις. (In a summary historical description.)

[34] Cf. *Epid. IV* 5.188.10 Li. = Per. 270 La. τὰ κρίνοντα, οἷα τὰ ἐμεύμενα, "the critical signs, e. g. vomit."

[35] *Epid. VI* 5.286.10 Li. = Per. 313 La. τὸ γονοειδὲς τὸ τοιοῦτον ὅτι κρίσιμον, καὶ τῶν ἤτρων τὰ τοιαῦτα ὅτι αἱ οὐρήσιες ῥύονται.

[36] *Epid. IV* 5.186.12–14 Li. = Per. 262–263 La. ἐν ἀρχῇσιν ὑπόγλισχρα ὑποχωρήματα, ἐξ οἵων τὸ παχὺ κρίσιμον. ἀγρύπνῳ μετὰ ταῦτα ὑπόγλισχρα ὑπόχολα πέπονα. χολώδεα μὴ λεπτὰ ἐπὴν δὴ ἄρξηται συνίστασθαι, ταχεῖαι αἱ κρίσιες. The punctuation as adopted in Langholf, Syntaktische Untersuchungen p. 164 (cf. 165) makes no good sense, because ὑπόχολα ... χολώδεα is contradictory there.

[37] *Epid. VI* 5.334.3–6 οἷσι φωναὶ ἀπερρήγνυντο ἐς τὸ βηχῶδες, τούτων οἱ πλεῖστοι οὐδὲν (οὐδὲν Manetti/Roselli: 'überhaupt nicht' Gal.: οὐδὲ MV) ἐπυρέτηναν, οἱ δέ τινες βραχέα· ἀτὰρ οὐδὲ περιπλευμονικὰ ἐγίνετο τούτων οὐδενὶ οὐδὲ παραπληγικὰ οὐδὲ ἄλλο οὐδὲν ἐπεσημάνθη (ἐπεσ- Pall.: ἐσ- MV), ἀλλ' ἐν τῇ φωνῇ ἐκρίνετο.

[38] *Epid. VI* 5.294.5–6 πᾶν τὸ ἐκπυέον ἀνυπόστροφον· οὗτος γὰρ πεπασμός, καὶ κρίσις ἅμα καὶ ἀπόστασις.

ulcers and swellings (*II* 1.11 ≈ *VI* 3.21);[39] segregation into the legs or feet (*IV* 27 in an individual case description).[40]

A passage particularly valuable for the reconstruction of what a *krísis* was thought to be is found in *I*, ch. 9 Li. (= ch. 19 Kw., Jones), a comprehensive account about groups of patients in a particular year: "In this situation [of the weather and the prevailing diseases], they [the patients] usually recovered under four disease signs: if there was either good nose-bleeding or if they excreted through the bladder much urine with much good sediment or through the bowels faeces well mixed with bile, or if they were seized with *dysenteríē*. Many [patients] had their *krísis* not under only one of the signs mentioned, but most went through all of them. Their condition seemed to be worse, but in fact all to whom this occurred recovered."[41] The passage evinces that although theoretically a *krísis* was thought to be possible with only one of the four symptoms, in reality this was the exception.

Perspiration is mentioned as an element of the *krísis* in a number of passages in the *Epidemics*. But there are likewise reports about cases of *krísis* without sweat; hence, perspiration was not an indispensable element: *IV* 2 "He had the *krísis* around the 9th day without sweat."[42] *II* 3.1 "Usually there was a complete *krísis* around the 14th day, in some cases with perspiration, in some with rigor ... In some cases around that season the *krísis* was with perspiration."[43]

Nowhere in the *Epidemics* or in other treatises of the Hippocratic Collection is there an exhaustive enumeration of the various kinds of *apóstasis* that may be present particularly at the *krísis*. The information is provided rather incidentally — a few casual remarks in case histories and in general statements, and some random notes. But when examining those passages in which *apóstasis* is explicitly connected with *krísis*, one comes

---

39 *Epid. II* 5.82.14–15 τὰ γενόμενα ἕλκεα {καὶ} κρίνοντα πυρετοὺς καὶ φύματα· οἷσι ταῦτα μὴ παραγίνεται, ἀκρισίη. ≈ *Epid. VI* 5.302.9–10 τὰ γινόμενα ἕλκεα καὶ (καὶ MV: om. Gal., Pall.) φύματα κρίνοντα πυρετούς· οἷσι ταῦτα μὴ παραγίνεται, ἀκρισίη.

40 *Epid. IV* 5.172.3–4 Li. = Per. 200 La. κοπιώδης ἐξ ἔργων. εἰκοσταῖος, ἐς πόδας, καὶ κρίσις. ἦρα τοῖσι κοπιώδεσιν ἐς ἄρθρα καὶ οὐκ ἐς ὀφθαλμόν;

41 *Epid. I* 2.656.7–658.6 Li. = 1.195.21–196.6 Kw. = 1.174 Jones ἐν δὲ ταύτῃ τῇ καταστάσει ἐπὶ σημείων μάλιστα τεσσάρων διεσῴζοντο· οἷσι γὰρ ἢ διὰ ῥινῶν καλῶς αἱμορραγῆσαι ἢ κατὰ κύστιν οὖρα πολλὰ καὶ πολλὴν καὶ καλὴν ὑπόστασιν ἔχοντα ἔλθοι ἢ κατὰ κοιλίην ταραχώδεα χολώδεσιν ἐπικαίρως, ἢ δυσεντερικοὶ γενοίατο. πολλοῖσι δὲ συνέπιπτε μὴ ἐφ' ἑνὸς κρίνεσθαι τῶν ὑπογεγραμμένων σημείων, ἀλλὰ διεξιέναι διὰ πάντων τοῖσι πλείστοισι καὶ δοκεῖν μὲν ἔχειν ὀχληροτέρως· διεσῴζοντο δὲ πάντες, οἷσι ταῦτα συμπίπτοι.

42 *Epid. IV* 5.144.15–16 Li. = Per. 72 La. κρίσις περὶ ἐνάτην ἄνευ ἱδρῶτος.

43 *Epid. II* 5.100.17–102.1 ἐκρίνετο πάντα τὰ πολλὰ περὶ τεσσαρεσκαίδεκα, ὀλίγα σὺν ἱδρῶτι, ὀλίγα σὺν ῥίγει ... καί τισιν (τισιν I ante corr., Li.: τοῖσιν I post corr., VHR, Gal.) ὑπὸ τοῦτον τὸν χρόνον καὶ ἐκρίθη ξὺν ἱδρῶτι.

to infer that any kind of *apóstasis* could occur at the *krísis*, i. e. could be an integral part of the *krísis*. There is admittedly no stringent proof for this assumption, but there are good reasons for it: First, the forms of *apóstasis* mentioned as occurring during the *krísis* coincide to a large extent with the 'categories' of *apóstasis* listed in *Epidemics II* 1.7 (cf. above p. 80 f.). In the majority of these 'categories,' examples are explicitly attested as being part of the *krísis*. Second, since certain mild forms of *apóstasis* like urine (with sediment), nose-bleeding, and discharge of menstrual blood were regarded as being constitutive elements of a *krísis*, this should be all the more the case with the stronger and more dramatic forms. Third, if one does not confine one's analysis of *apóstasis* to the case descriptions of final *krísis*, but includes also the many cases in which the *krísis* was incomplete (initiating a relapse), one finds considerably more examples of 'critical segregations' which cover almost all of the theoretical possibilities.[44]

It has been said above that any kind of *apóstasis* could be an integral part of the *krísis*. This must be formulated more precisely now. In the passage from *Epidemics II* 1.7 quoted above (p. 80 f.) it was stated that an *apóstasis* has to be "not inadequate to the size of the disease; for example, with the niece of Timenes, there occurred a segregation into a finger which was unable to receive the disease; it flowed back [into the body], and she died."

Another necessary qualification of a successful *apóstasis* is the state of 'coction' or 'ripeness' of the matters segregated. The contrary state is 'rawness.' In Greek, 'raw' (*ōmós*, and accordingly *ōmótēs*, 'rawness') has a double meaning, 'uncooked' as well as 'unripe.'[45] The ripening of fruits and vegetables was popularly considered a cooking process – namely, cooking in the sun. Several decades after the earlier books of the *Epidemics* were written, Aristotle, starting from such popular concepts inherent in the Greek language, established an elaborate system of the various kinds of 'cooking,' 'boiling,' 'ripening,' etc.[46] No such system is presented explicitly in the Hippocratic Corpus, but obviously the ideas underlying the Hippocratic doctrine of 'cooking' or 'ripening' were quite similar. The verb used in the Corpus is *péssō* which means 'to cook,' 'to boil,' and also 'to ripen,' 'to digest.' The substantive denoting the action or process is *pépsis*, 'cooking,' 'ripening,' 'digestion;' the substantive denoting the result is *pepasmós*, 'cookedness,' 'ripeness.' The corresponding adjectives are *pépōn* or *pépeiros*, 'cooked,' 'ripe.' These words all stand in a close etymological

[44] A list of incomplete crises in *Epid. I* and *III* will be given below p. 113 f.; cf. p. 110 f. and the general remarks p. 92 f.

[45] So has the German 'roh.'

[46] Arist., *Meteor. IV*, ch. 2–3, 379 b 10–381 b 22; cf. Düring, Aristoteles 383 f.

relationship which was still felt in the fifth and fourth centuries B.C.; such words as *péssō* and *pépsis* were normally used to signify cooking food in the household.

According to Aristotle, "human activity imitates nature insofar as the 'cooking' (*pépsis*) of the food inside the body is similar to cooking food on a fire (*hépsēsis*) because it happens ... through the warmth of the body." Less explicitly, the Hippocratic Collection expresses the idea that the 'cooking' of food and other matters in the human body is a function of the body heat,[47] of the 'inborn warmth' (*émphyton thermón*)[48] which, although this expression is used only rarely, is one of the most important physiological principles in the Hippocratic Corpus.[49] Just as unripe fruits or uncooked foodstuffs are harmful to the body[50] and are more easily 'cooked' within the body when they are 'ripe' or have been 'cooked' on fire, the pathogenic substance(s) or any harmful matter(s) within the body can, analogically, be more easily overcome when they are 'ripe' or 'cooked.' In fact, overcoming the harmful substance(s) to be excreted in an *apóstasis* means to 'cook' them to 'ripeness' within the body. The 'riper' the substances are, the better for a patient. As digesting the food was considered not only a 'cooking' process, but also a process of 'overcoming' the food, the harmful substance had to be 'overcome' by the body. The Greek verb for 'overcome' is *krateín* or *epikrateín*, a word borrowed from the sphere of social or political relations.[51] There are a number of passages in the Hippocratic Collection where the two verbs have almost the meaning of 'to digest.'[52] The same concept underlies *Epidemics VI* 5.15: "Some foods are overcome quickly, others slowly."[53] In the process of digestion,

---

[47] *Ibid.* 381 b 6–9; *Salubr.* 6.82.15–21 Li. = *Nat. Hom.* 216.12–17 Jouanna = *Salubr.* 4.54 Jones; *Vict. III* 6.616.20–21 Li. = 206.32–33 Joly = 4.396 Jones.

[48] *Aph. I* 14–15 (4.466.8, 15 Li. = 4.104–106 Jones); *Morb. I* 11 (6.158.18–19 Li. = 28.4–5 Wittern [M: om. θ]); *Cord.* 6 (9.84.9); cf. Joly (ed.), Hippocrate, Du régime, p. 280, on *Vict. II* 62 (6.576.15 Li. = 184.23 Joly = 4.350 Jones).

[49] Cf., e.g., *Epid. I* 2.638.5 Li. = 1.190.18–19 Kw. = 1.164 Jones πρεσβυτέροισι δὲ καὶ ὅσοις ἤδη τὸ θερμὸν κρατεῖται. *Epid. VI* 5.296.3–4, 310.6–7, 312.5, 312.14–314.2. More explicit in other treatises, e.g. *Nat. Hom.* (*passim*).

[50] Of the 5 occurrences of the word ὠμός in *Vict. II*, e.g., 3 are for 'unboiled' (6.556.20 Li. = 174.16 Joly = 4.328 Jones; 564.14 Li. = 178.11 Joly = 336 Jones; 566.11 Li. = 178.23 Joly = 338 Jones), while 2 are for 'unripe' (6.562.12 Li. = 176.25 Joly = 4.334 Jones; 564.1 Li. = 178.1 Joly = 334 Jones): this clearly illustrates that the two processes were considered the same.

[51] For other expressions taken from this sphere, see below p. 96, where recent literature is quoted, and p. 127.

[52] *VM* 1.578.4–7 Li. = 1.4.25–5.5 Kw. = 1.18 Jones; 580.4 Li. = 5.17 Kw. = 20 Jones; 582.2, 6 Li. = 6.15, 19 Kw. = 22 Jones; 584.12–16 Li. = 7.23–8.3 Kw. = 24 Jones; 594.9 Li. = 12.8 Kw. = 30 Jones; *Salubr.* 6.82.21 Li. = *Nat. Hom.* 216.17 Jouanna = *Salubr.* 4.54 Jones.

[53] *Epid. VI* 5.322.5 βρώματα τὰ μὲν ταχέως κρατεῖται, τὰ δὲ βραδέως (βραδέως Gal., Pall.: ἐναντίως MV).

either the body overcomes the food, or the food overcomes the body, as for example the author of *On Ancient Medicine* implies in ch. 14: "They [the early physicians who invented medical diet] thought that nutriment which is stronger than the human nature and cannot be overcome by it, is harmful, and they tried to eliminate it."[54] Equally, either the body overcomes the disease (i. e. the harmful matter), or the disease (the harmful matter) overcomes the body, *On Regimen in Acute Diseases, Appendix*, ch. 3 Li. (= ch. 5 Kw.): "If the body becomes weak, the disease overcomes it; and if the disease has overcome the body, it becomes incurable."[55] This concept appears also in *Epidemics I*, ch. 4 Li. (= ch. 9 Kw., Jones): "Some got [an *apóstasis*] ... into the hip-joint; with a few it ceased in a *krísis* and was overcome quickly, and they regained their previous shape."[56] Hence, body and disease (or, more precisely, body and harmful matter), just as body and food, are in a teleological relationship of strife and struggle, based on the principles of defeat and victory. The author of *On Regimen IV*, ch. 88 even contends that, if in contrast to one's daily activities one dreams of "fight or conflicts, this means tumult in the body."[57] The aphoristic formulation of *Epidemics I* quoted earlier (p. 1) expresses the same situation: "The art (*tékhnē*) [of medicine] has three [aspects]: the disease, the patient, and the physician ... Together with the physician, the patient must fight the disease." 'Cooking' or 'ripening' or 'digesting' (the English translation does not matter very much because the three words are the same or largely overlap semantically in the Greek texts) is an important principle in this action.

Two obscure passages of the *Epidemics* can now be simply explained and, in turn, elucidate a passage in *On Regimen in Acute Diseases*, ch. 13 (end) Li. (= ch. 49 Kw., Jones), where the following is stated as a general

---

[54] *VM* 1.602.4–6 Li. = 1.15.20–22 Kw. = 1.36–38 Jones τὸ κρέσσον τῆς φύσιος τῆς ἀνθρωπείης, οὗ μὴ ἠδύνατο κρατεῖν, τοῦτο βλάπτειν ἡγήσαντο, καὶ τοῦτο ἐζήτησαν ἀφαιρεῖν.

[55] *Acut. (Sp.)* 2.402.7–9 Li. = 1.148.19–22 Kw. = 70.13–15 Joly ἀσθενέος δὲ τοῦ σώματος γινομένου τὸ νόσημα ἐπικρατεῖ· ὅταν δὲ τὸ νόσημα ἐπικρατήσῃ τοῦ σώματος, τὸ τοιόνδε ἀνιήτως ἔχει. For the body overcoming the disease, see the same treatise 508.3 Li. = 174.6 Kw.

[56] *Epid. I* 2.628.14–630.3 Li. = 1.188.20–22 Kw. = 1.162 Jones ἔστι δ' οἷς ... κατὰ ἰσχίον, ὀλίγοισι κρισίμως ἀπολείποντα καὶ ταχὺ πάλιν ἐπικρατεύμενα ἐπὶ τὴν ἐξ ἀρχῆς ἕξιν. The form ἐπικρατεύμενα, which is attested by the codices AV, is a simple passive; Littré's ἐπικρατευόμενα is a mistake of some *recentiores*.

[57] *Vict. IV* 6.642.17–19 Li. = 220.5–7 Joly = 4.424 Jones (with Heidel's νείκη or νείκεα instead of the transmitted νίκη). — The first chapter of *On the Nature of Man* (*Nat. Hom.* 6.32.2–34.7 Li. = 164.3–166.11 Jouanna = 4.2–4 Jones) illustrates that the social relations among fifth and fourth century Greek philosophizing physicians often had the same typical agonistic character. See also below p. 243 on professional competition in medical prognosis.

truth: "Excessive insomnia has the effect that drink and food are incompletely digested; and excessive change to the other extreme [i. e. excessive sleep] makes the body languid and causes it to suffer from being cooked, and from headache."[58] This 'truth' is a direct consequence of a doctrine contained in *Epidemics VI* 4.12: "Evidently, when one is awake, one is warmer outside and colder inside; asleep, the opposite."[59] When the body is too cold inside, it cannot 'cook' the food which then remains undigested; and when the body is too hot inside, it is 'cooked' itself. When a fever is too strong, not only the harmful matter but the whole body is 'cooked.' In *Epidemics IV* 16 it is reported that certain fever patients were without appetite and seized with nausea and stomach-ache, and that they were 'cooked.'[60]

Coction of the harmful matter is not an *apóstasis* in itself. The term *apóstasis* always implies a *segregation* (evacuation) of that matter, either through excretion (excrement or other) or through isolation, e. g. in the form of an abscess (Latin *abscessus* is the literal translation of *apóstasis*) or of pain in the joints (e. g. of the hip), or of a rash (*exánthēma*). Of course, isolation can be followed by excretion. It is obvious that not every *apóstasis* is indicative of the 'cookedness' of the harmful matter excreted or isolated in the *apóstasis*. A rash or articular pain can be a good *apóstasis*, but whereas it makes perfect sense to the Hippocratic to speak of 'raw faeces' or 'ripe sputum,' it would be meaningless to call a rash or pain 'cooked' or 'ripe.' Similarly blood, whose outflow can be an excellent *apóstasis*, is never called 'ripe' or 'raw.'

Thus, we grasp the theoretical background of the statement in *Epidemics I*, ch. 5 Li. (= ch. 11 Kw., Jones) already quoted above (p. 79): "You should direct your attention to timely coctions of all substances excreted through all ways of excretion, or to good and critical segregations." The two parts of this sentence divided by 'or' are not mutually

---

58 *Acut.* 2.330.6–332.2 Li. = 1.134.4–6 Kw. = 2.104 Jones ἀγρυπνίη ἰσχυρὴ πόμα καὶ σιτίον ἀπεπτότερα ποιεῖ, καὶ ἡ ἐπὶ θάτερα αὖ μεταβολὴ λύει τὸ σῶμα καὶ ἑφθότητα καὶ καρηβαρίην ἐμποιεῖ. A consequence seems to be that abundant sleep helps to concoct the food particularly well and can, therefore, compensate for malnutrition; this is possibly implied in the fragment from the middle Attic comedy *Ganymedes* by Eubulus (17 Kock, Edmonds), ὕπνος αὐτὸν ὄντα κακόσιτον τρέφει. One might ask whether the fragment describes the habits of somebody (of the cup-bearer himself?) who lives on wine rather than solid food and, therefore, sleeps a lot.

59 *Epid. VI* 5.310.6–7 ἐμφανέως ἐγρηγορὼς θερμότερος τὰ ἔξω, τὰ ἔσω δὲ ψυχρότερος· καθεύδων τἀναντία. The reason may be implied in 320.6–7 τὸ αἷμα ἐν ὕπνῳ ἔσω μᾶλλον φεύγει. For the history of these doctrines, cf. the commentary by Manetti/Roselli; for the doctrinal context, see Cesare Marelli, Place de la Collection hippocratique dans les théories biologiques sur le sommeil, in: Formes de pensée 331–339, especially 335.

60 *Epid. IV* 5.154.9–13 Li. = Per. 119 La. βραχύτεροι οἱ πυρετοὶ ... καὶ ἀπόσιτοι καὶ ἑφθοὶ καὶ ἀσώδεες καὶ καρδιαλγέες.

exclusive alternatives, but complement each other, covering all possible forms of *apóstasis*.

Not every accumulation of liquids in the body or even in peripheral, 'isolated' parts of it is an *apóstasis*, as evinced by *Epidemics V*, ch. 48: A young man having run on rough ground felt pain at the heel, particularly at its lowest part, which, however, "did not receive any *apóstasis* while accumulating liquid." The liquid attracted by the hurt heel was no *apóstasis*, and the patient died from gangrene.[61]

Bodily excretions and harmful matters are 'cooked' or 'ripe' at the *krísis* as stated in *Epidemics I*, ch. 3, "The urine of most people ... was cooked after some time, around the *krísis*."[62] The passage quoted from *Epidemics I*, ch. 5 Li. (= ch. 11 Kw., Jones) goes on: "Coctions indicate quickness of the *krísis*, safety, and health." *Only* coction indicates that there will be a *krísis* with favourable results on one of the 'critical days' in the near future. The same text continues: "Substances raw and uncooked and turning into bad segregations indicate an absence of the *krísis* or [indicate] pain or delay or death or a return of the same," i. e. a relapse. Another text in *Epidemics I* (ch. 10 Li. = ch. 23 Kw., Jones) mentions more concisely the two alternative possibilities (unfavourable versus favourable outcome): "Segregations which turn towards the bad and towards the critical."[63]

On the preceding pages, only cases of complete *krísis*, or *krísis* generally, have been dealt with. Incomplete coction or incomplete segregation result in an incomplete or even a missed *krísis* (with the risk of a relapse) or at least in a continuation of symptoms after the *krísis*. A particularly instructive report is *Epidemics III*, 1st series, case 5: "Khairion ... caught a fever ... On the 7th day there was rigor, acute fever, he perspired all

---

[61] *Epid. V* 5.236.1–3 ἤλγεε τὴν πτέρνην, μάλιστα τὸ κάτω μέρος, ἀπόστασιν δὲ ὁ τόπος οὐκ ἐλάμβανεν οὐδεμίην ὡς ξυνάγων ὑγρόν (ξυνάγων (-ον M) ὑγρόν MV: στενυγρὸς ὢν coniecit Li.). To Littré, the text as transmitted did not make sense (see his note 1); it is, however, perfectly understandable. The participial construction ὡς ξυνάγων ὑγρόν is either causal ("because") or temporal ("while," cf. Langholf, Syntaktische Untersuchungen p. 94–95, where *Epid. VII* 5.380.20–21 ὡς ἀφοδεύων is quoted). For συνάγω 'accumulate (or collect) liquid' cf. *Aff.* 6.244.24–246.1 πεπαίνει δὲ (sc. τὰ καταπλάσματα) ὅσα θερμαίνοντα ξυνάγει. *Medic.* 9.214.3 Li. = 22.34–35 Heiberg τῷ ξυναγομένῳ κάτωθεν ἰχῶρι. *Epid. VII* 5.400.4 κατὰ τὴν καρδίην ἔφη (sc. a female patient) δοκεῖν τι ξυνάγεσθαι ἑωυτῇ. συνάγω in this sense also *Oss.* 9.186.24; 188.1; 192.11; 196.10. Sometimes the verb is used in contrast to διαχέω ('dissipate liquid'): *Aff.* 6.246.1, 14.

[62] *Epid. I* 2.610.7–9 Li. = 1.183.2–4 Kw. = 1.150 Jones οὖρά τε τοῖσι πλείστοισιν ... μετὰ χρόνον περὶ κρίσιν πεπαινόμενα.

[63] *Epid. I* 2.670.11–12 Li. = 1.199.20–21 Kw. = 1.180 Jones ἀποστάσιες ἐπὶ τὸ ὀλέθριον καὶ κρίσιμον. Here and in a number of other passages, 'critical' (*krísimos*) and *krísis* have a 'positive' meaning (opposite of 'death,' 'bad condition,' 'relapse' or the like), namely 'final *krísis* towards recovery.' This is a semantic evolution out of the original, neutral meaning 'judgement,' 'decision.'

over, *krísis*." Then it is explained that the patient continued to discharge bad urine, which improved only on the 8th day, and stool which was bad until the end of his disease. He relapsed on the 9th day. "On the 17th day, there was rigor, acute fever, he perspired, no fever, *krísis*." The urine was good after this, but the stool, as had been mentioned before, continued to be bad. On the 18th day he was a little feverish again and exhibited some other symptoms. On the 19th day, the fever was away, the urine was good, but he had a sore throat. "Complete *krísis* on the 20th day."[64] A continuation of symptoms after the final *krísis* is observed in *Epidemics I*, case 7: "On the 5th day there was ample nosebleeding on the left side with unmixed [i. e. unfavourable] blood, he perspired, *krísis*. After the *krísis* sleepless, wandering in his talk, thin and slightly black [i. e. bad] urine ..." After a bath, "he slept and regained his reason. He did not relapse but had frequent nosebleeds after the *krísis*."[65] Similar are case 10,[66] and *Epidemics III*, 1st series, case 1.[67] Further examples of incomplete crises in *Epidemics I* and *III* will be presented below.[68]

Days of a *krísis* in Treatises Other than the *Epidemics*

The other constitutive feature which, together with fever (sometimes also rigor) and *apóstasis*, makes up a *krísis*, is the time component. As has been said already (p. 82), a *krísis* occurs exclusively on certain days of the disease; happenings outside these days are never 'critical.' There are various schemes of sequences of critical days contained in the Hippocratic Collection. In order to reconstruct the specific doctrine of the *Epidemics*, it will be necessary first to study related beliefs in other treatises. This will help to clarify the very inexplicit doctrinal statements of the *Epidemics*.

If one leaves aside what is taught about the critical days characteristic of particular diseases, or about critical symptoms characteristic of particular critical days and thus considers only those doctrines which apply generally to the development of all diseases, one still finds a surprising variety of

---

64 *Epid. III* 3.46.10–48.21 Li. = 1.219.8–220.5 Kw. = 1.226–228 Jones Χαιρίωνα ... πῦρ ἔλαβεν ... ἑβδόμῃ ἐπερρίγωσε, πυρετὸς ὀξύς, ἵδρωσε δι' ὅλου, ἐκρίθη ... ἑπτακαιδεκάτῃ ἐπερρίγωσε, πυρετὸς ὀξύς, ἵδρωσεν, ἄπυρος, ἐκρίθη ... τελέως ἐκρίθη εἰκοστῇ (εἰκ. AR, Gal.: om. V).

65 *Epid. I* 2.700.11–702.8 Li. = 1.209.4–15 Kw. = 1.198–200 Jones πέμπτῃ ἐρρύη λάβρον ἐξ ἀριστεροῦ ἄκρητον, ἵδρωσεν, ἐκρίθη. μετὰ κρίσιν ἄγρυπνος, παρέλεγεν, οὖρα λεπτὰ ὑπομέλανα ... ἐκοιμήθη, κατενόει. τούτῳ οὐχ ὑπέστρεψεν, ἀλλ' ᾑμορράγει πολλάκις μετὰ κρίσιν.

66 *Epid. I* 2.704.15–708.5 Li. = 1.210.15–211.14 Kw. = 1.202–204 Jones.

67 See below p. 111.

68 p. 110 f. and 113 f.

numerical schemes presented in the various Hippocratic treatises. These are the principal examples (quoted without any regard to their mutual chronological relationship, which is problematic[69]):

A simple system is contained in *On Regimen in Acute Diseases*, ch. 4 Li. (= ch. 13 Kw., Jones). Although it is preoccupied with diet, it still allows some insight into the underlying numerical *krísis* theory, which, however, is perhaps referred to only incompletely by the author: "The more the patients discharge, the more [food] you must give them until the *krísis*, and particularly until 2 days after the *krísis* is overdue; at least to those whose *krísis* seems to be on the 5th or 7th or 9th day, in order to allow for the even and the odd."[70] (The problem of the even and the odd will be discussed shortly below, p. 102–123).

In *Koan Prognoses* 147–148 we find: "Deep sleep without restlessness indicates a safe *krísis*. But sleep with restlessness and with pain of the body is unsafe | on the 7th or 9th or 14th day | nose-bleeding generally makes fever disappear. Of the same effect are a bilious or dysenteric looseness of the bowels and pain of the knees or hip-joints and urine ripened towards the *krísis*."[71]

In *On Critical Days*, ch. 11 there is the following system: "The fevers get to their *krísis* on the 4th, 7th, 11th, 14th, 17th, 21st day, and apart from these acute diseases, on the 30th, then on the 40th, then on the 60th day. When the fever has continued beyond these (day-)numbers, it is

---

[69] Because the problem of relative chronology of the treatises hardly admits a solution for all of the texts, it is unnecessary for the present purpose to adduce every possibly relevant example. Cf. Sudhoff, Lehre von den kritischen Tagen; Thivel, Cnide 216–236.

[70] *Acut.* 2.250.10–252.1 Li. = 1.115.7–12 Kw. = 2.72 Jones καὶ ὅσῳ ἂν πλείων ἡ κάθαρσις γίνηται, τοσῷδε χρὴ πλεῖον διδόναι ἄχρι κρίσιος· μάλιστα δὲ κρίσιος ὑπερβολῆς δύο ἡμερέων, οἷσί γε (γε MV: δὲ A) ἢ πεμπταίοισιν ἢ ἑβδομαίοισιν ἢ ἐναταίοισι δοκεῖ κρίνειν, ὡς καὶ τὸ ἄρτιον καὶ τὸ περισσὸν προμηθὲς ᾖ.

[71] *Coac.* 5.614.15–616.2 ὕπνοι βαθέες μὴ (μὴ A: οὐ IR) ταραχώδεες βέβαιαν κρίσιν σημαίνουσιν· οἱ δὲ ταραχώδεες (βέβαιαν … ταραχώδεες A: om. IR) μετ᾽ ἀλγήματος σώματος ἀβέβαιοι | ἑβδομαίοισιν ἢ ἐναταίοισιν ἢ τεσσαρεσκαιδεκαταίοισιν | ῥύσιες ἐκ ῥινῶν λύουσιν ὡς ἐπὶ τὸ πολὺ τοὺς πυρετούς, ὁμοίως δὲ καὶ κοιλίης ῥύσις χολώδης ἢ (ἢ A: καὶ IR) δυσεντεριώδης καὶ πόνος γουνάτων ἢ ἰσχίων καὶ (καὶ AR: ἢ I) οὖρον πεπανθὲν πρὸς τὴν κρίσιν. The vertical strokes printed in the text and in the translation are intended to indicate a problem of punctuation which seems unsolvable. A syntactically similar text (Heraclit. 22 B 1, cf. A 4 Diels/Kranz) is quoted by Aristot. *Rhet. III* 1407 b 11–18 ("difficult to punctuate"). In *Coac.*, full stop can be put alternatively at either place. The Greek manuscripts have it at the second place, but their testimony as to punctuation cannot be taken as authentic because punctuation was rarely used at the time when the texts were composed. Probably it does not matter at all how we decide. Both paragraphs (147 and 148) seem to form one unit describing the main symptoms present in a *krísis*. The day numbers apply equally to both halves of the statement.

becoming chronic."[72] This treatise consists mostly of excerpts taken over from other books available within the Hippocratic Collection; several of its paragraphs, however, have no extant parallel elsewhere, and the text quoted is one such instance.

The numerical system displayed here closely resembles the one of *Prognostics*, ch. 20, especially with regard to the division of the series in two sub-groups. *Prognostics* seems, however, to represent a more developed stage of the doctrine and cannot have been the source of *On Critical Days* because of obvious discrepancies. It also poses new problems: "Fevers from which people recover and fevers from which they die get to their *krísis* on the same days. The most benign fevers with the safest symptoms cease on the 4th day or earlier; but the most malign ones with the most perilous symptoms kill on the 4th day or earlier. This is the end of their first attack. The second attack extends through the 7th day, the third through the 11th, the fourth through the 14th, the fifth through the 17th, the sixth through the 20th. In the most acute diseases, these attacks end with the 20th day by addition of 4. Nothing of this, however, can be calculated exactly in whole days, because not even the year and the months are apt to be reckoned in whole days. After that, likewise by the same addition, the first *períodos* has 34 days, the second 40 days, the third 60 days. It is very difficult to prognosticate, at the beginning of these days, those diseases that are going to get to their *krísis* within a longer time, because their beginnings are very much the same. In fact, you must think about it from the first day and make your observations at every addition of a unit of 4. Then it will not escape your notice where the disease will turn."[73]

---

[72] *Dieb. Judic.* 9.306.21–25 κρίνονται δὲ οἱ πυρετοὶ τεταρταῖοι, ἑβδομαῖοι, ἑνδεκαταῖοι, τεσσαρεσκαιδεκαταῖοι, ἑπτακαιδεκαταῖοι, εἰκοστῇ καὶ πρώτῃ. ἐκ δὲ τούτων τῶν ὀξέων· τριακοσταῖοι, εἶτα τεσσαρακοσταῖοι, εἶτα ἑξηκοσταῖοι· ὅταν δὲ τούτους τοὺς ἀριθμοὺς ὑπερβάλλῃ, χρονίη ἤδη γίγνεται ἡ (ἡ IR: om. M) κατάστασις τῶν πυρετῶν.

[73] *Prog.* 2.168.6–170.9 Li. = 1.100.8–101.8 Kw. = 2.42 Jones οἱ δὲ πυρετοὶ κρίνονται ἐν τῇσιν αὐτῇσιν ἡμέρῃσι τὸν ἀριθμόν, ἐξ ὧν τε περιγίνονται οἱ ἄνθρωποι καὶ ἐξ ὧν ἀπόλλυνται. οἵ τε γὰρ εὐηθέστατοι τῶν πυρετῶν καὶ ἐπὶ σημείων ἀσφαλεστάτων βεβῶτες τεταρταῖοι παύονται ἢ πρόσθεν· οἱ δὲ (δὲ C′: τε M: τε δὲ V) κακοηθέστατοι (post κακ. add. τῶν πυρετῶν C′: om. MV) καὶ ἐπὶ σημείων δεινοτάτων γινόμενοι τεταρταῖοι κτείνουσιν ἢ πρόσθεν. ἡ μὲν οὖν πρώτη ἔφοδος αὐτῶν οὕτω τελευτᾷ· ἡ δὲ δευτέρη ἐς τὴν ἑβδόμην περιάγει (-γει C′: -γεται MV), ἡ δὲ τρίτη ἐς τὴν ἑνδεκάτην, ἡ δὲ τετάρτη ἐς τὴν τεσσαρεσκαιδεκάτην, ἡ δὲ πέμπτη ἐς τὴν ἑπτακαιδεκάτην, ἡ δὲ ἕκτη ἐς τὴν εἰκοστήν. αὗται μὲν οὖν (οὖν MV: om. C′) ἐπὶ τῶν ὀξυτάτων νοσημάτων διὰ τεσσάρων ἐς τὰς εἴκοσιν ἐκ (ἐκ MV: om. C′) προσθέσιος (-ος MV: -ας C′) τελευτῶσιν. οὐ δύναται δὲ ὅλῃσιν ἡμέρῃσιν ἀριθμεῖσθαι οὐδὲν τούτων ἀτρεκέως· οὐδὲ γὰρ ὁ ἐνιαυτός τε καὶ οἱ μῆνες ὅλῃσιν ἡμέρῃσιν πεφύκασιν ἀριθμεῖσθαι. μετὰ δὲ ταῦτα ἐν τῷ αὐτῷ τρόπῳ κατὰ τὴν αὐτὴν πρόσθεσιν ἡ μὲν (μὲν C′: om. MV) πρώτη περίοδος τεσσάρων καὶ τριήκοντα ἡμερέων, ἡ δὲ δευτέρη τεσσαράκοντα ἡμερέων, ἡ δὲ τρίτη ἑξήκοντα ἡμερέων. τούτων δὲ ἐν ἀρχῇσίν ἐστι χαλεπώτατα προγινώσκειν τὰ μέλλοντα ἐν πλείονι

The fevers are described in this text as generally assaulting the patients in distinct 'attacks,' with the 'critical days' (4, 7, 11, 14, 17, 20, etc.) being the end of each 'attack.' Nothing is said about the intensity of each 'attack.' It is conceivable that 'attack' actually means only the span of time in which a febrile disease may (or may not) execute an 'assault' on the patient. The 'attacks' are organized in larger units called *períodos* (plural: *períodoi*). While there is no problem at all in understanding what an 'attack' is, the word '*períodos*' presents considerable difficulties. Its original meaning is 'way round,' 'circuit' (e. g. of substances in the body), but it also has the temporal sense of 'period.'[74] It is unclear whether *períodos* in the text quoted has only the temporal meaning or implies a circuit of the *materia peccans* in the body. Since numerous medical expressions of the Hippocratic Collection are taken over from the sphere of social activities,[75] one might think of the harmful substance(s) as performing 'campaigns' in the body and pushing an attack from time to time, with 'desertions' or 'secessions' (this is the meaning of *apóstasis* in the social and political sphere), defeat and victory. The clearest passage containing *períodos* is *On Diseases IV*, ch. 48, which deals with the 'critical days' of wounds. Although it is a special application of a *krísis* doctrine, it is useful for the present purpose because in spite of the special circumstances of wounds it may be exemplary: "Wounds get inflamed on the 5th day; furthermore, depending on the size of the wound, according to the following series of days: the 3rd, 5th, 7th, 9th, 11th. Then, after the end of the first *períodos*, the 3rd day is the beginning of the second *períodos*, i. e. the 14th day from the 1st day. The largest wounds get inflamed on the 14th day."[76] The second *períodos* begins with the 3rd after the 11th day, i. e. with the 14th as is explicitly stated. It is not said what the end of the first *períodos* is, either the 14th day (which

---

(πλείονι C': πλείστῳ MV) χρόνῳ (post χρ. add. ἢ ἐλάσσονι C': om. MV) κρίνεσθαι, ὁμοιόταται γὰρ αἱ ἀρχαὶ αὐτῶν εἰσιν· ἀλλὰ χρὴ ἀπὸ τῆς πρώτης ἡμέρης ἐνθυμεῖσθαι καὶ καθ' ἑκάστην τετράδα προστιθεμένην σκέπτεσθαι, καὶ οὐ λήσει ὅπῃ τρέψεται.

74 'Way round' in *Vict.*, e. g. 6.494.1 Li. = 138.29 Joly = 4.256 Jones. For further attestations, see Joly's *index verborum*. — Galen's concept of *períodos* (*De morbor. tempor.* 7.411–413 K., *Adv. eos qui de typis scrips.* 7.475 ff. K.) is not helpful.

75 Cf. above p. 89; below p. 127; Lichtenthaeler, La médecine hippocratique II–V, 91–114; Kudlien, Beginn 60 (cf. 62 f.); Giuseppe Cambiano, Pathologie et analogie politique, in: Formes de pensée 441–458; Mario Vegetti, Metafora politica e immagine del corpo negli scritti ippocratici, in: Formes de pensée 459–469.

76 *Morb. IV* 7.576.26–578.4 Li. = 104.9–15 Joly ἀποφλεγμαίνει δὲ τὰ ἕλκεα πεμπταῖα, καὶ κατὰ λόγον τούτων τῶν ἡμερέων, ὡς ἂν καὶ τὰ ἕλκεα μεγέθ⟨ε⟩ος ἔχῃ, καὶ τριταῖα καὶ πεμπταῖα καὶ ἑβδομαῖα καὶ ἐναταῖα καὶ ἑνδεκαταῖα· εἶτα ἀπηρτισμένης πρώτης περιόδου, πάλιν δευτέρης ἀρχὴ ἡ (ἀρχὴ ἡ codices recent.: ἀρχῆς M) τρίτη, ἥτις ἐστὶν ἀπὸ τῆς πρώτης τεσσαρεσκαιδεκάτη· τὰ δὲ μέγιστα αὐτῶν τεσσαρεσκαιδεκαταῖα ἀποφλεγμαίνει.

would then have a double function) or an earlier day (any out of the 11th, 12th, and 13th).[77]

To return to *Prognostics*: It is said there that the number system can be arrived at by continually adding units of 4. In fact this is possible if one bears in mind a peculiarity of counting in antiquity. There were two ways, either by exclusion (our usual method), or by inclusion of the element from which one started. A prominent example of inclusive counting is the modern terminology of musical harmonics. A 'third' is only two steps above the fundamental note, a 'fourth' three steps, and so on. This nomenclature is inherited from antiquity. A medical 'fossil' of the ancient mode are adjectives denoting types of intermittent fever, the tertian and quartan fever,[78] which, in spite of their names, afflict the patient every second and third day respectively.[79]

The sequence of critical days postulated in *Prognostics* can be arrived at by *combining* the two ways of counting. The text quoted above states that after the 20th day the same counting procedure starts anew (i. e. the historian needs to reconstruct only the sequence 1 to 20, the following day numbers being cyclic repetitions of it). The tetradic sequence 1 ... 20 to be reconstructed must fulfil the condition that the days no. 4, 7, 11, 14, 17, 20 are the end-points of the single attacks of 'four' days. Hence there is only *one* possible solution:[80]

1	2	3	*4*								*11*	12	13	*14*			*17*	18	19	*20*
			4	5	6	*7*	|	8	9	10	*11*			*14*	15	16	*17*			

All but one of the six tetrads are counted by inclusion, the sole exception being the third tetrad which does not start with the end of the preceding one.

[77] Lonie, in his thorough discussion of the passage (Hippocratic treatises 318–322), makes two assumptions: that the author of *Morb. IV* "ends his first period at eleven ..., and begins again at twelve" (cf. his diagram). Lonie gives no argument for the first assumption. The second one seems to contradict his Greek text (p. 328) as transmitted by the *recentiores* and followed by the editors (see the preceding note), and to contradict even his own translation (p. 32): "The second period begins with the third day [after the end of the first period], i. e. on the fourteenth day from the first." If, however, one keeps the reading of M (which, *pace* Lonie, p. 328, clearly has τρίτη according to my photograph), one can understand it as: "Then, after the end of the first period, [the wounds get inflamed] again on the 3rd day of the second commencement, which is the 14th day from the 1st day." τρίτη would then be the usual orthographical variant for τρίτῃ (*dativus temporis*). In this case, the absence of the article before τρίτῃ would be parallel with two more cases of lacking article in the same sentence (περιόδου, ἀρχῆς).

[78] *Febris tertiana, quartana* < *tritaíos, tetartaíos pyretós.*

[79] On the two ways of counting in antiquity and for the difficulties due to their combinations, see Adolf Schmidt, Handbuch der griechischen Chronologie, Jena, 1888, 95–120.

[80] Cf. Grensemann (ed.), Hippokrates, Achtmonatskinder, p. 99 ff.

This scheme is not logical. The author of *Prognostics* was aware of that, and he explained the irregularity by adducing an analogy only too well-known to the Greeks of his time who had to live with a multitude of local calendars. Since not even the year and the months, although they are governed by celestial bodies, could be calculated in whole days, resulting in the frequent intercalations of days and months, it is all the more explicable that the time units underlying the crises are not exactly whole days either.[81]

How do the *períodoi* fit into the scheme? The wording is vague: "After that, likewise by the same addition, the first *períodos* has 34 days, the second 40 days, the third 60 days." But when do they start? Clearly the author presupposes a basic knowledge of the theory on the part of the reader. Unfortunately, the modern interpreter does not have this knowledge. For a possible solution, the question has to be divided: When does the first *períodos* start? When do the other *períodoi* start?

The first question has two possible solutions. The days 1 ... 20 are either counted outside any of the *períodoi*, and the first *períodos* starts after the 20 days; or the days 1 ... 20 are part of the first *períodos*. In either case the 34 days of the first *períodos* would be achieved with the 14th day of one of the cycles 1 ... 20, namely in the case of the first possibility with the 14th day of the third cycle; in the case of the second possibility with the 14th day of the 2nd cycle.[82]

With regard to the second question, since the first *períodos* is shorter than the second, which in turn is shorter than the third one (34 : 40 : 60), it is not quite impossible that they all start together (i. e. either with the 1st or the 21st day):

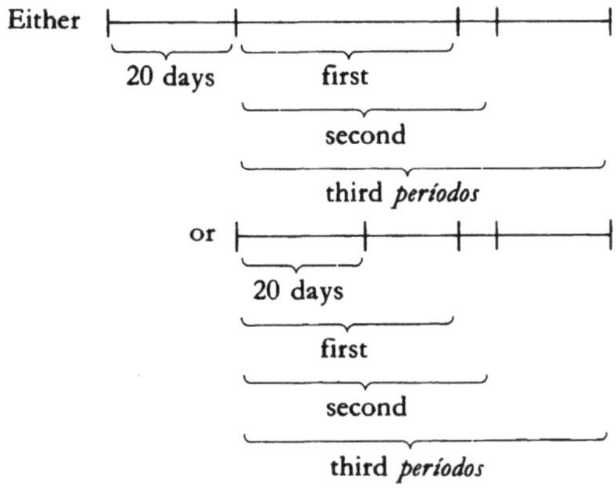

[81] For another *a fortiori* argument see below p. 171, note 202.

[82] This calculation presupposes *exclusive* addition of the cycles of 20 days.

This interpretation would accord fully with the text of *Prognostics* where *períodos* is used only with ordinal numbers. Yet it seems untenable because in other Hippocratic texts, *períodoi* (plural) are counted with cardinal numbers:[83] this clearly implies for those texts that the *períodoi* follow one upon the other. By analogy, one feels inclined to interpret *Prognostics* the same way. Again it remains uncertain when the first *períodos* begins:

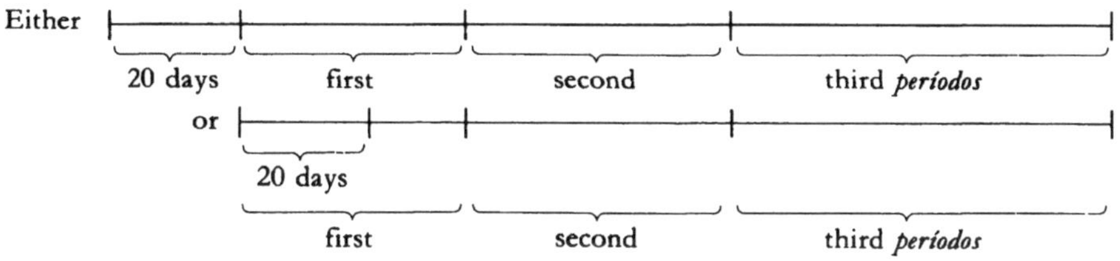

Since one does not see any reason why the first 20 days should play an extra rôle outside the *períodoi*, it seems more plausible to include them in the first *períodos*.[84]

The scheme of *Prognostics* must have been unsatisfying for some physicians because of its lack of logic. There is at least one logical system of critical days in the Collection. Grensemann, in his edition of several Hippocratic embryological texts,[85] comments extensively on a passage which he thinks has intruded into them at a later stage of the textual transmission, and which he consequently eliminates. But Joly, the subsequent editor, considers it authentic.[86] The passage in question is found in *On the Foetus in the Seventh Month* ch. 9 Li. (= *On the Foetus in the Eighth Month* ch. 1 Grensemann = ch. 9 Joly) and reads: "The same calculation [as in gynaecology, embryology, and infant development] applies also to the critical days ... If you want to restore without blunder the health of the sick, you have, in your observation, to pay attention to all odd days; and of the even ones, to the 14th, the 28th, and the 42nd, because this interval [i. e. the third made up out of the uneven numbers] and the perfect and complete number [i. e. the number 7] is applied to harmony [i. e. theory of musical harmony] by some [authors, or scholars] ... One must

[83] For references, see below p. 105.

[84] A secondary problem is the question how the counting should be continued after the 34 days of the first *períodos*: should one continue the respective cycle of 20 days until it is complete, or should one disrupt it after the 34th day, and begin a new cycle of 20 days? The answer is of no practical consequence because in any case the ends of the second and third *períodos* fall on critical days.

[85] Grensemann (ed.), Hippokrates, Achtmonatskinder, p. 99 f.

[86] Joly (ed.), Hippocrate, De la génération, p. 171–173, 179 f.

see it as a sequence of units of 3 [i. e. triads] and units of 4 [i. e. tetrads], with the triads always being conjunct, and with the tetrads being conjunct two by two and being separated two by two."[87] In the natural sequence of days, there are two distinct cycles; the critical days fall at the end of each 'third' and each 'seventh' (to use musical terminology). 'Conjunct' as used here means inclusive counting, 'separated' exclusive counting:

Triadic cycle

1	2	*3*		*5*	6	*7*		*9*	10	*11*		*13*	14	*15*	…
		3	4	*5*		*7*	8	*9*		*11*	12	*13*		*15*	

Tetradic cycle

1	2	3	4							11	12	13	*14* |	15	… *42*
			4	5	6	*7* |	8	9	10	11				

This system with the critical days occurring on all odd days and on all days numbered by 7 or its multiples is strictly logical in itself, although its premises cannot be verified by modern medicine. Obviously the analogy of musical harmony was a sufficient proof of correctness for the ancient physician.[88]

The translation given differs from those hitherto published, principally in the sentence "because ... by some," which gives the theoretical explanation of the preceding instruction. All translators agree that the argumentation is borrowed from musical theory, but it has not been recognized that, grammatically, the expressions "this interval"[89] and "the perfect and complete number"[90] are constructed parallel to each other, both together forming the 'subject' (or 'nominal phrase') of the sentence.[91] "This interval" refers, in musical terminology, to the pattern formed by the odd numbers 1, 3, 5 ... 41, 'thirds' (inclusive counting). The "perfect and complete number" is 7, itself an odd number and therefore, according to the author's system, to be respected anyhow; only the even multiples of 7 had to be mentioned as critical days: 14, 28, 42.

---

[87] *Sept*. 7.448.11–21 Li. = *Oct*. 80.3–12 Grensemann = *Oct*. 171.17–172.9 Joly ὁ δὲ αὔτὸς λόγος καὶ ἐπὶ κρισίμων. ... σκοπεῖν γὰρ χρὴ τὸν μέλλοντα {ἰητρὸν} ὀρθῶς στοχάζεσθαι τῆς τῶν καμνόντων σωτηρίας θεωροῦν⟨τα⟩ τὰς μὲν περιτ⟨τ⟩ὰς πάσας, τῶν δὲ ἀρτίων τὴν τεσσαρεσκαιδεκάτην καὶ τὴν ὀγδόην εἰκοστὴν καὶ ⟨τὴν⟩ τεσσαρακοστὴν καὶ δευτέρην. οὗτος γὰρ ὁ ὅρος τίθεται τῷ τῆς ἁρμονίης λόγῳ πρός τινων καὶ ὁ ἀρτιφυής τε καὶ τέλειος ἀριθμός. ... θεωρεῖν δὲ χρὴ οὕτως· τριάσι τε καὶ τετράσι, ταῖς μὲν τριάσι συνημμέναις (codd. recc.: συνηγμέναις M) ἁπάσαις, ταῖς δὲ τετράσι δύο μὲν παρὰ δύο συνημμέναις, δύο δὲ παρὰ δύο διεζευγμέναις (Gr.: συνεζευγμέναις M).

[88] On analogy as a heuristic tool and as an argument of proof cf. below p. 215–222.

[89] οὗτος ὁ ὅρος.

[90] ὁ ἀρτιφυής τε καὶ τέλειος ἀριθμός. For the proposed new translation of this expression, see shortly below.

[91] The sentence is in the passive voice; Joly, in his French rendering, has transformed it into the active.

There is ample evidence from Greek and Roman antiquity that 7 was a number of perfection and completion; the adjective *téleios*, "complete," as used in the text quoted is found repeatedly with 7 in contexts outside the Hippocratic Collection.[92] The other adjective paraphrased in the translation by "perfect" is *artiphyḗs*. The word has been rendered as 'even' by Littré, Joly, and Liddell/Scott/Jones, but 'even' prevents the correct interpretation and is linguistically improbable, as one would expect another word form.[93] In fact, the adjective is derived from a first element *arti-*, which in compounds means 'well fitted,'[94] and *-phyḗs*, '-natured,' the literal translation of the compound being 'with a well-fitted nature,' 'excellent,' 'perfect,' almost synonymous to 'complete.'[95] This quality is suitable for a number that plays a prominent rôle in Hippocratic systems of critical days, as the examples quoted make evident.[96]

It is impossible to determine whether the 'logical' system of the embryological text or the illogical one of *Prognostics* reflects a more original stage. Lichtenthaeler[97] contended that the author of *Prognostics*, though starting from musicology, did not feel obliged to follow it strictly. No proof is possible here. The paucity of the extant medical text material precludes a solution of this problem which would illuminate a rather important detail of the development of Greek medicine. In any case, considering the widespread use of numerical speculation in antiquity, it is not unreasonable to assume that musicology was but one out of many topics which were to exert their influence on Greek medical theories.

---

92 It is called τελεσφόρος and/or τέλειος in later sources, see Roscher, Hebdomadenlehren 116 (cf. 109 ff.). Roscher's suggestion that the texts which he quotes are derived from Poseidonios cannot be verified; the texts are accordingly omitted in Edelstein/Kidd, Posidonius, and in Theiler, Poseidonios. More attestations in Roscher, Die enneadischen ... Wochen 48, note 154; Roscher, Enneadische Studien 71.

93 *ἀρτιοφυής, which, although not attested in any Greek text, could have been formed easily according to the rules of Greek word formation.

94 For more detailed information and for literature cf. Lexikon des frühgriechischen Epos, Fasc. 8, Göttingen, 1976, s. v. ἀρτιεπής, ἀρτίπος, ἀρτίφρων. Nadia van Brock, Recherches sur le vocabulaire médical du grec ancien (Études et comm., 41), Paris, 1961, 190–192.

95 In some compounds, *arti-* has the temporal meaning that something has 'just' happened. *artiphyḗs* would then mean 'just born' (see Liddell/Scott/Jones for references), a sense which is impossible here.

96 See also below p. 103. Outside the Hippocratic Collection, the number 7 *as such* was credited with having the peculiar qualities of 'right measure,' 'right (or decisive) moment,' cf. Theophr. *De causis plant. VI* 4.2 (as part of an argumentation why there are seven odours): ὁ δὲ ἀριθμὸς ὁ τῶν ἑπτὰ καιριώτατος καὶ φυσικώτατος. (Cf. Roscher, Hebdomadenlehren 98.) The Pythagoreans called the seven καιρός, καιροφυής, κρίσις: Roscher, Die enneadischen ... Wochen 48, note 154. Roscher, Sieben- und Neunzahl 30, note 66. Roscher, Hebdomadenlehren 28–30, notes 39–44. Burkert, Lore 40, 467, 475. Cf. also Wellmann, Die Fragmente der sikelischen Ärzte p. 41 ff.

97 Lichtenthaeler, Quatrième série 133–135.

A system similar to, and in its practical result completely compatible with, those of the embryological text and of *Prognostics* is formulated in *Aphorisms II* 24. No musicological influence can be seen in it. The passage intimates the reasons why the days are critical and seems to imply that the day 4 and day 7, even if not counted from the beginning of the disease, are important for calculating a *krísis*; 3 does not play any rôle in this reasoning: "The 4th day is indicative of the 7 days.[98] The 8th is the beginning of another series of 7 days. One has to pay attention to the 11th day because it is the 4th day of the second series of 7 days. Again one has to pay attention to the 17th day because it is the 4th day reckoned from the 14th day and the 7th from the 11th."[99]

Days of a *krísis* in the *Epidemics*

There are two general lists of critical days in *Epidemics I* and *III*, books which, because of their obvious similarities in content, disposition, and language, have been regarded by most critics ancient and modern as the works of one author,[100] and as perhaps even one work divided and/or otherwise mutilated through the vicissitudes of the textual transmission. Uniting the two lists, one gets the following sequence: 3, 4, 5, 6, 7, 8, 9, 10, 11, 14, 17, 20, 21, 24, 27, 30, 31, 40, 60, 80, 120. It is difficult to see any system in this series. None, of course, can be detected in 3 ... 11 because all numbers are represented there. As to the rest, multiples of 7 are included only until 21; after 31, only even numbers occur, all of them being divisible by 20, and all but the number 60 being also divisible by 40.

In comprising all days from the 3rd to the 11th, the combined two series differ from all other systems of critical days, but closely resemble the number lore of an ancient nosological treatise which, although not yet containing the *krísis* doctrine, admitted of being re-interpreted to some extent in the light of this later doctrine: *On Diseases II*, ch. 12–75.[101] The

[98] "The 7 days" seems to mean "the result of the 7 days" or simply "the 7th day." On the oscillation between cardinal and ordinal numbers, cf. p. 61–65.

[99] *Aph.* 4.476.11–15 Li. = 4.114 Jones Τῶν ἑπτὰ ἡ τετάρτη ἐπίδηλος. ἑτέρης ἑβδομάδος ἡ ὀγδόη ἀρχή (ἀρχή C'V: ἄρχει M)· θεωρητὴ δὲ (δὲ C'M: πάλιν V) ἡ ἑνδεκάτη· αὕτη (αὕτη C'V: ἡ αὐτὴ M) γάρ ἐστι τετάρτη τῆς (τῆς C': ἀπὸ τῆς MV) δευτέρης ἑβδομάδος· θεωρητὴ πάλιν ἡ ἑπτακαιδεκάτη· αὕτη γάρ ἐστι τετάρτη μὲν ἀπὸ τῆς τεσσαρεσκαιδεκάτης, ἑβδόμη δὲ ἀπὸ τῆς ἑνδεκάτης. Cf. Stephanus Atheniens. *Comm. in Hp. Aph.*, ed. Leendert G. Westerink, Berlin, 1985 (Corpus Medic. Graec. XI 1.3.1), *ad loc.* (p. 188–190).

[100] Deichgräber, Die Epidemien *passim*. Lichtenthaeler, Le troisième Épidémique 27–30.

[101] Cf. above p. 67 f.

following list contains the two kinds of day indications of this treatise, viz. the periods of *n* days as well as single *n*th days. For the reasons stated above,[102] no attempt has been made to distinguish between the two ways of expression. Thus, 1, 2, 3 ... in the vertical column mean both a period of 1, 2, 3 ... days and the 1st, 2nd, 3rd ... days. The other figures in the list are the chapter numbers. The list does not contain the (spans of) days for which only a treatment is prescribed.[103]

1: 22; 47.	11: 14; 44.
2: 47.	12: –
3: 20; 22; 56.	13: –
4: 54 = 58; 56.	14: 40; 44; 45; 47; 56; 57; 63.
5: 17; 22; 27; 41; 61.	15: 47; 53.
6: 17; 61.	16: –
7: 14; 16; 20; 21; 40; 41; 44;	17: –
47; 54 = 58; 56; 64; 65; 67.	18: 25; 47; 63.
8: 47.	19: –
9: 12; 14; 41; 47.	20: 12; 25; 46; 64.
10: 47; 64.	40: 12; 57; 64.

It is obvious that, although certain (spans of) days, particularly 7 and 14, are mentioned more often (because they were, as may be inferred, considered more important) than others, no system of days is followed in the nosological treatise. Nevertheless it is remarkable that the numbers 12, 13, 16, 19 are missing both there and in *Epidemics I* and *III*. This can scarcely be coincidence because the same numbers are missing also in the other lists of critical days quoted in the preceding section of this chapter (with the exception of *On the Foetus in the Seventh Month*, where all odd days are regarded as critical).

Epidemics I and *III* evince a dogmatic schematism in that the odd – even principle absent from the *Prognostics* system plays a prominent rôle there. In fact, the two lists combined above for the sake of a comparison with *On Diseases II*, ch. 12–75 are strictly kept apart from each other and are, in 'theory' at least, never mixed up together. Here is the complete text of the relevant passage dealing with critical days, *Epidemics I*, ch. 12 Li. (= ch. 26 Kw., Jones): "Diseases which get to their paroxysms [i. e. aggravations, or severe fits] on even days get to their crises on even days; and diseases whose paroxysms are on odd days get to their crises on odd

102 Cf. note 98.

103 For the sake of completeness, here are the nosological 'decisive periods' expressed in units other than days; they are all in years: Ch. 12 "Sometimes the disease returns in the seventh or fourteenth year." (*Morb. II* 7.20.6–7 Li. = 143.4–5 Jouanna ἐνίοτε δὲ ὑπ' οὖν ἔστρεψεν ἡ νοῦσος ἑβδόμῳ ἔτει ἢ τεσσερεσκαιδεκάτῳ.) Ch. 49 "This disease lasts seven or nine years." (*Morb. II* 7.76.6–7 Li. = 186.8–9 Jouanna αὕτη ἡ νοῦσος γίνεται ἑπτὰ ἔτεα ἢ ἐννέα.) Ch. 57 "For many, the disease lasts one year." (*Morb. II* 7.90.6 Li. = 197.6–7 Jouanna πολλοῖσι δὲ καὶ ἐνιαυσίη γίνεται ἡ νοῦσος.)

days. The first *períodos* of diseases which get to their crises on even days are the 4th, 6th, 8th, 10th, 14th, 20th, 24th, 30th, 40th, 60th, 80th, 120th. And of the diseases which get to their crises on odd days, the first *períodos* are the 3rd, 5th, 7th, 9th, 11th, 17th, 21st, 27th, 31st. In addition, one must know that, if crises which do not conform with the above-mentioned pattern occur, there will be relapses and the outcome may even be fatal. That is why one has to concentrate one's attention [on them] and be aware that at these times there will be crises in the direction of recovery or death, or tendencies to the better or the worse."[104]

The list with the even days is longer (it comprises 12 particular days) and covers a considerably more extended space of time (days no. 4 ... 120) than the one with the odd days (9 particular days, covering days no. 3 ... 31). Both lists are expressly said to present the days of the "first *períodos*." As the text stands, it can only mean that the first *períodos* of the even days is almost four times longer than the one of the odd days (120:31). The text transmitted is absolutely clear in that respect.[105] The difference seems to be rather large, although one might expect some limited discrepancies. It has been shown above how dissimilar in length the *períodoi* in other systems of critical days of the Hippocratic Collection are from each other. In *On Diseases IV*, ch. 48 the "first *períodos*" covers a space of time whose precise length must be between 11 and 14 days (see above p. 96 f.). In *Prognostics*, the "first," "second," and "third" *períodoi* cover 34, 40, and 60 days respectively (p. 95). But is it believable that in

---

[104] *Epid. I* 2.678.5–680.9 Li. = 1.201.18–202.8 Kw. = 1.184 Jones τὰ δὲ παροξυνόμενα ἐν ἀρτίῃσι κρίνεται ἐν ἀρτίῃσιν· ὧν δὲ οἱ παροξυσμοὶ ἐν περισσῇσι, κρίνεται ἐν περισσῇσιν. ἔστι δὲ (ἡ post δὲ add. Gal.: om. AVIR) πρώτη περίοδος τῶν (περίοδος τῶν A, Gal.: κρίσιμος τῶν περιόδων VIR) ἐν τῇσιν ἀρτίῃσι κρινόντων τετάρτη, ἕκτη, ὀγδόη (ὀγδ. AVIR, Gal. in lemm.: om. et damnavit Gal. in explic.), δεκάτη (δεκ. AVIR: om. Gal.), τεσσαρεσκαιδεκάτη, εἰκοστή, τετάρτη καὶ εἰκοστή, τριακοστή (post τριακ. add. τετάρτη καὶ τριακοστὴ Gal. in explic.: om. Gal. in lemm.), τεσσαρακοστή, ἑξηκοστή, ὀγδοηκοστή, εἰκοστὴ καὶ ἑκατοστή. τῶν (τῶν AVIR: ἐκ τῶν Gal.) δ' ἐν τῇσι περισσῇσι κρινόντων περίοδος πρώτη· τρίτη, πέμπτη, ἑβδόμη, ἐνάτη, ἑνδεκάτη, ἑπτακαιδεκάτη, εἰκοστὴ πρώτη, εἰκοστὴ ἑβδόμη, τριακοστὴ πρώτη. εἰδέναι δὲ χρὴ ἔτι (ἔτι Kw.: ὅτι AVIR, Gal.), ἢν ἄλλως κριθῇ (ἢν ... κριθῇ AVIR: τὰς ἄλλας κρίσεις Gal.) ἔξω τῶν ὑπογεγραμμένων (ὑπο- AVIR: προ- Gal.), ἐσομένας ὑποστροφάς· γένοιτο δὲ ἂν καὶ ὀλέθρια. δεῖ δὴ προσέχειν τὸν νόον καὶ εἰδέναι ἐν τοῖσι χρόνοισι τούτοισι τὰς (τὰς AVIR: om. Gal.) κρισίας ἐσομένας ἐπὶ σωτηρίην ἢ τὸ (ἢ τὸ VIR: εἴτε A: ἢ Gal.) ὀλέθριον (ὀλέθριον AVIR: ὄλεθρον Gal.) ἢ ῥοπὰς ἐπὶ τὸ ἄμεινον ἢ τὸ (τὸ AVIR: om. Gal.) χεῖρον.

[105] The word πρώτη at the beginning of the odd list refers to περίοδος and does not mean a day. This interpretation is supported by two arguments: *(1)* After the expression πρώτη περίοδος of the even list, something corresponding is needed in the odd one. *(2)* It is not attested anywhere else that the first day is critical. Unfortunately Galen's explanations, in which he criticizes the expression περίοδος, are partly mutilated; Wenkebach in his edition did not succeed in restoring them plausibly.

Epidemics I the first *períodos* alone almost reaches the extension of all three *períodoi* of *Prognostics*, ch. 20 added together? Some scepticism is permissible. A possible, though speculative explanation of the striking discrepancies is that the text of the first list of critical days (even days) has suffered during its textual transmission, at a stage before Galen (because he read the same text), but otherwise not determinable. Even if this assumption is correct, it cannot be proved and there is still no way of *correcting* the possible mistake. With some imagination, one might suggest that the "first *períodos*" of the first list originally comprised the days no. 4 ... 30, and that an expression like "after the first *períodos*" or "after this" has been mistakenly omitted before "40th." The second list might be transmitted in its original form. As will be shown shortly below, the author concentrates more on the even days, about which he has something new to say. Perhaps the reader was supposed to know about the subsequent *períodoi* of odd days. This is, however, mere speculation which should not — and will not — be an integral part of any further argumentation.

It must be taken as a fact that in each of the two lists as they are transmitted, only the "first *períodos*" is mentioned, whereas elsewhere in *Epidemics I períodoi* (plural) are either counted with cardinal numbers higher than 1 (ch. 4 Li. = ch. 6 Kw., Jones "from the first attack four *períodoi*; in seven *períodoi* ..."[106]) or are used in the plural (ch. 3 Li., Kw., Jones "After the relapses they had the *krísis* in the same *períodoi*;"[107] ch. 12 Li. = ch. 26 Kw., Jones "One must investigate, within which *períodoi* [certain kinds of fever] get to their *krísis*"[108]). Hence it is obvious that the two lists of even and odd critical days in *Epidemics I* do not present the whole doctrine but only part of it, and possibly in a textual version mutilated in the course of the transmission.[109]

The same doctrine of even and odd critical days underlies the historical case descriptions of individual patients, and it is instructive to see the relationship between the doctrine and 'reality.'[110] Before examining this particular relationship, it is essential to determine the possible ways in

---

[106] *Epid. I* 2.620.7—9 Li. = 1.186.3—5 Kw. = 1.156 Jones ἀπὸ τῆς πρώτης λήψιος τέσσαρας περιόδους· ἐν ἑπτὰ δὲ τελέως ἔκριναν.

[107] *Epid. I* 2.612.9—10 Li. = 1.183.15—16 Kw. = 1.152 Jones ἐκ δὲ τῶν ὑποστροφέων ἐν τῇσιν αὐτῇσι περιόδοισιν ἐκρίνοντο.

[108] *Epid. I* 2.682.1—2 Li. = 1.202.9—10 Kw. = 1.184 Jones ἐν τίσι (τίσι scripsi: τῇσι A: ᾗσι VIR) περιόδοισι κρίνονται, σκεπτέον.

[109] Further passages in other books of the *Epidemics* where *períodoi* are counted or referred to in the plural are *II* 5.74.13, 14, 76.1, 116.12; *IV* 5.188.9—10 Li. = Per. 270 La.; *VI* 5.344.10, 348.16, 17.

[110] For the relationship between the doctrine and the individual case histories with regard to the critical days cf. Deichgräber, Die Epidemien p. 17—23, 44. Nikitas, Untersuchungen 80 f.

which the numbering of days was originally arrived at in the individual case descriptions.

When reading through these reports, one immediately notices that most of the days mentioned by number occur also in the two lists of *Epidemics I.*[111] This is all the more astonishing since only a small minority of them is reported in the case descriptions to have actually occasioned a *krísis*. Most of the days referred to in the reports by number are those for which the physician mentions non-critical symptoms.

In the 42 individual histories of *Epidemics I* and *III*, approximately 310 indications of particular numbered days are made, the days being mostly — but not always[112] — counted from the beginning of the disease. Out of these approximately 310 numerical indications,[113] only 24 refer to days which, in the historical cases, actually did occasion a *krísis* (i. e. ca. 7.7%); all but 54 (i. e. ca. 82.6%), however, concern the days comprised in the two lists of potentially critical days. More precisely: Out of these 54 indications pertaining to days not included in the two lists (i. e. ca. 17.4% of the whole of ca. 130 indications), 33 (i. e. almost two thirds, or ca. 10.6% of the whole) refer to the important first two days of the disease, and 21 to other days not included in the lists (i. e. ca. 6.8% of the whole).[114]

Thus the vast majority of numerical day indications refer to the important days 1 and 2 and to days which were considered potentially critical without, however, actually being critical in the historical cases observed. When evaluating this ratio, one must take into account the fact that several of the disease cases ended quickly and therefore fell within the first two days and days 3 ... 11 (the latter series being completely comprised in the two lists). But even with this reservation, the predominance of the potentially critical days is striking: the ancient physician obviously had a strong bias towards onesidedly envisaging these days and neglecting the ones outside the scheme. There are essentially two possibilities which could account for it. One of them can be dismissed immediately, namely that 'in reality' little or nothing worth describing occurred on the days outside the scheme of potentially critical days. Probability is against this assumption.

There remains the second possibility, namely that the reason is not inherent in the 'reality' observed but in the technique of observing 'reality'

[111] The fact has already been mentioned by Deichgräber, Die Epidemien p. 12.

[112] Cf. shortly below p. 108—112.

[113] This is an approximate figure because the Greek text has variant readings here and there.

[114] The 54 indications concern the days no. 1 (14 times), 2 (19 times), 12 (twice), 13 (once), 15 (twice), 16 (5 times), 18 (3 times), 19 (twice), 29 (once), 34 (3 times including one real *krísis, Epid. III*, 2nd series, case 8 [cf. below p. 112, note 130]), 70 (once), 100 (once).

and/or of presenting the results of this observation.[115] Little is known about the way in which the individual case descriptions of *Epidemics I* and *III* (and of other books of the *Epidemics*) were written down. It seems unlikely that they are identical with the material of notes as taken at the patient's bedside or shortly after the examinations. Their sometimes careful composition[116] seems to be the result of a redactional revision by the author(s). So there are, again, two explanations for the concentration on the potentially critical days. Either the original raw-material (written as rough drafts, or memorized, or both) on which the reports were based comprised much more data than the ultimate reports, and the indications about the potentially critical days were subsequently filtered out for the literary presentation, or the original observation itself concentrated on the potentially critical days.

The recommendation quoted above in the context of the two lists (p. 104), "one has to concentrate one's attention [on the days contained in the lists]" allows either interpretation. The author of *Prognostics* formulates more clearly: "You must ... make your observations at every addition of a unit of 4. Then it will not escape your notice where the disease will turn." (Above p. 95 f.) Similarly the embryological text quoted above (p. 99) recommends: "You have, in your observation, to pay attention to all odd days; and of the even ones, to the 14th, the 28th, and the 42nd." Although these counsels do not discourage visits on other days not critical according to the respective schemes, they seem to favour visits on critical days; at least, they could be understood in this sense by other physicians who used the texts as handbooks for their daily work. The *Epidemics* do not contain much information as to the dates of the visits.[117] It is, therefore, impossible to determine which is the correct explanation of the phenomenon that the days mentioned in the case reports coincide so largely with

---

115 Quotation marks are used here, for two reasons: first, because the very word and concept of 'reality' is never mentioned or discussed by the Hippocratic authors and was possibly unknown to them; second, because its opposition to 'theory' cannot, even today, be determined unambiguously.

116 Rainer Hellweg, Stilistische Untersuchungen zu den Krankengeschichten der Epidemienbücher I und III des Corpus Hippocraticum (Habelts Dissertationsdrucke, Reihe Klass. Philol., 35), Bonn, 1985.

117 The term used in *Epid. IV, V, VI, VII* for a physician's visit is *esérkhomai*, 'to enter.' Rarely the days of visits are indicated in the individual case descriptions. Except for a sporting accident whose treatment began already "on the next day," *Epid. VI* 8.30 (5.354.13 Li. = Per. 333 La.), all these visits were made on days which, according not only to the scheme of *Epid. I* but also that of *Prog.*, were potentially critical: *Epid. IV* 25 (5.166.5 Li. = Per. 173 La.) "on the 7th day;" *Epid. V* 53 = *VII* 74 (5.238.6–7 = 432.23) "on the 4th day," where symptoms of the 3rd day are nevertheless described, perhaps after information obtained from others); *Epid. VII* 80 (5.436.6) "on the 17th day," with a note already on the 7th day.

the days of the two lists. In fact, there is no need to start from a strict alternative. Both explanations may be true, perhaps to a varying degree for the various case descriptions.

The complexity of the problem can be seen from the following individual case descriptions. These texts about single patients all present the remarkable phenomenon that the day counting does not proceed directly (day 1 ... n) but contains one or more breaches (day 1, 2 ... n | day n, n + 1, n + 2 ... n + n_1 | ...). One cannot detect the precise motives for these recommencements in day-counting; still it is worth-while to examine briefly the case descriptions containing this feature.

A normal childbirth was not within a physician's province. He intervened only if there were complications which the midwife could not cope with. In this case, the day numbering began anew with the first day of the additional complication and of the doctor's activity. The individual report in *Epidemics I*, case 11 is about the wife of Dromeades:[118] she "gave birth to a daughter, and everything else went as it should." But on the 2nd day rigor and acute fever occurred. "2nd day" means, of course, after the delivery. Here the day-counting switches over to a new starting-point, namely to the day on which the first disease symptoms appeared: "On the 1st day she began suffering around the *hypokhóndrion* [i. e. the upper stomach]." The 2nd day after the delivery is the 1st day of the disease (puerperal fever), and the days of the disease proper are then counted forth until the 6th day on which the woman died. No reason can be discovered for the breach in counting except the one mentioned: that the childbirth as such was not considered part of the disease (we do not know whether it was thought to have provoked the disease). Probably the doctor was called only after the first symptoms (fever etc.) occurred. In this case, the new start in counting has no consequences as to the days considered potentially critical: even had the first way of counting been continued, all days for which observations are recorded would still fall within the first two days and days 3 to 7 (critical according to the two lists).

The following case (*Epidemics I*, case 4)[119] is different in this respect. On Thasos, the wife of Philinos had been delivered of a daughter, and the placenta and the lochia had been discharged without trouble. But on the 14th day after the delivery, she caught a fever with rigor. Now the day counting switches over to a new start. The 14th day (first day with fever) becomes the 1st day of the disease, and observations are then recorded for the 6th, 7th, 8th, 9th, 10th, 11th, around the 14th, around the 17th, and for the 20th day. All of these days are potentially critical according to the two lists. Had the medical author instead counted from

---

118 *Epid. I* 2.708.6–710.11 Li. = 1.211.15–212.14 Kw. = 1.204–206 Jones.
119 *Epid. I* 2.690.11–694.2 Li. = 1.205.14–206.16 Kw. = 1.192–194 Jones.

the day of the childbirth, he would have arrived at the days no. 19, 20, 21, 22, 23, 24, ~27, ~30, 33, of which the nos. 19, 22, 23, 33 are not contained in the lists. Probably the physician saw the patient not before the 1st day of her disease and quite naturally counted from then on — perhaps visiting the patient only on the potentially critical days.

In another case, the delivery itself was not quite without problems: The wife of Epikrates (*Epidemics I*, case 5),[120] "when she was about to give birth," was seized with violent rigor and could not be warmed up, "as they said." The physician was not yet present and knew it only from hearsay. "On the next day" the condition was unchanged. "On the 3rd day" she brought forth a daughter, and everything connected with the birth proceeded without complications. Here ends the first series of counting the days. Then the report continues: "On the 2nd day after the delivery she caught an acute fever, pain of the *kardíē* [heart or stomach] and of the genitals," etc. This is the second start of counting the days, and it is significant that fever was not mentioned before it. The counting goes on in the way already known from the other cases, namely the "2nd day after the delivery" becomes the 1st day of the disease proper. This is implicitly expressed: "During the night of the 6th day after the fever had begun, she became delirious." The days mentioned subsequently, besides the 6th, are the 7th, 8th, 9th, 10th, 11th, 14th, 15th, 16th, 18th, 20th (approximately), 21st (approximately), 27th (approximately), 31st (approximately), 40th, 80th. All of these days except the nos. 15, 16, and 18 are contained in the lists of potentially critical days. If the author had counted from the rigor two days before the delivery, many more days would have fallen outside the scheme of the lists: nos. 12, 13, 18, 19, ~23, ~34, 43, 83; had he counted from the delivery, the following days: nos. 12, 15, 16, 19, ~22, ~28, ~32, 41, 81 would have done so.

A fourth case is not so clear by itself, but the analogy of the three other cases helps to clarify it, *Epidemics III*, 2nd series, case 2:[121] "The woman who, on Thasos, lay near The Cold Water and had given birth to a daughter and had not yielded the necessary discharge [placenta, blood, and lochia], was seized with acute fever and rigor on the 3rd day. Already a long time before the delivery she had been febrile, confined to bed, and without appetite. After the rigor, the fever became continuous, acute, and with shivering; on the 8th day she was very delirious ...," etc. This 8th day is probably reckoned from the day on which she felt the rigor, i. e. from the 3rd day after the childbirth, and so accordingly would be the

[120] *Epid. I* 2.694.3–698.5 Li. = 1.206.17–208.4 Kw. = 1.194–196 Jones.
[121] *Epid. III* 3.108.5–112.12 Li. = 1.234.3–235.6 Kw. = 1.260–262 Jones.

subsequent ones, nos. 11, 20, 27, 40, 60, 80, which are all contained in the two lists.[122]

Another class of individual reports presenting a breach in day-counting consists of cases featuring an incomplete *krísis* which initiates subsequently a relapse. The days are, in such cases, numbered until the *krísis*, after which the counting starts anew. In other cases, however, there is only one series of numbers in spite of an incomplete *krísis*.

Herophon (*Epidemics I*, case 3)[123] fell ill with acute fever and other symptoms. There are descriptions of the 5th, 6th, 7th, 8th day, and of the 9th day on which there was a *krísis*. The patient's recovery in this *krísis* was only deceptive. On the 9th day, reckoned from the *krísis* (9th = 1st day), he had a relapse of the fever. If the original counting had been perpetuated, this would have occurred on the uninteresting 13th day, which is not in the lists. Again a new, third counting starts with the relapse: On the 3rd day after the beginning of the relapse (i. e. on the uninteresting 15th day according to the original counting), he feels better.

---

[122] In *Epid. III*, 2nd series, case 14 (3.140.15–142.4 Li. = 1.243.13–25 Kw. = 1.280–282 Jones), the account mentions the 1st, 6th, 11th (approximately), 14th, 16th, 17th (death). An event prior to the 1st day is described as follows: Ἐν Κυζίκῳ γυναικὶ θυγατέρας τεκούσῃ διδύμας καὶ δυστοκησάσῃ καὶ οὐ πάνυ καθαρθείσῃ τῇ πρώτῃ πυρετός ... The same words to identify a patient occur in *Epid. II* 2.20 (5.92.8–12 Li. = Per. 29–31 La.). It is possible that the two case descriptions are about the same patient. This would imply that the post-natal complications of *Epid. II* occurred before those of *Epid. III*, hence that in *Epid. III* the 1st day did not follow immediately on the delivery. A clear instance of two case descriptions identifying an anonymous male patient by using literally the same phrase are *Epid. IV* 53 (5.192.15–194.4 Li. = Per. 290–292 La.) and *Epid. VI* 8.10 (5.342.5–9), where a patient is called "the one to whom Kyniskos introduced me," πρὸς ὃν Κυνίσκος εἰσήγαγέ με. The identity, however, of the two women in childbed is by no means certain. In historical case reports, there are several other striking instances of literal repetitions which must be explained otherwise (but how?); e. g. in the individual case descriptions *Epid. I*, case 4 (2.690.17–692.1 Li. = 1.205.19–20 Kw. = 1.192 Jones) προσθεμένῃ δὲ ταῦτα μὲν ἐκουφίσθη, κεφαλῆς δὲ καὶ τραχήλου καὶ ὀσφύος πόνοι, and *Epid. I*, case 5 (2.694.9–10 Li. = 1.206.22–24 Kw. = 1.194 Jones) προσθεμένῃ δὲ ταῦτα μὲν ἐκουφίσθη, κεφαλῆς δὲ καὶ τραχήλου καὶ ὀσφύος πόνος. *Epid. III*, 2nd series, case 12 (3.136.10–11 Li. = 1.242.4 Kw. = 1.278 Jones) γυναικεῖα κατέβη πρῶτον τότε· παρθένος γὰρ ἦν, and *Epid. II* 2.8 (5.88.7–8 Li. = Per. 16 La. περὶ γυναικείων κατάρρηξιν, καὶ ἴσως τότε πρῶτα γενόμενα· παρθένος γὰρ ἦν. Compare also *Epid. I* 2 (2.604.5–6 Li. = 1.181.15–16 Kw. = 1.148 Jones) τοῖς ἐνδοιαστῶς ἔχουσι πολλοῖσιν ἐβεβαίωσε, and *Epid. VI* 7.10 (5.342.6–7) τοῖσιν ἐνδοιαστοῖσιν ἐβεβαίωσεν. *Epid. I*, ch. 4 Li. (= ch. 9 Kw., Jones) (2.628.11–12 Li. = 1.188.17–18 Kw. = 1.160 Jones) ἐξανθήματα σμικρὰ καὶ οὐκ ἀξίως τῆς περιβολῆς τῶν νοσημάτων, and *Epid. II* 1.7 (5.78.5–8) ἐξανθήματα ... μὴ ἀναξίως τῆς περιβολῆς τῆς νούσου. *Epid. III* 7 (3.84.7–8 Li. = 1.228.6–7 Kw. = 1.246 Jones) καὶ ἄλλα, ἃ σήψ καλεῖται, ἐκθύματα μεγάλα, and *Epid. VI* 8.3 (5.344.1–2) καὶ ἐκθύματα (ἐκθύματα Pall.: ἐκφ- codd.), ἃ σήψ καλεῖται. Can these parallel formulae be interpreted as vestiges of either oral or written medical texts, which were learned and memorized by heart?

[123] *Epid. I* 2.688.9–690.10 Li. = 1.204.20–205.13 Kw. = 1.190–192 Jones.

The final *krísis* with a definite recovery was "around the seventeenth day," and it is a moot question as to where this no. 17 is counted from.

The case to be quoted next has a similar arithmetic structure. First series of days: beginning of the disease until *krísis*. Second series: *krísis* until relapse. Last series: beginning of relapse until the definite end of the disease. This last series is subdivided into two sub-series: Third series, beginning of relapse until a day with delirium. Fourth series, day with delirium until death (*Epidemics III*, 1st series, case 6):[124] The daughter of Euryanax contracted a fever. On the 6th day, she had a *krísis* which apparently was definite because her anus suppurated and the pus erupted from the ulcer. This is regarded as a favourable critical sign.[125] Perhaps the physician considered the disease terminated. A new counting begins: On the 7th day after the *krísis* (6th = 1st day), she relapsed and perspired. The beginning of this relapse is the commencement of a third series of counting days (7th = 1st day): "Around the 10th day after the perspiration she became delirious ... After being free from symptoms for one day,[126] she became very delirious again on the 12th day." Now an additional fourth counting starts: "On the 7th day after being delirious the second time, she died." Had the original counting been continued throughout the development of this disease, the numbers arrived at would have been: 6 (*krísis*), 12 (relapse), ~21 (first delirium), 23 (second delirium), 29 (death). All but two of these numbers are missing in the two lists.

There is a further case of a recommencement in counting days after a *krísis*, and this case is considerably simpler than the two preceding ones. Pythion (*Epidemics III*, 1st series, case 1)[127] was seized with a tremor that started from his hands. The report continues: "On the 1st day there was acute fever and delirium." (It remains unclear whether the tremor happened on the 1st day or before.) Subsequently, the 2nd, 3rd, 4th, 5th, 6th, 7th, 8th, and 10th day are described. On the 10th day, a *krísis* occurred; around that day, however, the urine was relatively thin (i. e. did not contain a sufficient amount of the *materia peccans*), a less favourable prognostic sign (cf. *Prognostics*, ch. 12).[128] In fact, a twofold segregation of the harmful matter was formed: a suppuration at the anus, and strangury. This double *apóstasis* happened "after the *krísis*, 40 days later." According to the original day-counting, it would have been on the non-critical 49th day.

---

124 *Epid. III* 3.50.1–52.9 Li. = 1.220.6–221.2 Kw. = 1.228–230 Jones.

125 Cf. *Epid. IV* 5.182.14–15 Li. = Per. 248 La., with the commentary *ad loc*. Cf. below p. 191 f.

126 This is the technical sense of διαλιποῦσα.

127 *Epid. III* 3.24.3–28.6 Li. = 1.215.2–13 Kw. = 1.218 Jones.

128 *Prog.* 2.142.4–6 Li. = 1.90.17–21 Kw. = 2.26 Jones ὁκόσοι δὲ οὖρα λεπτὰ καὶ ὠμὰ οὐρέουσι ..., τούτοισιν ἀπόστασιν δεῖ προσδέχεσθαι ἐς τὰ κάτω τῶν φρενῶν χωρία. This is exactly what happened in this case.

Any attempt to determine why the individual reports quoted above contain the breaches in counting the days seems futile. Did the physician establish some sort of ideal 'time-table' in advance for each of the cases, paying most of his visits on the days he regarded as potentially critical and readjusting his 'time-table' of visits when there was an apparent end and a recommencement of the disease after an incomplete *krísis*? Or did he pay his visits regardless of any such preconceived 'time-table' but, when composing his reports on the basis of more extended raw-material, pick out the days contained in the lists, adjust others numerically to this scheme by introducing the breaches into his counting, and omit those days that did not fit either way?

As has been said above, the two explanations are not mutually exclusive. Perhaps they are both true. The physician may have followed the 'time-table' for his visits, and when composing the reports he may, in addition, have modified the arithmetic form of his material (i. e. changed the day-counting) in order to present it in conformity with his theory of critical days.[129] A more precise answer is not possible; the surviving text material simply does not contain any hints useful for a solution.

The discussion already provides, however, answers to part of the following complex of questions: How has the doctrine of the two lists, and in particular the doctrine of odd and even, been established? Did this doctrine exist before the individual case reports were written? Was the doctrine 'induced' from the reports? Or did the author(s) possess part of the doctrine which was then, by some kind of 'induction,' revised and completed on the basis of the individual case observations?

It is evident that the potentially critical days as such, which are contained in the two lists, already played a prominent rôle when the individual disease cases were observed and/or described, because the descriptions concentrate on these days. Although the days are seldom actually critical in the reports, they seem to have been of particular interest. In the reports of *Epidemics I* and *III*, an actual *krísis* (complete or incomplete) occurs only on the following days: Even numbers, 4th (once), 6th (twice), 10th (once), 14th (once), 20th (5 times), 24th (once), 34th (once), 40th (once), 80th (once), 120th (once). Odd numbers, 3rd (once), 5th (once), 7th (once), 9th (once), 11th (twice), 17th (twice), 27th (once).

Out of the list of even critical days, the 8th, 30th, and 60th day are not represented in the individual case descriptions; there occurs, however, a 34th critical day which, although probably not part of the list,[130] yet

[129] The physicians even felt entitled to adapt the facts to the doctrine with regard to days with a high number, see below p. 209 f.

[130] Poorly attested in part of the Greek (but not in the Arabic) tradition of Galen, cf. Gal. *In Hp. Epid. I comm.* p. 123.21–22 Wenkebach, reproduced above p. 104, note 104.

belongs to the system of critical days of *Prognostics*. Out of the list of odd critical days, the 21st and 31st are not represented in the descriptions. Most of the even and odd critical days occur in the cases only once. All this makes it quite obvious that the two lists are not 'induced'[131] from the case descriptions as we have them.

A particular question concerns the alleged regular correlation of paroxysms (aggravations) on even days with *krísis* on even days, and paroxysms on odd days with *krísis* on odd days. Could this constituent of the doctrine have been 'induced' from the reports? The answer is again "no."

Among the 42 individual case descriptions of *Epidemics I* and *III*, there are 13 (cf. list I) which mention one or more paroxysms on even days but no paroxysms on odd days.[132] In these 13 cases,

- complete crises are mentioned 2 times (both on even days);
- incomplete crises are mentioned 3 times (2 on even days, 1 on an odd day);
- fatal outcomes are mentioned 9 times (4 on even, 5 on odd days).

In the following synopses, the numbers followed by symbols indicate the days, P stands for 'paroxysm,' K for 'complete *krísis*,' (K) for 'incomplete *krísis*,' † for 'death.'

List I (Paroxysms on Even Days)

Epidemics I,	case 1:	2P	4P	6†
	case 7:	4P	5(K)	(Additional symptoms follow.)
	case 8:	2P	5†	
	case 10:	6P	20(K)	(Additional symptoms follow.)
Epidemics III,	1st series, case 2:	6P	20(K)	27† (The 14th day features symptoms which might be called critical, but the word is not used there.)
	case 4:	4P	5†	
	case 7:	4P	5†	
	case 8:	2P	7†	
	case 12:	4P	10P	14†
Epidemics III,	2nd series, case 3:	4P	6P	10†
	case 6:	2P	4K	
	case 10:	2P	24K	
	case 16:	14P	24†	

[131] For the concept of 'induction,' which was unknown to the Hippocratic authors and even to Aristotle in its modern sense, see Kurt von Fritz, Die ἐπαγωγή bei Aristoteles, in: *idem*, Grundprobleme der Geschichte der antiken Wissenschaft, Berlin/New York, 1971, 623–676. Cf. below p. 164, 213–224.

[132] In *Epidemics III*, 1st series, case 4, a paroxysm of pain is mentioned to have occurred before the 1st day, on a day not specified.

In 3 case descriptions (cf. list II), a paroxysm falls on an odd day, and none on an even day. In these cases,
- a complete *krísis* is mentioned once (on an odd day);
- an incomplete *krísis* is mentioned once (on an odd day);
- fatal outcomes are mentioned twice (on even days).

List II (Paroxysms on Odd Days)

Epidemics I,	case 3:	5P	9(K)	17K
Epidemics III,	2nd series, case 1:	7P	120†	
	case 4:	3P	4†	

In 9 cases (cf. list III), paroxysms fall on even as well as on odd days in each description, and
- complete crises are mentioned 4 times (3 or 4 on even days, 1 or 0 on an odd day);[133]
- incomplete crises are mentioned 3 times (1 on an even day, 2 on odd days);
- fatal outcomes are mentioned 4 times (1 on an even day, 3 on odd days).

List III (Paroxysms on Even and Odd Days)

Epidemics I,	case 2:	3P	4P	11†		
	case 5:	7P	16P	80K (The 27th day features symptoms which might be called critical, but the word is not used there.)		
	case 6:	πῦρ πεπλανημένως, οἱ πυρετοὶ παροξυνόμενοι ἄλλοτ' ἀλλοίως, ἀτάκτως ... οἱ παροξυσμοὶ ἐν κρισίμοις μάλιστα. 80K				
	case 12:	7P	10P	11†		
Epidemics III,	1st series, case 1:	2P	5P	8P	10(K) (Another symptom follows.)	
	case 5:	5P	6P	7(K)	17(K)	19 or 20K
	case 11:	5P	6P	7†		
Epidemics III,	2nd series, case 2:	πυρετοὶ πεπλανημένως παροξυνόμενοι, τὰ μέν, τὰ δ' οὔ. 80†				
	case 9:	πυρετὸς ἄλλοτε ἀλλοίως παροξυνόμενος, τὰ πλεῖστα ἀτάκτως. 120K				

These lists and the rudimentary statistics suffice to prove that the doctrine of the regular correlation of odd and even paroxysm days and

[133] Dependent on which variant reading one chooses in *Epid. III* 3.48.20 Li. = 1.220.5 Kw. = 1.228 Jones, where εἰκοστῇ is omitted by VI but read in R; Galen, who knew both readings, expressly preferred the one with εἰκοστῇ.

krísis days cannot have been 'induced' from the 42 reports of *Epidemics I* and *III*. Among the 13 cases with paroxysms exclusively on even days, only 2 have a complete *krísis* on an even day; among the 3 cases with paroxysms exclusively on odd days, only 1 has a complete *krísis* on an odd day; but among the 9 cases in which paroxysms occur on even as well as on odd days, 4 have a complete *krísis*, i. e. almost half of them. All this, if taken statistically, is in marked contradiction to the rule. Furthermore, there are as many as 17 cases among the 42 which do not feature any paroxysm at all; and in 9 out of these 17, not even a *krísis* is mentioned.

There is more likelihood in the assumption that the doctrine formulated in the context of the two lists existed before the case-reports were written, and that the doctrine provided the framework for the observation and/or description of 'reality.'

The doctrine of odd/even paroxysm days and odd/even critical days in *Epidemics I* served prognostic purposes. The physician observing the paroxysms did not need (or believed he did not need, although the extant case records contradict any such belief) to wait for the *krísis* but could prognosticate beforehand "where the disease will turn."[134]

Epidemics I contains another prognostic remark which, although not claiming to be universally true, is said to have been valid for one particular *katástasis* (i. e. one particular historical system, or combination, of season, weather, and diseases at one particular geographic place): ch. 9 Li. (= ch. 20 Kw., Jones)[135] "The circumstances of the crises,[136] from which we recognized [the outcome], were either similar or dissimilar.[137] For instance, the two brothers who began [being sick] together at the same time of the day[138] ..., brothers of Epigenes. The elder one had a *krísis* on the 6th, the younger one on the 7th day. Both relapsed simultaneously at the same time of the day, and there was an intermission of 5 days.[139] After the

---

[134] As the author of *Prognostics* formulates, cf. above p. 95. The arithmetical method applied there is, however, different.

[135] *Epid. I* 2.660.6–664.10 Li. = 1.196.23–197.23 Kw. = 1.176–178 Jones.

[136] For τὰ περὶ *c. acc.* cf. Langholf, Syntaktische Untersuchungen 108–111.

[137] ἢ ὅμοια ἢ ἀνόμοια seems to allude to *Epid. VI* 5.298.4–9, cf. 352.16–354.2. For more details, see below p. 205, note 362; 206, note 367.

[138] The word might even mean 'hour' here, Langholf, Hermes 101 (1973), 382–384. Langholf, Syntaktische Untersuchungen 140.

[139] According to Galen (*In Hp. Epid. I comm.*, ed. Wenkebach, p. 98–99), there was a scholarly discussion in antiquity about this intermission. Galen and unnamed predecessors took "there was an intermission" (διέλιπεν) in a pluperfect sense (= "there had been ..."), which is possible grammatically but forces the interpreter to postulate a text corruption. Galen thought that some words had been mistakenly omitted, and proposed to insert ἓξ τῷ μὲν ἑτέρῳ, τῷ δ' ἑτέρῳ between the transmitted ἡμέρας and πέντε. If one extended Galen's conjectural insertion, one would even get a perfect homoioteleuton:

[second] relapse, both had the *krísis* simultaneously on the 17th day altogether." It seems as though this impressive double case of the two brothers[140] was only the starting point for the following observations, because the day numbers in the case of the brothers are incomplete: "both relapsed ..., there was an intermission of 5 days," but it is not stated when the relapse began, and when the ensuing intermission began and ended. Perhaps the physician had not paid attention to these dates, and perhaps it was not before the definite end of the two cases that the physician became aware of the numerical congruences. He continues by mentioning 5 more sub-groups of patients from the same *katástasis* who all had a final *krísis* on the 17th day, and adds that "most of the patients in this *katástasis* were sick in this manner, and I do not know anyone who recovered without experiencing the relapses in this manner; and all whom I know, to whom the relapses happened according to this type, recovered." They never had a further relapse (i. e., all patients who exhibited this chronological structure of the disease, and all patients who recovered, formed one and the same group). Since even the *majority* of cases followed that scheme during the season described and at the geographic place considered (city of Thasos),[141] the physician had a highly efficient method of prognosis. Here are the details of the sub-groups:

i. "The two brothers," they began simultaneously, *krísis* 6th/7th day respectively, relapse simultaneously xth day, intermission yth day, end of the intermission (= second relapse) (y + 5)th day, final *krísis* 17th day simultaneously.[142]

ii. "Most," *krísis* 6th day, intermission for 6 days, final *krísis* 5th day after the relapse.

διέλιπεν ἡμέρας ⟨ἓξ τῷ μὲν ἑτέρῳ, τῷ δ' ἑτέρῳ ἡμέρας⟩ πέντε. But this seems too drastic a modification. The text should not be changed. — Poseidonios (see following note) seems to have had a text different from ours, because he explains that the brothers were twins. He probably read ἑτέρῳ ... ἑτέρῳ instead of πρεσβυτέρῳ ... νεωτέρῳ.

140 Poseidonios (frg. 384, 386 Theiler = 311, 104 Edelstein/Kidd) interpreted this passage in terms of his doctrine of συμπάθεια.

141 The modern reader used to precise medical statistics cannot help but feel suspicious of these statements. With all probability, they are largely exaggerated. One might thus conclude that they were not published on Thasos (where people would have remembered what had happened during the *katástasis*), but at another place; perhaps in order to impress a city's officials who had to appoint a 'public physician' out of several itinerant candidates? On the mode of election Cohn-Haft, Public Physicians 5–6, 21–22 *et saep.*; cf. Langholf, Kallimachos 26–27.

142 The structure of this double case is similar to the one numbered *v* (see shortly below): two intermissions, two relapses. But in the case of the two brothers, a calculation is impossible because there are at least two unknown quantities, perhaps even three, since it is not explicitly stated that the second intermission (of 5 days) occurred to them simultaneously.

iii. "Some," *krísis* 7th day, intermission for 7 days, final *krísis* 3rd day after the relapse.
iv. "Some," *krísis* 7th day, intermission for 3 days, final *krísis* 7th day after the relapse.
v. "Some," *krísis* 6th day, intermission for 6 days, sick again for 3 days, intermission for 1 day, sick for 1 day, final *krísis* ("e. g. in the case of ..." [1 name follows]).
vi. "Some," *krísis* 6th day, intermission for 7 days, final *krísis* 4th day after the relapse ("e. g. in the case of ..." [1 name follows]).

The striking case of the two brothers, although perhaps still observed incompletely because the definite viewpoints were not yet found, seems to have become the starting-point for further and more precise observations with the result that "the circumstances of the *krísis*," although being "dissimilar" in detail, proved to be "similar" as far as the main features were concerned.[143] None of these cases of a *krísis* on the 17th day is included in the case reports of *Epidemics I* and *III*.[144] Possibly the medical author made his discovery about the relevance of the 17th day without inducing it from any previously formulated individual case reports like those transmitted in *Epidemics I* and *III*.

To conclude this section of the present chapter, let us briefly consider an intricate and probably unsolvable problem: What was the function of the descriptions of individual disease cases? One gets the impression that they do not form a random collection of reports that were written in accordance with the doctrine and happened to be at hand when the two books were compiled. They seem, at least partly, to have been collected after a theoretical plan. This can be concluded from the striking ratio between the 13 cases with paroxysms on even, and the only 3 cases with paroxysms on odd days. It seems as though the author's (or authors') interest was more absorbed by the even than the odd days. This conclusion is supported by what has been remarked above[145] concerning the two lists: the one of the even days is longer and covers a considerably longer space of time (almost four times) than the list of odd days. An additional trace

---

143 Periods of 17 days had some importance in meteorology. R. Böker calls this space of time a *Streuungsfrist*, i. e. a period within which certain weather phenomena occur with varying temporal distribution (cf. the literature quoted by him in Pauly/Wissowa, Suppl. IX, 1703 f. s. v. 'Windfristen'). In fact the 17 days in the *Epidemics* text are nothing but a *Streuungsfrist* for the features pseudo-*krísis*, intermission, relapse, final *krísis*. Did the author(s) project a meteorological scheme on the cases observed (cases which were thought to be influenced by the weather, cf. below p. 164–179)?

144 But there is a similar remark in *Epid. I* 2.620.3–5 Li. = 1.185.20–22 Kw. = 1.156 Jones ἔκρινε τούτοισι πάνυ εὐτάκτως, τοῖσι πλείστοισι σὺν τῇσι διαλειπούσῃσιν ἐν ἑπτακαίδεκα ἡμέρῃσιν.

145 p. 104 f.

of this bias in interest appears in four explicit statements that "the paroxysms happened on even days," statements which are completely missing for the odd days: *Epidemics I*, ch. 9 Li. (= ch. 18 Kw., Jones); *ibid.*, case 1; *III*, ch. 6; 2nd series, case 10.[146] Their stereotyped wording suggests that they are formulaic answers to a recurring routine problem. A similar formula, also without any corresponding statement about the odd days, is "the pain was on the even days:" *Epidemics III*, 2nd series, cases 3, 10, 12.[147]

An interest in the general odd/even problem (which had older historical roots, cf. the beginning of the following section of this chapter), seems to have been *one* incentive for composing the individual case reports. There must have been other motives. The fact that the cases collectively contradict the doctrine on the odd/even correlation between paroxysms and crises could even be taken as an indication that the case material was gathered in order to falsify this particular correlation rule, were it not for the relatively numerous cases which do not feature a paroxysm (or not even a *krísis*) and which would remain unexplained this way. Perhaps there is no single and simple formula that could exhaustively explain the *raison d'être* of the collection of case reports.

2. *Precursors and Applicability of the* krísis *Doctrine*

That the author(s) of *Epidemics I* and *III* onesidedly emphasized the paroxysms and the pains on even days (cf. the preceding section of this chapter) need not be interpreted to the effect that he (or they) deemed the even days more dangerous than the odd ones. It is more probable that he (or they) paid (and called) special attention to the even days because traditionally it had been the odd days which played a prominent rôle.[1]

---

146 *Epid. I* 2.652.4–5 Li. = 1.194.23 Kw. = 1.172 Jones οἱ παροξυσμοὶ ἐν ἀρτίῃσιν. 684.9 Li. = 203.9–10 Kw. = 186 Jones οἱ παροξυσμοὶ ἐν ἀρτίῃσιν. *III* 3.82.1–2 Li. = 1.227.5–6 Kw. = 1.244 Jones οἱ παροξυσμοὶ τοῖσι πλείστοισιν ἐν ἀρτίῃσι. 132.4–5 Li. = 240.22–23 Kw. = 274 Jones οἱ δὲ παροξυσμοὶ ... ἐν ἀρτίῃσιν ἦσαν μᾶλλον.

147 *Epid. III* 3.116.12–13 Li. = 1.236.10 Kw. = 1.264 Jones ἐν ἀρτίῃσιν οἱ πόνοι τούτῳ. 132.4–5 Li. = 240.22–23 Kw. = 274 Jones (cf. preceding footnote). 136.13 Li. = 242.7 Kw. = 278 Jones οἱ πόνοι ἐν ἀρτίῃσιν. Less clear are expressions like "The pains occurred on the critical days," *Epid. I* 2.622.14 Li. = 1.186.24 Kw. = 1.158 Jones παροξυνόμενοι ἐν κρισίμοισι (ἐν κρ. IR, Gal. interpret. Arab.: om. AV, Gal.). 624.1–2 Li. = 187.1 Kw. = 158 Jones ἐν κρισίμοις ὡς ἐπὶ τὸ πολὺ κακούμενοι. 698.11–12 Li. = 208.9–11 Kw. = 198 Jones τὰ μὲν πλεῖστα ἐπεσήμαινον οἱ παροξυσμοὶ ἐν κρισίμοις μάλιστα (μάλιστα AV, Gal.: μᾶλλον IR).

1 Cf. Kudlien, Bedeutung des Ungeraden; Thivel, Cnide 216–236.

They do so, for example, in *On the Foetus in the Seventh Month*: "If you want to restore without blunder the health of the sick, you have, in your observations, to pay attention to all odd days; and of the even ones, to the 14th, the 28th, and the 42nd" (see above p. 99 f.). Even less differentiated in presenting the traditional doctrine is *On Diseases IV*. In ch. 46 it says, "It is on the odd days that man either recovers or dies,"[2] and in ch. 47: "This is well-known to absolutely everybody."[3] The author considers this doctrine self-evident but refers to a by-gone epoch when its therapeutical consequences were still unknown and patients died because the doctors purged them on the odd days, thus aggravating their condition.[4] Several chapters of *On Diseases IV* are devoted to a 'physiological' aetiology of the cycle of odd days. Robert Joly, in the preface to his edition of the treatise,[5] rightly says that none of these numerical explanations seems to be based on rational reasons, but that it is the old number-lore which reappears, superficially rationalized, and whose authority annihilates any endeavour of serious verification. Joly regards that as typical of the 'level' ("niveau") of ancient science in general. 'Level,' a metaphor taken from geodesy, is a term which provokes the question, "in relation to what?," and here difficulties of standpoint begin. Comparing standards of ancient science and medicine to later or modern ones is, of course, an unhistorical procedure, and the historian may find it questionable. On the other hand, the student of history is constantly comparing the subject matter of his research to the world in which he is living, often without being aware of his doing so. Hence it might be heuristically important and help to sharpen the historian's methodological awareness if questions involving the 'level' of ancient science are asked. Some questions contain the 'level' problem only implicitly. In such cases, it is useful to recognize that the problem is nevertheless present. The internal cohesiveness of ancient treatises, for instance, cannot be assessed without implicitly measuring them by modern standards. Even *comparing* treatises to each other in this respect ("treatise A is more coherent than treatise B" *et sim.*) implies an unhistorical evaluation because we do not know how tolerant the ancient authors, and the readers they wrote for, were when they noticed inconsistencies, self-contradictions, etc. Such a comparison is still more problematical in the case of Hippocratic treatises because many of them

---

[2] *Morb. IV* 7.572.1–2 Li. = 100.23–24 Joly ἐν δὲ τῇσι περισσῇσι τῶν ἡμερέων καὶ ὑγιὴς γίνεται ὁ ἄνθρωπος καὶ θνήσκει.

[3] 574.23–24 Li. = 103.2 Joly τοῦτο πᾶς οἶδεν ὅς τίς ποτε.

[4] In *Morb. II* 12–75, e. g., the doctrine is still unknown, see ch. 40 (7.56.11 Li. = 171.18–19 Jouanna), where purging on the 9th day is recommended. For other recommendations to purge on odd days, see Lonie, Hippocratic treatises 326.

[5] p. 32; cf. also Thivel, Cnide 229 f.

can be dated only with a precision of several decades and are, moreover, rather inexplicit as to their doctrines.

The aetiology of the cycle of odd critical days as constructed by the author of *On Diseases IV* seems more objectionable today than do, for example, the (partly compatible) physiological systems of *On the Nature of Man* (including *On Healthy Regimen*) or *On Regimen I–IV*. Both of these works contain in themselves certain minor self-contradictions which do not affect the nucleus of the argument, but in *On Diseases IV*, the very basis of the discussion is self-contradictory.[6] According to *On Diseases IV*, ch. 32–48,[7] fever is developed whenever there is a quantitative disproportion (ch. 44–45) of the four humours, bile, phlegm, water, and blood. These four humours are usually contained in food and drink, and the body draws them out of the content of the belly just as the plant draws the appropriate humours out of the soil (ch. 32–34). There are, besides the belly, four cisterns in the body, namely the gall-bladder for the bile (and no other humour), the head for the phlegm, the spleen for the water, and the heart for the blood (the latter three cisterns contain also smaller quantities of other humours) (ch. 35–40). Whereas the roughage of the food leaves the belly on the next day, the four humours, after having been attracted by the four cisterns on the first day, stay there during the second day and are 'cooked,' i.e. concocted into a more fluid, less viscous state.[8] On the same day, the thinner humours are expelled from the cisterns back into the belly by the new, raw (i.e., thicker) humours which mechanically push out the old (thinner) ones while streaming into the cisterns. The old concocted humours then concoct the food in the belly and are excreted on the third day. This mechanism presupposes that food is taken in *every day*, that on the first day fresh humours are sucked into the cisterns, and that on the second day the cooked humours are driven back into the belly (ch. 42) by the fresh, uncooked humours. By a mistake in reasoning, the author abandons this presupposition when trying to explain why the odd days are critical. He suddenly postulates (ch. 46) that "on the even days the body [i.e. the cisterns] draws from the belly, and on the odd days it releases [the humours into the belly], and the belly excretes them." This is incompatible with the first assumption. Obviously the author did not notice the self-contradiction.[9] His modern reader is more accustomed to thinking in complex functional systems.

---

[6] Cf. the discussion in Lonie, Hippocratic treatises 304–310, 322–324; more generally on inconsistencies of this treatise *ibid.* 47 f.

[7] *Morb. IV* 7.542.3–578.8 Li. = 84.1–104.20 Joly.

[8] According to *VM* 1.614.6–10 Li. = 1.21.7–11 Kw. = 1.46 Jones, ripening thickens the humour. For such contrary effects of heat, cf. Lonie, Hippocratic treatises 156 f., 307 f.

[9] Lonie, Hippocratic treatises 323.

Perhaps the author's reasoning was regarded as less objectionable by somebody sharing the basic doctrine about the critical nature of the odd days. As a matter of fact, the author does not intend to prove *that* these days are critical; he presupposes it and only tries to make out the reasons *why* they are so. For a reader believing in the doctrine, the author's expositions might have contained elements useful for an understanding of the 'why' of the facts. As the doctrine was an unquestionable truth, at least for that author and consequently for part of his readers – could not any explanations of its reasons be true, even though they contradicted each other in certain points?

That the critical functions of the body are different on odd and even days is also stated in *On Humours*, ch. 6:[10] On odd days, critical excretions appear 'above' (i. e. through the openings of the head), and on even days 'below' (through intestines and bladder). This is supposed to happen if the paroxysms are on even days, as they are said usually to be. In the rarer cases in which the paroxysms are on odd days, the direction of the excretions is inverse, and the crises are then less reliable. Nothing is said in this context about any internal mechanism, and it is vain to speculate today, in the absence of further hints provided by the text, whether any such aetiological explanation of the doctrine of *On Humours* did ever exist. Of course, the alleged regularity of the 'phenomena' described must have been attractive to speculative individuals. It is even possible that aetiological speculations were at the origin of the 'phenomena.' All of these modern reflexions equally apply, *mutatis mutandis*, to the doctrine of the two lists of even and odd days in *Epidemics I*, with which there might be some historical relationship. In *Epidemics I*, ch. 12 Li. (= ch. 26 Kw., Jones), the even days are not considered more dangerous than the odd ones; they are only paid more attention (cf. above p. 104 f.; 117 f.). In *On Humours*, ch. 6, disease 'systems' (*katástasis*) with paroxysms on odd days have "less reliable crises" (*dyskritōteros*), i. e. they are more dangerous. Is this assertion only a thoughtless and schematic continuation of the doctrine contained in *Epidemics I*? We cannot know at present.

Another formulation of the traditional doctrine that the odd days are critical is found in *On Regimen in Acute Diseases, Appendix*, ch. 9 Li. (= ch. 21 Kw.): "You should be particularly concerned about the odd number, because these days let the sick slide in either direction."[11]

According to Aristoxenos (fourth century B. C.), it was a doctrine of Pythagoras (or rather of the Pythagoreans) that the crises of the diseases

[10] *Hum.* 5.486.4–15 Li. = 4.74–76 Jones.

[11] *Acut. (Sp.)* 2.436.3–5 Li. = 1.157.7–9 Kw.; cf. 448.3–6 Li. = 160.17–19 Kw. For further attestation of the doctrine in the Hippocratic Collection, see Kudlien, Bedeutung des Ungeraden.

occur on the odd days, and that it is on the odd days, too, that one disease is transformed into another. The reason for both was seen in the obscure 'fact' that the odd numbers have a beginning, a middle, and an end, and that, accordingly, the odd days have a beginning, culmination, and abatement.[12]

This kind of 'argumentation' reveals that the Pythagorean doctrine of the odd and even[13] did not need a proof, just as in *On Diseases IV* the alleged fact that the odd days were particularly decisive needed not be proved. An explanation, however, of the causes of the 'fact' must have been welcome.

One of the objectives of the author(s) of *Epidemics I* seems to have been to find out whether the traditional doctrine of the (almost) exclusive importance of the odd days for the crises was correct or not. This was done by collecting material and interpreting it in the framework of that doctrine. The doctrine was modified as a result: its applicability was extended to the even days.

It becomes, however, sufficiently clear that the author(s) of *Epidemics I* did not pave the way in this question. The number-lore of critical days as contained in some treatises other than *Epidemics I* and *III* comprises odd as well as even days, as was noted in the preceding chapter. Although the chronological relationship between these other doctrines and *Epidemics I* and *III* cannot be established precisely, there do not seem to be any convincing reasons to suppose that they are *all* younger than *Epidemics I* and *III*. Indeed, the day number doctrines contained in some of these treatises may be more ancient than the treatises themselves. To repeat the main features of the other doctrines: In *On Critical Days*, ch. 11, the crises occur "on the 4th, 7th, 11th, 14th, 17th, 21st day, and apart from these acute diseases, on the 30th, then on the 40th, then on the 60th day."[14] In *Prognostics*, ch. 20, the critical days are the 4th, 7th, 11th, 14th, 17th, 20th, etc.[15] Number systems in which the 7th day plays a prominent rôle admit that the even multiples of 7 also constitute critical days. This is the case in *Koan Prognoses* 147–148[16] and in the embryological text quoted above.[17]

---

12 Diels/Kranz, vol. 1, p. 451.29–31; Fritz Wehrli, Die Schule des Aristoteles, vol. 2 (Aristoxenos), 2nd ed., Basel/Stuttgart, 1967, frg. 23, cf. p. 54; Burkert, Lore 32–34.

13 For further attestation from Pythagorean sources, cf. Diels/Kranz, vol. 3, Wortindex, *s. v.* ἄρτιος and περιττός; Burkert, Lore 32–34, 264 f., 427 f., 434–438, 468–472; Roscher, Hebdomadenlehren 207 (bottom) f.; Roscher's references prove how firmly the doctrine of the critical nature of the odd days was upheld also in later antiquity. Cels. *III* 4.11–15 (p. 106 f. Marx).

14 Cf. above p. 94 f.

15 Cf. above p. 95.

16 Cf. above p. 94.

17 Cf. p. 99 f.

Obviously, the research on odd and even days undertaken in *Epidemics I* and *III* was not intended to lead into *terra incognita*: it concerned only a very marginal point of the doctrine and did not question the basic importance of the 'categories' odd and even.

Studying the historical background against which *Epidemics I* and *III* outlined their theory of critical days can thus help to clarify some of the objectives and methods of these books; the same holds true of the background of the closely interwoven complex of *krísis*, *pépsis*, and *apóstasis*. The preceding sections of the present chapter attempted to reconstruct some essential features of this doctrine. How coherent the 'theory' once was is unknown to us because we do not know all its particulars. Some details may, even within the *Epidemics*, have differed from book to book without our being able to recognize this, because these treatises are extremely inexplicit.[18] It might be meaningful for certain special purposes to discuss the 'level' of *On Diseases IV* and of other Hippocratic works because some of them are explicit enough concerning their theoretical premises and the conclusions they draw. As to the *Epidemics*, it seems useless to discuss their 'level.' These writings are so fragmentary (books *II, IV,* and *VI* even more than *I* and *III*) and reveal so little about their basic theoretical assumptions that questions as to their internal cohesiveness cannot reasonably be answered.

Thus an inquiry into the historical background of the *krísis*, *pépsis*, and *apóstasis* doctrines of the *Epidemics* should not start from the idea frequently expressed in modern literature that the scientific 'level' of the *Epidemics* was in any respect higher than that of other, or earlier treatises (e. g. *On Diseases II*, ch. 12—75). We shall try to trace scientific evolutions, but the question whether the development was in an upward or downward direction will not be asked.

It has been stated above that *On Diseases II*, ch. 12—75, one of the oldest texts of the Hippocratic Corpus,[19] contains certain doctrines which, although they are not identical with those of later treatises (e. g. *Epidemics I* and *III*), yet can, to a certain extent, be re-interpreted in the sense of their more recent doctrines;[20] that is to say, later Hippocratic authors, even though probably quite aware that their own doctrines represented a later stage of a scientific development, must have been able to use the older doctrines at least eclectically and to interpret them in the light of their own more developed theories. We do not know whether the author(s) of *Epidemics I* and *III* knew the treatise *On Diseases II*, ch. 12—75, nor, in particular, is there any proof that the author(s) of these later books re-

---

[18] Cf. below p. 136—149.

[19] p. 25, 52 f.

[20] Cf. above p. 67.

interpreted passages of that specific work through the filter of their own doctrines. *On Diseases II*, ch. 12–75 is but *one*, in fact a relatively old, surviving textbook representative of a nosological approach that is also found in some other treatises derived from a nosological literary source now lost.[21] The nosological approach, however, had not only a literary history traceable in the Hippocratic Collection, but above all a professional history of practical application in the medical craft. This non-literary history of the 'Hippocratic' nosology is less clearly recognizable but must have been more important than the literary one.

As Jouanna[22] and Grensemann[23] have demonstrated, the group of nosological and gynaecological books contained in the Hippocratic Collection testifies to a process of repeated re-interpretations of traditional nosological texts and doctrines; for example, the younger part of *On Diseases II* (the chapters 1–11) and the treatises *On Affections* and *On Diseases I* are in part re-interpretations and expansions of a common heritage in the light of a more recent binary theory centred on the two physiological humours phlegm and bile.[24] For the non-gynaecological treatises in particular, Jouanna's book gives a good idea of how some concepts recognizable only *in nuce* in the old *On Diseases II*, ch. 12–75 were subsequently developed in later treatises representative of the same nosological doctrinal and textbook tradition. The humoral pair phlegm/bile is but one example. Since the common literary source and the common professional origin of the nosological treatises comprised only a few elements that could not be observed directly through the senses,[25] and since in particular no complex physiological theory was underlying these source texts, this common literary and professional tradition was apt to be used as a background for any new physiological or pathological theory. This may be the reason why *On Diseases II*, ch. 12–75, in spite of being so archaic in comparison to other treatises, maintained its place as a textbook.

Perhaps the author(s) of *Epidemics I* and *III* did not use *On Diseases II*, ch. 12–75; but he (or they) stood in a literary as well as a non-literary tradition kindred to *On Diseases II*, ch. 12–75. Hence it is not surprising that *On Diseases II*, ch. 12–75 is largely compatible with *Epidemics I* and *III*. To the modern historian of medicine, this compatibility might seem less conspicuous because the 'historisch-kritische Methode' has educated him to look at the differences rather than at the similarities that exist

---

21 Cf. above p. 25, 52 f.
22 Jouanna, Archéologie *passim*.
23 Grensemann, Knidische Medizin *passim*.
24 Jouanna, Archéologie 141–142, 292–293, 347–348.
25 Cf. above p. 53 ff.

between two texts. For the ancient medical practitioner, however, the similarities between the doctrines of *On Diseases II*, ch. 12–75 and of *Epidemics I* and *III* must have been striking.[26]

As demonstrated above,[27] it is frequently expressed in *On Diseases II*, ch. 12–75 that a disease takes its course according to a particular time scheme, which is measured mostly in units of days. For many diseases, it is stated: "He dies within *n* days (or: on the *n*th day); if he survives them (or: it), he recovers."[28] An expansion of this type is a formula also repeatedly encountered: "He recovers if this or that happens; otherwise he dies within *n* days (or: on the *n*th day)."[29] In some passages single days are mentioned (indicated by ordinal numbers), but it would be incorrect to speak of 'critical days.' It is not single days which are critical but the period of *n* days or the period terminated by the *n*th day.[30] Although the event by which the patient is saved consists sometimes of a discharge of (harmful?) matters,[31] the modern historian of medicine would not call the event 'critical' in the sense of the *Epidemics* because the formulas employed do not express the point of time at which the event takes place, or at which the patient either dies or begins to recover. Even the expression "he dies on the *n*th day" must not, as has been demonstrated above,[32] be taken at face value. There are strong arguments in favour of the assumption that "on the *n*th day" is actually equivalent to "on the *n*th day or earlier," and hence is but a linguistic variant of "within *n* days."

Nevertheless, an ancient follower of the doctrine underlying *Epidemics I* and *III* (and the other *Epidemics*) could, to a certain extent, read his theory of *krísis*, *pépsis* ('cooking' or 'ripening') and *apóstasis* ('segregation' or 'evacuation' of the harmful substances) into the text of *On Diseases II*, ch. 12–75. This was possible for the same reason that certain inferable source texts of the ancient stage of nosology could again and again be re-interpreted in the light of new theories: they scarcely contained any indications about the internal pathological or physiological process but described the outward phenomena that could be perceived by the senses.

On Diseases II, ch. 16 is a good example.[33] It is about a disease of the head, in the course of which the patient has rigor, fever, and headache, especially pain in his ears, temples, forehead, and eyes. If somebody moves him, he vomits. Among other symptoms, it is stated that his teeth feel

---

[26] Langholf, Kompatibilität.
[27] Cf. above p. 61–68.
[28] Cf. p. 62–65.
[29] Cf. p. 65–67.
[30] Cf. p. 61–65.
[31] Cf. p. 65–67.
[32] Cf. p. 65.
[33] *Morb. II* 7.28.22–30.17 Li. = 150.8–151.16 Jouanna.

rough (as from acid), and that the blood vessels of his head are swollen and throb. "If this [patient] has an eruption through the nose or ears, there flows slightly purulent water, and he recovers: otherwise he generally dies within seven days."[34] For the author(s) of *Epidemics I* and *III* and for any other ancient physician sharing a doctrine kindred to the one of the *Epidemics*, the nosological process underlying *On Diseases II*, ch. 16 must have been absolutely clear: harmful humours which have concentrated in the head either 'ripen' there ('are cooked') until they are discharged in a thin, i. e. cooked, form (purulent water, *apóstasis*) through the nose or ears, or they remain more or less 'unripe,' 'uncooked,' and cause the patient's death.

Ch. 12 also describes a disease of the head:[35] The patient's head is benumbed, he urinates frequently, and for the rest he exhibits the symptoms of *straggūríē*. He suffers this for 9 days, and if water or mucus breaks through his nose or ears, he recovers, mostly on the 40th day.[36] As in ch. 16, this description can very well be interpreted in the sense of the doctrine contained in *Epidemics I* and *III*, according to which the harmful humours of the head, in this kind of disease, 'are cooked' or 'ripen' during 9 days, then leave the body as an *apóstasis*. (Two more chapters of *On Diseases II*, ch. 12–75, which permitted a re-interpretation, namely 40 and 41, have been quoted above, p. 67.)

The reason why the *pépsis*, *apóstasis*, and *krísis* doctrine of the *Epidemics* could so easily be applied to so many pathological processes (either to 'factual' disease descriptions like the ones contained in *On Diseases II*, ch. 12–75, or to observations in the daily routine of the ancient practitioner) lies in the fact that all of these three concepts were defined only vaguely. *Pépsis*, 'cooking,' 'ripening' was thought to be wrought by the internal heat, and to render the liquid substances (body humours) thinner and easier to overcome.[37] The origin of the concept is clearly popular, not theoretical. *Apóstasis* was the 'segregation' or 'evacuation' of the harmful matter "through all ways of excretion."[38] "Segregations occur either through the veins or the sinews or the bones or the tendons or the skin or other outlets. The segregations beneath the disease [beneath the diseased region] are good, [segregations] such as varicose veins or heaviness of the loin; the best ones are ... the ones through outflow, such as blood out of the nose, pus out of the ear, urine ... Those [patients] to whom this does

---

[34] Cf. above p. 65.

[35] *Morb. II* 7.18.19–22.17 Li. = 142.1–145.12 Jouanna. The words ὅταν πλήρης ... τούτων διαθερμανθεῖσα form part of the preceding chapter, cf. Jouanna (ed.), Hippocrate, Maladies II, p. 141.

[36] Cf. above p. 65 f.

[37] Cf. above p. 89, 120.

[38] *Epid. I* (cf. above p. 79).

not occur have segregations wrought in the teeth, eyes, nose, sweat ... [a list of a lot of other possible forms of *apóstasis* follows]."[39] Like other medical terms,[40] the word *apóstasis* was originally a political expression. Its meaning was 'defection,' 'revolt.' The body endeavours to banish the harmful substance and is not too particular about the ways of excretion.

The substance to be segregated from the body did not possess a generic name,[41] and nowhere is it systematically explained how it was contained in, or represented by, the various substances leaving the body during the *apóstasis.*[42] This vagueness does not seem to be just coincidence. Obviously the physicians of the fifth and fourth centuries B. C., who operated with the concept, were not able and/or not willing to be very explicit. A theory which is vague has a wider range of applicability. In fact, these same theoretical concepts of *pépsis* and *apóstasis* were considered appropriate to describe pathological 'reality' until the beginning of the nineteenth century A. D.[43]

The same applies to the third central concept, *krísis*, which was equally vague, and was necessarily so because it was thought to be a function of *pépsis* and *apóstasis.* (*krísis* and *krī́nō* never signify 'excretion,' 'to excrete;' in this sense, the compounds *apo-* and *ek-* are used.) As has been demonstrated above, there is no agreement among the various lists of 'critical days' contained in some treatises of the Hippocratic Collection. The very chronology of the days potentially critical in the course of the diseases seems to have been controversial, although there are no overt polemics in the Collection about that point; *quot capita tot sententiae.* The word *krísis* itself and the kindred verb *krī́nō* were not coined by medical theorists to designate a well-defined process; they were, like other medical words, taken over from the sphere of daily life, more especially of social and political activities.[44] How vaguely *krísis* was 'defined' can be recognized by studying the verb *krī́nō* in *Epidemics I* and *III.* Since a verb form in Greek, as in many other languages, usually contains some information about the person(s) or thing(s) involved in the action ("who or what acts or is acted upon?"), we can learn something about the elements regarded as being constitutive of a *krísis* in *Epidemics I* and *III.*[45]

The verb *krī́nō*, which originally means 'to put asunder,' 'to judge,' 'to decide,' is used in various grammatical ways, even within the stylistically

---

[39] *Epid. II* (cf. above p. 80).

[40] Cf. above p. 89, 96, and the following remarks on *krísis* and *krī́nō*.

[41] Cf. above p. 80.

[42] Except for the cases where humours like bile, phlegm etc. are said to leave the body.

[43] This was due to the influence of Galen; cf. Owsei Temkin, Galenism: Rise and decline of a medical philosophy, Ithaca/London, 1973.

[44] Cf. above note 40.

[45] The topic is briefly discussed in Thivel, Cnide 180 f.

quite homogeneous text of *Epidemics I* and *III*. The variety of grammatical constructions reflects the uncertainty of the author(s) as to what is really happening during a *krísis*. A similar variety of the construction of *krī́nō* can be encountered in texts by other Hippocratic authors, as will shortly be demonstrated; the uncertainty was not confined to *Epidemics I* and *III*.

The verb is used in the active and in the passive voice. When used in the active, *krī́nō* can have as its grammatical subject either the disease or a symptom of the disease. In *Epidemics I*, ch. 4 Li. (= ch. 6 Kw., Jones), the tertian fevers "judged" (something), but it is not expressed here whom or what they judged since there is no object connected with the verb.[46] *III*, ch. 12 says that "the segregations which happened to these [patients] did not judge," again without an accusative.[47] Cf. *IV* 41 "The segregations judge."[48] A dative is added in *I*, ch. 4 (= ch. 8 Kw., Jones): (Certain aforesaid symptoms) "judged *for* some of them," i. e., judged *on behalf of* some patients.[49] In passages outside *Epidemics I* and *III*, grammatical objects in the accusative are given; in two texts, certain symptoms 'judge' diseases: *Epidemics VI* 3.21 "The occurring ulcers and swellings which judge the fevers."[50] And *On Crises* 15 = *Aphorisms* 4.36, "These perspirations judge diseases."[51] In *Articulations*, ch. 69 a reflexive construction is used: "[The gangrenous limbs] judge themselves."[52]

In the active, it was also possible to say in the *Epidemics*, "[he, she, it] judged," without an object and probably with the disease to be supplied as the agent, e. g. *I*, ch. 9 Li. (= ch. 20 Kw., Jones).[53]

Similarly it is expressed in the passive voice that diseases are judged, but the word 'disease' is not used. The agent of the judgement is not mentioned in this construction: *Epidemics I*, ch. 12 Li. (= ch. 26 Kw., Jones) "That which has the paroxysm(s) on even days is judged on even

---

46 *Epid. I* 2.620.9 Li. = 1.186.5 Kw. = 1.156 Jones ἔκριναν (VIR: ἔκρινον A).

47 *Epid. III* 3.92.10–11 Li. = 1.229.25–230.1 Kw. = 1.250 Jones οὐδὲ γὰρ αἱ γινόμεναι τούτοισιν ἀποστάσιες ἔκρινον ὥσπερ ἐπὶ τοῖσιν ἄλλοισι.

48 *Epid. IV* 5.182.6 Li. = Per. 244 La. αἱ ... ἀποστάσιες ... κρίνουσι.

49 *Epid. I* 2.626.8–9 Li. = 1.187.21–22 Kw. = 1.160 Jones ἔστι δ' οἷσιν ἔκρινεν αὐτῶν ὀλίγοισιν.

50 *Epid. VI* 5.302.9 = 72 Manetti/Roselli τὰ γινόμενα ἕλκεα καὶ φύματα, κρίνοντα πυρετούς.

51 *Judic.* 9.280.25–26 ≈ *Aph.* 4.516.1 Li. = 4.144 Jones οὗτοι οἱ ἱδρῶτες νούσους κρίνουσιν. Cf. also *Aph.* 4.540.4–5 Li. = 4.162 Jones ≈ *Liqu.* 6.134.15–136.1 Li. = 170.18–20 Joly τὸ θερμὸν φίλιον καὶ κρῖνον, τὸ δὲ ψυχρὸν πολέμιον καὶ κτεῖνον.

52 *Art.* 4.286.11–12 Li. = 2.223.16–17 Kw. = 3.364 Withington αὐτὰ γὰρ ἑωυτὰ κρίνει μοῦνον.

53 *Epid. I* 2.660.9, 662.3 Li. = 1.197.3, 7 Kw. = 1.176 Jones ἔκρινεν ἑκταίῳ ... ἔκρινε δὲ τοῖσι πλείστοισιν ... More cases of the active are found in this chapter, where also the passive voice is used indiscriminately.

days."[54] (In the same chapter, the active voice is used indiscriminately.) The patient can be mentioned in the dative. Again no mention of the agent: *Epidemics I*, ch. 9 Li. (= ch. 20 Kw., Jones) "For both patients [it] was judged at the same time on the 17th day."[55] Cf. *IV* 7 "On the 6th day it [neuter plural] was judged for the young girl, on the 6th day [it] returned, all [neuter plural] was judged on the 6th day. During these times [of the year], all [neuter plural] was judged on the 6th and 8th day."[56] Similarly it can be said in the passive voice that patients 'are judged:' *I*, ch. 9 Li. (= ch. 19 Kw., Jones), literally, "Many [patients] happened not to be judged during [only] one of the symptoms."[57] The agent of the judgement is not expressed here either; "during" (*epí* with genitive) is much more vague than, e. g., "by" would be. Also in the following passages from outside the *Epidemics I* and *III* no agent is indicated: *Epidemics II* 3.11 "On the next day, he was judged, and he was without fever."[58] *IV* 20 "Another one out of those who came from Leokydes was judged on the 7th day."[59] *Koan Prognoses* 586 "Patients whose urine gets a sediment quickly are judged quickly."[60] In numerous passages it is only stated ambiguously, "[he?, she?, it?] was judged." Since the Greek verb form *ekríthē* does not contain any indication of a gender, it may refer to the patient ("he, she was judged") as well as to the disease ("it"); examples are found at the end of the cases no. 3, 5, 6, 7, 13 of *Epidemics I* and in many other passages of *Epidemics I* and *III*. (This passive construction is again used indiscriminately together with the active one, "[he, she, it] judged.") Although active constructions may mention an agent, there is no passage which expresses in the passive that a symptom or a disease or a patient is judged *by* anything.

The variety of grammatical constructions with incompatible and even contradictory meanings is indeed remarkable: Diseases or segregations judge (whom? or what?); segregations judge diseases; gangrenes judge themselves; (he?, she?, it?) judges (whom? or what?); diseases are judged (by what? or by whom?); 'it,' viz. the disease, is judged for a patient; the

---

54 *Epid. I* 2.678.5–6 Li. = 1.201.18–19 Kw. = 1.184 Jones τὰ δὲ παροξυνόμενα ἐν ἀρτίῃσι κρίνεται ἐν ἀρτίῃσι.

55 *Epid. I* 2.662.2–3 Li. = 1.197.6–8 Kw. = 1.176 Jones ἐκρίθη ἀμφοτέροισιν ὁμοῦ … ἑπτακαιδεκαταίοισιν.

56 *Epid. IV* 5.148.13–14 Li. = Per. 89 La. ἕκτῃ τῇ παρθένῳ κριθέντα, ἕκτῃ ὑπετροπίασεν, ἐκρίθη δὲ δι' ἕκτης πάντα. ἐν τούτοισι τοῖσι χρόνοισιν ἑκταῖα ὀγδοαῖα ἐκρίνετο.

57 *Epid. I* 2.658.2–3 Li. = 1.196.3–4 Kw. = 1.174 Jones πολλοῖσι δὲ συνέπιπτε μὴ ἐφ' ἑνὸς κρίνεσθαι τῶν … σημείων.

58 *Epid. II* 5.114.4 Li. = Per. 56 La. τῇ δ' ὑστεραίῃ κριθεὶς ἀπύρετος.

59 *Epid. IV* 5.158.17–18 Li. = Per. 143 La. ἄλλος τῶν παρὰ Λεωκύδεος ἐκρίθη ἑβδόμῃ, ἄλλος τετάρτῃ.

60 *Coac.* 5.720.9–10 οἷσιν οὖρα ταχέως ὑπόστασιν ἴσχει, ταχέως οὗτοι κρίνονται. (This is the reading of the only relevant codex, A.)

patient is judged (by what? or by whom?); finally, "(he?, she?, it?) is judged" (by what? or by whom?) with ambiguous reference either to the disease or to the patient. No medical 'term' produced by a systematic theory would have been employed so unsystematically.

Obviously the author(s) of *Epidemics I* and *III* did not coin the expressions *krísis* or *krī́nō* but inherited them from a traditional professional environment which included medical literature. Although the substantive *krísis* is practically unheard-of in the more conservative nosological treatises of the Hippocratic Collection (it is absent from *On Diseases II*, ch. 12–75; *On Diseases II*, ch. 1–11; *On Affections; On Diseases I*; in *On Internal Diseases* it is used only once, ch. 27[61]), the verb *krī́nō* is not infrequent in these works and is used mostly in the passive voice, "the disease is judged," e. g. *On Affections*, ch. 7 "The disease is judged at its shortest on the 7th, at its longest on the 14th day."[62] Ch. 10 "The disease is judged at its shortest on the 7th, at its longest on the 11th day."[63] Similarly ch. 11.[64]

Some grammatical usages of *krī́nō* found in *Epidemics I* and *III* and in kindred works are innovations in comparison to the usage in the more conservative nosological books. Two (old?) technical expressions with *krī́nō*, however, were not taken over by the authors of *Epidemics I* and *III* and of other texts. In the nosological treatise *On Internal Diseases* it is stated on several occasions that a certain number of days "judge whether the disease is deadly or not," e. g. ch. 24, "He should abstain from food during the first 10 days; because they judge whether it [the disease] is fatal [other possible translation: whether he is to die] or not."[65] Ch. 35 "Do not boil honey together with it [the gruel] before 10 days are over; because they judge whether it [the disease] is fatal or not."[66] More explicit is ch. 49: "From this disease the patient recovers when 30 days are over, because they judge whether it is fatal [other possible translation: whether he is to die] or not. The disease is serious."[67] Along with this type of expression, the same treatise has another one; e. g. in ch. 21, "It is judged in 30 days

---

[61] *Int.* 7.238.24 Li.; see Jouanna, Archéologie 432, and his footnote 1.

[62] *Aff.* 6.214.23–216.2 κρίνεται δὲ ἡ νοῦσος ἡ μὲν βραχυτάτη ἑβδόμῃ, ἡ δὲ μακροτάτη τετάρτῃ καὶ δεκάτῃ.

[63] *Aff.* 6.218.9–10 κρίνεται δὲ ἡ μὲν βραχυτάτη ἑβδόμῃ (ἑβδόμῃ θ: ἑβδομαίη M), ἡ δὲ μακροτάτη ἑνδεκάτῃ (ἑνδεκάτῃ θ: ἑνδεκαταίη M).

[64] *Aff.* 6.218.23–220.1 κρίνεται δὲ ἡ μὲν βραχυτάτη ἐνάτῃ (ἢ δεκάτη post ἐν. add. M: om. θ), ἡ δὲ μακροτάτη τεσσαρεσκαιδεκάτῃ.

[65] *Int.* 7.228.9–10 σιτίων δὲ ἀπεχέσθω τὰς πρώτας ἡμέρας δέκα· αὗται γὰρ κρίνουσιν εἰ (εἰ θ: ἢ M) θανάσιμος ἢ οὔ.

[66] *Int.* 7.254.5–7 μὴ συνεψεῖν τὸ μέλι, ἕως ἂν τεσσερεσκαίδεκα (τεσσ. θ: αἱ δεκατέσσαρες M) ἡμέραι παρέλθωσιν· αὗται γὰρ κρίνουσιν ἢν θανάσιμον (κρ. ἢν θαν. M: κρίνουσι θανασίμους θ) ἢ οὔ.

[67] *Int.* 7.290.20–22 ταύτῃ τῇ νούσῳ ἢν τριήκοντα ἡμέραι παρέλθωσιν, ὑγιαίνεται ὁ ἄνθρωπος· αὗται γὰρ κρίνουσιν εἰ θανάσιμος ἢ οὔ· ἡ δὲ (δὲ θ: γὰρ M) νοῦσος χαλεπή.

whether it [the disease] is fatal or not."[68] And more explicitly ch. 27: "He should abstain from food until the disease is judged; it is judged within 7 days mostly, because within these days it becomes clear whether it is fatal [other possible translation: whether he is to die] or not."[69] Ch. 39 "For this [patient] the disease is judged within 7 or 14 days ... If he escapes them, he is healthy; for within these days it becomes clear whether it [the disease] is fatal [other possible translation: whether he is to die] or not."[70]

The usage of *krī́nō* in *On Internal Diseases* is quite simple and unproblematic if the English translation 'to judge' is replaced by 'to decide' (which is not appropriate for all passages in *Epidemics I* and *III*).[71] In this nosological treatise and in the other conservative ones, it is not single days which usually bring a decision but spaces of several days, even where ordinal numbers are used for the days ("on the *n*th day" = "on the *n*th day or earlier," cf. above p. 61 ff.). The expression "so-and-so many days judge (or: decide) whether the disease is deadly or not" is nothing but a mode of expression popular in ancient Greek and still in modern languages, a metonymy instead of "in so-and-so many days it is decided whether ..." There is no mystery as to any agent of a *krísis* in those treatises because there is no *event* that could reasonably be called a *krísis*. As soon as so-and-so many particularly dangerous days are over, one knows about the outcome of the disease — that is it. The fact that in the group of more conservative nosological treatises of the Hippocratic Collection the word *krísis* occurs but once, whereas the verb *krī́nō* is rather frequent is, therefore, no coincidence.

On Affections, ch. 8 has a general description of what it means 'to be judged' or 'to be decided' (the word *krísis* is not used): "To be decided is, in the diseases, when the diseases increase or diminish or turn into another disease or are terminated."[72] This passage is not a definition of a *krísis* (although the more elaborate *pépsis*, *apóstasis*, and *krísis* doctrine of *Epidemics I* and *III* and of other treatises could be read into it), but a description of what may happen during the particularly dangerous days of a disease.

---

68 *Int.* 7.220.9—10 κρίνεται δὲ ἐν τριήκοντα ἡμέρῃσιν εἰ (εἰ edd.: ἢ θΜ) θανάσιμον ἢ οὔ.

69 *Int.* 7.238.12—14 σιτίων δὲ ἀπεχέσθω τέως (τέως θ: ἕως Μ) ἂν κριθῇ ἡ νοῦσος· κρίνεται δὲ μάλιστα ἐν ἑπτὰ ἡμέρῃσιν· ἐν (ἐν θ: om. Μ) ταύτῃσι γὰρ ἀποδηλοῖ (ἀπ. θ: δηλοῖ Μ) εἰ (εἰ θ: ἢ Μ) θανάσιμος ἢ οὔ.

70 *Int.* 7.262.10—13 τούτῳ ἡ νοῦσος κρίνεται ἐν ἑπτὰ ἡμέρῃσιν ἢ τεσσερεσκαίδεκα (τεσ. θ: δεκατέσσαρσιν Μ) ... ἢν οὖν ταύτας ἐκφύγῃ (ἐκφ. θ: διαφύγῃ Μ), ὑγιής ἐστιν (ἐστιν θ: ἔσται Μ)· ἐν γὰρ (γὰρ θ: δὲ Μ) ταύτῃσι τῇσιν ἡμέρῃσι διαδηλοῖ εἰ (εἰ θ: ἢ Μ) θανάσιμος ἢ οὔ.

71 The verb *krī́nō* means both, cf. above p. 67, 81.

72 *Aff.* 6.216.4—5 κρίνεσθαι δέ ἐστιν ἐν τῇσι νούσοισιν ὅταν αὔξωνται αἱ νοῦσοι ἢ μαραίνωνται ἢ μεταπίπτωσιν ἐς ἕτερον νόσημα ἢ τελευτῶσιν.

For the modern historian of medicine, it is tempting to speculate that not only the various grammatical usages of *krī́nō* found in *Epidemics I* and *III*, but the whole concept of the reciprocal functions of *pépsis*, *apóstasis*, and *krísis* have one of their roots (but there must have been more roots[73]) in doctrines like the ones contained in the nosological treatises, where recurrent types of expression are, "He dies within so and so many days; if he survives them, he recovers"[74] or "It is decided in so and so many days whether the disease is deadly or not."[75] They reflect phenomena which are in fact typical of the processes observable in many acute diseases. An early extension is the formula already encountered in *On Diseases II*, ch. 12–75: "He recovers if this or that happens; otherwise he dies within so-and-so many days."[76]

It is but a small step intellectually to attribute to "this or that" a decisive power, i. e. to see in the very event the turning point of the patient's fate (*post hoc, ergo propter hoc*), particularly if the 'event' consists of an excretion or expulsion of foul or morbid matter. As soon as a theory about 'harmful substances' gained influence on medical thinking, the causal connection of the 'segregation' with the event of the turning point became inevitable.[77] The postulate of a 'ripening' of the 'harmful substance' was a further step to account for the usually observable delay between the beginning of a disease and the 'event.'

Only after the 'decision' about the outcome of the disease was no longer identical with the favourable or fatal result of an especially dangerous *space* of time, but had become a function of a 'harmful substance' 'segregated' or 'evacuated' in a (more or less) 'ripened' or 'cooked' state during an 'event' which happened at a *point* of time, did it become meaningful to speak of a *krísis*, of 'critical days,' 'critical segregations,'

---

[73] Another root of the doctrine concerning *krísis* and critical days must have been the speculation about particular days of good or bad omen (cf. Hes. *Op.* 765–828) and about numbers, in particular odd numbers, seven, etc. (cf. above p. 93 ff.). Kindred to this speculation about days is the one about the influence of astronomical events such as solstices, equinoxes and the risings and settings of stars (cf. below p. 164 ff.). Still another origin of the concept of *krísis* may lie in expressions like νόσημα ... ἀποκεκριμένον, 'localized disease' (as opposed to the more unfavourable case, namely a disease spread over the whole body) Pl. *Resp. III* 407 cd, cf. ἀποκρίνω and ἐκκρίνω 'to secrete' in *Morb. I* 6.190.14–192.10 Li. = 74.1–76.1 Wittern. There is some semantical overlapping between 'segregation' (ἀπόστασις, ἀφίστασθαι) and 'secretion' (ἀπο-, ἐκκρίνω), because the latter may be a special form of ἀπόστασις.

[74] Cf. above p. 62–65.

[75] Cf. above p. 130 f.

[76] Cf. above p. 65–67.

[77] The 'harmful substance' acting within the body is familiar to the medical imagination of many 'primitive' peoples. Rudiments of the concept are found in old nosological books of the Corpus such as *On Diseases II*, ch. 12–75, e. g. "wood-worm in the bone," "water in the brain," "dropsy in the lung," cf. above p. 55 f.

even of a 'pseudo-*krísis*,' an event which apparently *is* critical because it consists of a 'segregation' on a potentially 'critical day,' but after which the disease continues; that is, a *krísis* which is not a *final krísis* (e. g. because the matters segregated are not sufficiently 'ripe' or 'cooked'). And only after the event, *krísis*, had come into an artificial existence through the process of reification just outlined, did it become meaningful to look for crises in any kind or instance of disease, even if the patient did not exhibit any morbid excretions. Since every organism continuously discharges substances such as stool, urine, sweat, it became meaningful to ask questions as to the 'critical' significance of certain forms of these discharges, and to the agent of a *krísis*.

This stage of development was already reached in *Epidemics I* and *III* and in kindred treatises (e. g. in the other *Epidemics* and in the *Prognostics*). The development cannot be traced step by step in the extant treatises of the Hippocratic Collection. We see what appears to be an early stage in some conservative nosological texts and a final stage in the *Epidemics* and similar writings.[78] Therapeutics may have played a considerable rôle in the re-interpretation of the 'decisive space of time:' a recurrent, typical feature of the nosological and other treatises of the Collection is the prescription of liquid foodstuff (drinks, gruels) until the dangerous days are over, and then to switch over to solid food.[79] This change of diet after the decisive period must, from a practitioner's point of view, have been an 'event' and may perhaps also have contributed to the interpretation of the final day of the period as an 'event.'

The 'decisive space of time' characteristic of the nosological treatises prior to the *Epidemics* has, however, left linguistic traces in these latter works. An oscillation between cardinal and ordinal numbers similar to that observed in *On Diseases II*, ch. 12–75[80] can be found in the *Epidemics*, where expressions like "around *n* days" are rather frequently used synonymously instead of "around the *n*th day" (e. g. *Epidemics I*, ch. 3 "around the 80 days;"[81] *Epidemics V* 73 ≈ *VII* 1 "around the 12 and 14 days ... ; around the 15 days"[82]). It is possible to account for this mode of expression

[78] Deichgräber was not right when he wrote about *krísis* (Die Epidemien p. 42): "Dieses Wort hat innerhalb des hippokratischen Corpus und insbesondere innerhalb der Epidemien keine Geschichte, es wird hier als ein bekannter Begriff der Krankheitsbeschreibung verwandt, ohne daß man seine historische Quelle fassen könnte."

[79] Lonie, A structural pattern *passim*.

[80] Cf. above p. 61–65.

[81] *Epid. I* 2.612.6 Li. = 1.183.12 Kw. = 1.152 Jones περὶ τὰς (τὰς V Gal.: om. IR) ὀγδοήκοντα (ὀγδ. VR: π′ I).

[82] *Epid. V* 5.246.15–17 περὶ δὲ τὰς δεκαδύο καὶ δεκατέσσαρας ... περὶ τὰς δεκαπέντε. ≈ *Epid. VII* 5.364.10–13 περὶ δὲ τὰ⟨ς⟩ δώδεκα καὶ τεσσαρεσκαίδεκα ... περὶ δὲ τὰς πεντεκαίδεκα.

in purely linguistic terms,[83] but linguistics, although offering some valuable insight into the phenomenon, cannot describe it exhaustively. The evolution of the medical *krísis* doctrine as outlined above must likewise have played a rôle in the formation of the expression "around *n* days," which can best be explained as an idiomatic 'fossil' reflecting the ancient doctrine of 'decisive periods' during a more recent epoch when the physicians' interest had already concentrated on the end-points of these periods, namely on the 'critical days.' The linguistic explanation and an explanation in terms of medical history are not mutually exclusive.[84]

One can observe that the doctrines contained in the nosological texts are, to a very large extent, compatible with the ones of the later books, more precisely, that the doctrines of *Epidemics, Prognostics*, and kindred texts can largely be read into the earlier treatises. Thus, to the ancient physician, the older treatises not only did not essentially contradict those more recent, but they could even be used to support the later doctrines.

Moreover, daily routine was the best proof that the doctrine of *Epidemics I* and *III* and of other kindred treatises was defensible. For *krísis, pépsis*, and *apóstasis* can apparently be observed through the senses. 'Critical' symptoms can be seen, felt, touched, etc.: potentially critical days can be counted; thinner (i. e. 'cooked') body substances can be distinguished from thicker (i. e. 'raw'). One of the major achievements of the early nosological approach of Greek medicine, such as is reflected in *On Diseases II*, ch. 12–75, had been to rely more or less exclusively on symptoms which were observable through the senses, and at first sight a modern reader of the *Epidemics* might believe that this was still the standard and basic procedure in the latter treatises, which seemingly upheld the tradition; for example, *Epidemics VI* 8.17: "It is necessary to use the body for observation: sight, hearing, nose, touch, tongue, intelligence."[85]

As soon as one looks closer, however, one recognizes that *krísis, pépsis*, and *apóstasis* were not only vaguely defined but could not even be observed. The very formation of the three Greek words shows that they are abstracts, substantives denoting actions. These actions or processes were conceived of as happening *inside* the body. All that could be observed were outward phenomena believed to be related to the inward process. Their observation implied an interpretation of what was supposed to be going on within.[86]

---

[83] This has been done in Langholf, Syntaktische Untersuchungen p. 97–102, where a complete collection of the relevant material is found.

[84] Perhaps it was possible to apply the older 'petrified' expression to the more modern doctrine because of a latent tendency in Greek to use cardinal instead of ordinal numbers. For 'fossils' see also p. 45, 54 f., 253 f. For traces of the jargon of *Morb. II* in *Epid.*, see below p. 152, note 90.

[85] Cf. above p. 51, where more passages are quoted.

[86] Cf. above p. 75 f.

In *Epidemics I* and *III* and in the treatises related to them (the other *Epidemics, Prognostics*), there is doubtless a large amount of observation but it is less unbiased than in *On Diseases II*, ch. 12–75.

The development outlined so far proceeded from popular speculation on what happens inside the body, and from traditional word usage (e. g. Homeric *khólos* 'gall,' 'wrath,' 'anger;' *phrḗn* 'contents of the chest,' 'mental function (of these organs);' *kradíē* 'heart,' 'function of the heart') towards a narrowing of the meaning of such words. The semantic fields of words used by Greek professional physicians were narrower also in comparison to contemporary (fifth and fourth centuries B. C.) colloquial usage (e. g. in Aristophanes' comedies).[87] The narrowing was towards a concrete meaning. The oldest nosological texts extant in the Hippocratic Collection testify to a stage at which observation through the senses, but without an underlying detailed theory about what goes on inside the patient's body, was prominent. Certain traditional expressions and names identifying some of the disease entities are perhaps remnants of a still earlier, more speculative phase.[88] In the *Epidemics*, observation through the senses continues to be prominent; but this observation is to a large extent governed by underlying physiological and pathological theories, particularly the *krísis*, *pépsis*, and *apóstasis* doctrine. Speculation has re-entered Greek medicine.

3. Research Methods Traceable in the Epidemics

Let us now consider the conditions under which "speculation re-entered medicine," and the nature of this speculation. It is not unreasonable to speak of a 'system' with regard to some of the theories or concepts underlying the *Epidemics* treatises, for instance *krísis, pépsis*, and *apóstasis*, because they are clearly complementary. Any attempt, however, to reconstruct such a 'system' in its entirety would be futile: first because the *Epidemics* are never explicit about the underlying theories; second because the *Epidemics* are composite treatises, whose literary origin is only vaguely known to us. Books *I* and *III* are probably by the same author, or one closely organized group of authors. As to *II, IV, V, VI*, and *VII*, it is possible that they are comprised of materials from various sources and perhaps by various authors.

---

87 Cf. above p. 37–51.

88 Cf. above p. 55 f.

Lack of Explicitness in the *Epidemics*

All texts contained in the *Epidemics* seem to fit together doctrinally, but this apparent mutual compatibility might to some extent be the result of their inexplicitness. For example, there are statements which suggest that the theory of four humours as expounded in *On the Nature of Man* underlies the *Epidemics*. At *VI* 5.8 we find: "The tongue indicates the humour: Yellow tongues are *bilious*, and the *bile* is from greasy food. Red ones are from *blood*. Black ones are from *black bile* (dry ones from sooty burning and from the uterus). White ones are from *phlegm*."[1] A passage in *Epidemics III* (ch. 14) suggests the same scheme of four humours.[2] On the other hand, more humours are mentioned in the *Epidemics* as being operative in the human body, e. g. various kinds of mucus (apart from phlegm),[3] fluxes of viscous consistency,[4] serous[5] and salty[6] liquids. Moreover, black bile, which functions as an independent humour in the scheme of *On the Nature of Man*,[7] appears as a putrefied or otherwise corrupted product of the blood, or of blood plus bile.[8] A particularly interesting passage in this respect is *Epidemics VI* 6.14: "The bilious and sanguineous body becomes affected with black bile if it has no evacuations."[9] The text seems to be a re-interpretation of a very similar passage contained in

---

[1] *Epid. VI* 5.318.5–8 γλῶσσα ὀρὸν (γλ. ὀρὸν sec. Gal. ci. Jouanna (ed.), Hippocrate, La nature de l'homme, p. 49 n. 6: γλ. οὖρον MV Gal.: οὖρον γλ. Pall.: lingua urinam Joh.) σημαίνει· γλῶσσαι χλωραὶ χολώδεις, τὸ δὲ χολῶδες ἀπὸ πίονος. ἐρυθραὶ δὲ ἀφ' αἵματος. μέλαιναι δὲ ἀπὸ μελαίνης χολῆς – αὖαι δὲ ἀπὸ ἐκκαύσιος λιγνυώδεος (ἐ. λ. MV: λ. ἐ. Gal.: λιγνύος Pall.: ab exustione. fuliginose vero Joh., i. e. ἀπὸ ἐκκαύσιος· λιγνυώδεες) καὶ μητρῴου μορίου –. λευκαὶ δὲ ἀπὸ φλέγματος.

[2] *Epid. III* 3.96.4–98.5 Li. = 1.231.12–18 Kw. = 1.254 Jones, cf. below p. 200 f., note 343.

[3] *Epid. IV* 5.144.3 Li. = Per. 66 La. τὰ ... βλεννώδεα. 148.5 Li. = Per. 87 La. κόρυζαι.

[4] *Epid. IV* 5.156.2–3 Li. = Per. 125 La. ὠτὸς ῥεῦμα ... γλίσχρον παχύ. 156.11 Li. = Per. 129 La. ἐκ ῥινῶν παχέα ῥεύματα.

[5] *Epid. II* 5.72.5 ἰχῶρες. *Epid. VI* 5.288.5 αἵματος ... ἰχωροειδέος.

[6] *Epid. IV* 5.178.11–12 Li. = Per. 230 La. ἁλμῶδες ἐκ τῶν ὀφθαλμῶν ἦλθε δάκνον δάκρυον, καὶ κατὰ ῥῖνα καὶ κατὰ φάρυγγα καὶ οὖς ἀριστερόν. Cf. Langholf, Syntaktische Untersuchungen *ad loc.* Saltiness of the body is also mentioned in *Epid. II* 5.82.9–10; *Epid. VI* 5.326.4–5.

[7] Although some statements in that treatise suggest that the black bile was not yet completely distinguished from bile in general, cf. Jouanna (ed.), Hippocrate, La nature de l'homme, p. 49. – For the possible origin of the concept of black bile see above p. 46–50.

[8] *Epid. VI* 5.322.9–10 says that the little vessels excrete yellow bile if greasy matters dominate, and black bile if the blood dominates. The underlying theory can be recovered from a similar one outlined in *Aer.* 2.50.12–14 Li. = 1.52.2–6 Kw. = 1.102–104 Jones. For the relationship between bile and black bile, cf. throughout Müri, Melancholie; Flashar, Melancholie 21–49.

[9] *Epid. VI* 5.330.7–8 τὸ ἐπίχολον καὶ ἔναιμον σῶμα μελαγχολικὸν μὴ ἔχον ἐξεράσιας (ἐξ. ci. Manetti/Roselli: Entleerungen Gal.: extractiones Joh.: ἐξερώσιας MV Pall.).

Epidemics II 3.15: "I believe that the sanguineous and bilious [body] is affected with heartburn. Perhaps it results in 'the black' with these [patients]."[10] "The black" is ambiguous. It can mean the black bile or the 'black disease,' whose nosological description in *On Diseases II*, ch. 73 contains or implies all the elements mentioned in the *Epidemics II* passage (vomit of blood, of bile, and of acrid matters[11]). Perhaps "the black" means both. For a physician believing in black bile as an important body humour, the 'black disease' was plausibly caused by an excess of this liquid. It is needless to emphasize that the four humours theory is not necessarily incompatible with the postulate of more than four humours. Indeed, the authors of the *Epidemics* might have assumed that the other humours were secondary deformations of the four, or they might have believed that a multitude of more or less separate and autonomous humours existed, and might all the same in certain contexts and for purposes unknown to us (perhaps for didactic purposes?) have analytically singled out the four well-known ones.

When reading the *Epidemics*, particularly books *II, IV*, and *VI*, one intuitively gets the impression that these texts were originally scattered notes, possibly by various authors, jotted down for private, perhaps even personal, use, or for use within a small group of people closely working together (for instance, teachers and students). Galen repeatedly expresses this opinion when trying to explain why the language and style of the *Epidemics* are so concise and, therefore, so difficult to understand. Exemplary here is his statement in his commentary on *Epidemics VI*: "Hippocrates seems to have written this [a particular passage] as a short summary for himself and in order to aid his memory, therefore the passage is rather obscure."[12] In such a situation not only the language could omit much that under other circumstances would have been indispensable syntactically and semantically,[13] but also on the level of the doctrine much could be presupposed without even giving the slightest hint as to what was meant. This doctrinal as well as linguistic inexplicitness must have made it hard for the authors' contemporaries to understand the *Epidemics*,

---

[10] *Epid. II* 5.116.3–5 οἶμαι τὸ ἔναιμον καὶ τὸ ὑπόχολον ὀξυρεγμιῶδες· ἴσως δὲ ἐς μέλαιναν τούτοισι τελευτᾶν.

[11] *Morb. II* 7.110.14–112.12 Li. = p. 109 Jouanna. Cf. Kudlien, Beginn 77–88.

[12] Gal. *In Hp. Epid. VI comm.* p. 29.34–35 Wenkebach/Pfaff. This is merely a conjecture by Galen or by his learned predecessors, which cannot be proved correct. Galen's belief that the Great Hippocrates himself was the author of this text lacks support through testimony. More passages from Galen are quoted in Langholf, Syntaktische Untersuchungen 11 f.

[13] Deichgräber, Die Epidemien 64–74, 143 f. Langholf, Syntaktische Untersuchungen *passim*. López Férez, Historia 633–637. For examples from the *materia medica* (Κνίδιος κόκκος etc.), see above p. 29 f.

particularly books II, IV, and VI, unless they were members of their circle. Galen's commentaries on books II and VI written more than half a millennium later bear unintentional witness to these difficulties. For the modern historian of medicine, the obstacles are still greater because he no longer participates in the living tradition of ancient medicine as Galen did. Our advantage, however, as compared to the situation of ancient commentators, is that we are not obliged to follow any theoretical system, if such a system does not impose itself in single Hippocratic treatises. For example, Galen read his own systematic medical doctrines into those Hippocratic treatises which he regarded as authentic works of Hippocrates, or as worthy of the Master, in order to corroborate his own system.[14] This is the reason why in the present investigation Galen's works are scarcely quoted for their interpretations of Hippocratic texts. We do not, furthermore, feel obliged to reconstruct a 'Hippocratic system,' but always have to consider the possibility that some doctrines surfacing in the *Epidemics* did not form a 'system' but coexisted unreconciled or isolated.

Inexplicitness is sometimes stated explicitly. Here are some examples: *Epidemics II* 3.2, "*We know* the properties of drugs, and which [effects] arise out of which [properties]. For not all [properties] are adequate, but each of them [viz. of the properties] in its way and at its place; [drugs differ when] taken earlier or later; [drugs differ] through the processes such as drying or pulverizing or boiling, *and so on: I omit most of it*; and ..., *and so on*."[15] The text mentions some of the details although the user is supposed to know them already. *IV* 57: "Kritias, during a fever, suffered from dreams *which we know*."[16] Here the text gives no hint as to their content. *VI* 1.13 [Certain conditions of the eye are bad signs,] "and also the other ones *which have not been mentioned*."[17] The user of the text is supposed to know these "other" conditions. Sometimes expressions like "and so on" or "of the kind" occur without an indication as to what might be referred to by them. Examples are: *Epidemics II* 2.12 "One can prognosticate that they [the patients] get a greenish complexion after an outflow of blood; and other [predictions] of this kind. As regards moistening and drying and warming and cooling, many predictions of the kind

[14] On this complex, see Smith, Hippocratic tradition.

[15] *Epid. II* 5.104.6–12 φαρμάκων τε τρόπους ἴσμεν, ἐξ ὧν γίνεται ὁποῖ' ἄσσα (scripsi: ὁποῖα ἄσσα VIH: ὁποῖα καὶ ἄσσα H)· οὐ γὰρ πάντες, ἀλλ' ἄλλοι ἄλλως εὖ κεῖνται καὶ ἄλλοθι· πρωΐτερον ἢ ὀψίτερον ληφθέντα· διαχειρισμοῖσιν, οἷον ἢ ξηρᾶναι ἢ κόψαι ἢ ἑψῆσαι, καὶ τὰ τοιαῦτα· ἐῶ τὰ πλεῖστα· καὶ ... καὶ τὰ τοιαῦτα.

[16] *Epid. IV* 5.196.8–9 Li. = Per. 305 La. Κριτίας ἐν πυρετοῖς ὑπὸ ἐνυπνίων ὠχλεῖτο ὑφ' οἵων οἴδαμεν.

[17] *Epid. VI* 5.274.2–3 καὶ τἄλλα ὅσα παρεῖται. The verbal form is a resultative perfect, with the meaning: "(which) have been passed over in silence and are, therefore, missing in this list."

could be made."[18] *VI* 2.16 "[Cases] where eructation is useful, and other [phenomena] of the kind."[19] *VI* 7.4 "You should cut the dropsical promptly, cauterize the patients with *phthísis* immediately, trepan the heads [quickly], and so on."[20] *VI* 8.5 "... and other [signs] of the kind that occur during the sleep."[21] Occasionally an analogy is suggested, but no hint is given what the analogy is thought to consist of: *Epidemics VI* 7.6 "... and the other [signs] analogously." "... and likewise the other [signs]."[22]

The general problem whether Hippocratic authors were at times intentionally inexplicit in order to conceal their professional knowledge is difficult to solve, although for specific passages such as the ones quoted above the answer must be negative. In the *Oath*, the physician swears to instruct his sons, the sons of his teacher, and certain other pupils, "and nobody else." A similar precept is given in *Law*, ch. 5.[23] This professional usage is likely to have concerned rather those elements of the curriculum which could not be learned from books, namely practical skill. In all probability, it did not concern physical theory, for instance humoral doctrine, because these more modern topics were discussed widely in the general public.[24] Perhaps, however, the fact that in the extant treatises pharmaceutical prescriptions are sometimes referred to only summarily (see the instances quoted above p. 29 f.) can be interpreted as attesting intentional obscurity: the members of the author's group knew these preparations already, whereas outsiders were not supposed to know them. In another field of instruction and for other motives, Plato appears to have laid comparable restraints on himself in his writings.[25]

---

[18] *Epid. II* 5.88.18–20 ῥητέον ὅτι αἵματος ῥυέντος ἐκχλοιοῦνται, καὶ ὅσα ἄλλα τοιαῦτα· ὅ τι πρὸς τὸ ὑγραίνειν καὶ ξηραίνειν καὶ θερμαίνειν καὶ ψύχειν, πολλὰ ἄν τις τοιαῦτα εἴποι (ὅ τι ... τοιαῦτα om. IR: τὸ ... εἴποι om. H, sed suppl. in marg.: habet V).

[19] *Epid. VI* 5.286.1–2 ὅπῃ ἔρευξις λυσιτελέει, καὶ ἄλλα τοιαῦτα.

[20] *Epid. VI* 5.340.3–4 ὑδατώδεας θᾶσσον τάμνειν, φθίνοντας καίειν αὐτίκα, πρίειν κεφαλάς, καὶ τὰ τοιαῦτα.

[21] *Epid. VI* 5.344.6 καὶ τἄλλα ὅσα περὶ ὕπνον τοιαῦτα.

[22] *Epid. VI* 5.340.10, 12 καὶ τἄλλα κατὰ λόγον ... καὶ τἄλλα οὕτως.

[23] *Jusj.* 4.630.1–6 Li. = 4.8–12 Heiberg = 1.298 Jones ... διδάξειν τὴν τέχνην ταύτην ... υἱοῖσί τε ἐμοῖσι καὶ τοῖσι τοῦ ἐμὲ διδάξαντος καὶ μαθηταῖσι συγγεγραμμένοις τε καὶ ὡρκισμένοις νόμῳ ἰητρικῷ, ἄλλῳ δὲ οὐδενί. *Lex* 4.642.3–4 Li. = 8.15–17 Heiberg = 2.264 Jones τὰ δὲ ἱερὰ ἐόντα πρήγματα ἱεροῖσιν ἀνθρώποισι δείκνυται, βεβήλοισι δὲ οὐ θέμις, πρὶν ἂν τελεσθῶσιν ὀργίοισιν ἐπιστήμης. Burkert, Epoche 46.

[24] See, for instance, *Nat. Hom.* 1–2 (6.32.2–36.16 Li. = 164.3–170.7 Jouanna = 4.2–8 Jones), where such public debates are described, and Jouanna p. 222 ff. *ad loc.*

[25] Thomas A. Szlezák, Platon und die Schriftlichkeit der Philosophie, Berlin/New York, 1985, *passim*.

Purpose of the *Epidemics*

The phenomenon of the inexplicitness of the *Epidemics* treatises should be studied in the broader context of the question: What was the original purpose of these texts, which, at least partly, look like notes? The answer can, of course, not be given for the books of the *Epidemics* in their entirety, since they are composite works into which manifold texts of various origins seem to have been incorporated,[26] but for some passages an answer is within reach. It is useful for heuristic reasons not to start from the *Epidemics*, but from a particularly clear text contained in *On Humours*, a treatise which, although not belonging to the *Epidemics*, nevertheless has so much in common with them (in content and style) that Littré felt inclined to call it the "Eighth book of the *Epidemics*."[27] Chapter 2 contains a long list of substantives in the genitive: "... of vomit, intestinal evacuation, sputum, mucus, cough, eructation, hiccups, gas, urine, sneezing, tears, itching, plucking, touching, thirst, hunger, repletion, sleep, exercises [or: pains], absence of exercises [or: pains], body, intelligence, comprehension, memory, voice, silence."[28] In this compendium of the foremost categories related to symptoms, the genitives are dependent on a substantive in the nominative which immediately precedes them and which opens the whole sentence — a substantive for which two variant readings are transmitted in the two relevant manuscripts. The *Marcianus Ven.* 269 (= M), a codex notorious for its numerous conjectural emendations and simplifications of passages corrupt or difficult to understand, has a very familiar word that means 'education,' 'instruction' (*paídeusis*), hence: "Instruction about vomit ...," etc. The *Parisinus Graec.* 2253 (= A) is more conservative than M and tends to keep a wording even where it is nonsensical or hard to understand. It reads: "Passing (*paródeusis*) of vomit ...," etc., which makes sense only with part of the substantives following.[29] "Passing" may be a slight misspelling of another word (*parádosis*) meaning again 'instruction.'[30] Accordingly, the synonymous word in M (*paídeusis*)

---

[26] Langholf, Die parallelen Texte; Langholf, Generalisationen.

[27] Vol. 5, p. 470; cf. Deichgräber, Die Epidemien p. 75 f., who agrees. Since the *Epidemics* are of a mixed origin themselves, it is not much less objectionable to interpret the *Epidemics* by using the *Epidemics*.

[28] *Hum*. 5.478.9–13 Li. = 4.66 Jones ... ἐμέτου, κάτω διεξόδου, πτυάλου, μύξης, βηχός, ἐρεύξιος, λυγμοῦ, φύσης, οὔρου, πταρμοῦ, δακρύων, κνησμῶν, τιλμῶν, ψαυσίων, δίψης, λιμοῦ, πλησμονῆς, ὕπνων, πόνων, ἀπονίης, σώματος, γνώμης, μαθήσιος, μνήμης, φωνῆς, σιγῆς.

[29] Cf. Jones *ad loc.*

[30] M has παίδευσις, A has παρόδευσις, a word attested only in very late Greek, an additional reason for suspecting that it is wrong here; παράδοσις might have been the original reading of A. On the characteristics of the manuscripts cf. J. Ilberg, Zur Überlieferung des Hippokratischen Corpus, Rhein. Mus. 42 (1887), 436–461. J. Ilberg, Prolegomena I, in: Kühlewein (ed.), Hippocratis opera, vol. 1, p. XXV–XXVIII. Jouanna (ed.), Hippocrate, La nature de l'homme, p. 91–94.

might be an explanatory note which has subsequently replaced[31] the original word *parádosis* still traceable in A. The sense of the substantive introducing the series of genitives in *On Humours*, ch. 2 thus seems quite certain; the genitives suggest a teacher who has a certain curriculum of medical instruction to present and knows the doctrine so thoroughly that he does not need lecture notes on its contents, but merely uses a list of the topics to be discussed in the lecture so as not to leave any of them out.

A passage contained in *Epidemics II* 3.17 further supports the contention that parts of these treatises originally were the lecture notes of one or several medical teachers: "What has to be known about the embryo of seven months. Whether the nine months [namely of a normal pregnancy] have to be reckoned from the menstruation or from the conception, and whether they consist of 270 days like the Greek months, or something has to be computed to them."[32] The sentence on the regular (not premature) birth apparently refers to the complex problem of how to prognosticate the date of delivery. A normal pregnancy, according to modern statistics, may extend from 263 to 270 days. If the day of conception is not known, the modern mode of calculation starts from the first day of the last regular menstruation and adds 280 days to it. Perhaps the *Epidemics* passage implies something similar. If reckoned from conception, the pregnancy extends for 9 Greek months at 29½ days[33] (= 265½ days) or at 30 days (= 270 days), which corresponds to modern observations. If reckoned from the last normal menstruation, "something has to be computed to them." As it is transmitted, the text passage cannot have been the notes of a student attending lectures: a pupil would not just have listed the topics, omitting so much positive information; nor can the text have been intended for direct publication: the inexplicitness of the passage precludes any such interpretation. For the same reason it is also unlikely that the passage was part of a book-author's preliminary collection of material: notes of such briefness would not be of any use to somebody leisurely writing a book. The passage, however, could have been useful to an expert who knows

[31] This process of a replacement of original words by ancient explanatory glosses can be observed quite often in the Hippocratic Collection, cf. J. Ilberg, Die Ärzteschule von Knidos, Berichte über die Verhandlungen der Sächsischen Akad. d. Wiss., Phil.-hist. Klasse, vol. 76 (1924), fasc. 3, Leipzig, 1925, p. 24.

[32] *Epid. II* 5.118.1–5 Ἃ δεῖ εἰδέναι ἐς τὸν ἑπτάμηνον (ἑπτάμηνον VHIR: 'Achtmonatigen' Gal. comm.)· εἰ (εἰ Li., 'ob' Gal. comm.: ἢ VHIR) ἀπὸ τῶν γυναικείων ἀριθμητέοι οἱ ἐννέα μῆνες ἢ ἀπὸ τῆς ξυλλήψιος, καὶ εἰ (εἰ V: 'ob' Gal. comm.: ἐς HR: εἰς I) ἑβδομήκοντα καὶ διακοσίῃσιν (-ησιν HIR: -οισιν V) ⟨ἧσιν⟩ οἱ Ἑλληνικοὶ μῆνες γίνονται ἢ (ἢ scripsi: 'oder' Gal. comm.: καὶ VHIR) εἴ τι προσέτι τούτοισι.

[33] Cf. *Sept.* 7.436.5–6 Li. = 88.20–21 Grensemann (with important commentary, p. 110 ff., also 48 ff.) = 164.5–6 Joly.

all the details but wants to make sure in lecturing that he does not leave out any important topics, and that his lecture is well structured.

There are several other passages which, for similar reasons, are likely to have been teacher's notes: *Epidemics II* 2.24, "Arrangements concerning the patient, and inquiry about the disease: What he says, what kind of things he says, how to react to it. Information [viz. to be given by the physician]: to the patient, to those present, to those outside."[34] *VI* 4.7, "Comfort for patients: for instance, to act cleanly with regard to beverage and food, and to other things he [the patient] sees; and [to act] smoothly with regard to what he feels. Other [comforts]: Those therapeutic measures that do not harm much or can easily be corrected: for instance, cold [water?] only where it is necessary; visits, talk, appearance, clothes, haircut, fingernails, perfume [of the physician]."[35]

VI 4.12–16 are perhaps notes of a medical instructor who was going to teach about the effect of sleep and food on people too 'warm' by constitution. Since *little* sleep cools the body when no food has been taken in, but *more* sleep warms it, whether one has eaten or not,[36] patients with too much warmth can be treated by either artificially reducing their sleep, or by reducing the warmth that builds up during the sleep. The notes, which form a coherent thought, read: "Evidently, when one is awake, one is warmer outside and colder inside; asleep, the opposite.[37] For a person warm by constitution, [therapeutic measures for] cooling: Water as beverage,[38] rest.[39] Sleep in a cold place, covered [with a blanket].[40] Sleep while sitting, nap in an upright position.[41] Weak foodstuffs are cooling,

---

[34] *Epid. VI* 5.290.4–6 Ἡ περὶ τὸν νοσέοντα οἰκονομίη καὶ ἐς τὴν νοῦσον ἐρώτησις· ᾇ διηγεῖται, οἷα, ὡς ἀποδεκτέον· οἱ λόγοι· τὰ πρὸς τὸν νοσέοντα, πρὸς τοὺς παρεόντας, πρὸς τοὺς ἔξω (πρὸς τοὺς ἔξω MV: καὶ τὰ ἔξωθεν Gal.).

[35] *Epid. VI* 5.308.13–16 αἱ τοῖσι κάμνουσι χάριτες, οἷον τὸ καθαρείως δρᾶν ἢ ποτὰ ἢ βρωτὰ ἢ ἃ ἂν ὁρᾷ, μαλακῶς ὅσα ψαύει. ἄλλαι (ἄλλαι M: ἄλλα vel ἀλλὰ Gal.: om. V)· ἃ μὴ μέγα βλάπτει ἢ εὐανάληπτα, οἷον ψυχρὸν ὅκου τοῦτο δεῖ· ἔσοδοι, λόγοι, σχῆμα, ἐσθής, {τῷ νοσέοντι,} κουρή, ὄνυχες, ὀδμαί.

[36] *Vict. II* 6.572.18–21 Li. = 182.21–24 Joly = 4.346 Jones ὕπνοι δὲ νῆστιν μὲν ἰσχναίνουσι καὶ ψύχουσιν, ἢν μὴ μακροὶ ἔωσι ...· ἢν δὲ μακροὶ ἔωσι μᾶλλον, ἐκθερμαίνοντες συντήκουσι τὴν σάρκα ...· βεβρωκότα δὲ θερμαίνοντες ὑγραίνουσι ...

[37] Cf. *Epid. VI* 5.320.6–7 τὸ αἷμα ἐν ὕπνῳ ἔσω μᾶλλον φεύγει. "During sleep, the blood withdraws more to the interior."

[38] Water as a beverage is an agent for cooling, cf. *Vict. II* 6.554.7 Li. = 172.17 Joly = 4.324 Jones ὕδωρ ψυχρὸν καὶ ὑγρόν. "Water is cooling and moistening."

[39] As opposed to full sleep.

[40] Cf. *Epid. II* 5.102.13–15 τὸ ἐν ψύχει κεῖσθαι ἐπιβεβλημένον (ἐπι- V: ὑπο- HIR), ὡς ἕλκῃ μὲν τὸ ψυχρόν, θάλπῃ δὲ τὸ τοιοῦτον εἶδος. "Reclining in the cold with a cover, so that he inhales the cold, while the way of reclining keeps him warm."

[41] So as to avoid *deep* or *much* sleep which warms the body, while *little* sleep cools it, just as 'rest' does, cf. above.

strong warming."[42] For the reasons mentioned, these notes do not seem to have been a student's short version of what he heard from a teacher. If they were not a preliminary sketch of somebody intending to write a medical paper, a treatise or something similar — and for this purpose, they seem to be too short —, they were probably notes of a teacher who listed some topics on which he was going to expand. The extant list of topics is, of course, much less interesting to us than what the Master would have had to say about each of them in his oral instruction.

Also the following passage is likely to have been a teacher's note. It begins elliptically with a "That ..." Again, the implicit doctrinal context is extremely complex; each term used in the passage would have needed considerable expansion in a lecture: *Epidemics VI* 7.3, "That in each case many correct prescriptions can be made, some of them having the same effect, others not; of this kind are: dispersing, concentrating, expelling, solidifying, ripening [of humours] ..."[43] The thought expressed is similar to that at *Epidemics VI* 8.25, "Forms of regimen: [Only] as far as one understands — but without understanding thoroughly; because many of them are useful."[44] A full discussion of the topic is found in *On Places in Man*, ch. 41—43, where several examples are adduced to prove that one and the same therapeutic measure can have opposite effects, and that opposite measures can have the same effect.[45]

In the 8th section of *Epidemics VI*, a large number of sentences begins with "That ..."[46] Particularly interesting are the paragraphs 7—26.[47] They seem to form a coherent text unit, by style as well as (partly) by content. §§ 7 ff. seem to concentrate on regimen including the bodily and psychic effects of smells, sounds, words, exercise, leisure, sleep, insomnia. §§ 11 ff. obviously concentrate on 'meteorological' conditions (weather and season,

---

[42] *Epid. VI* 5.310.6—11 ἐμφανέως ἐγρηγορὼς θερμότερος τὰ ἔξω, τὰ ἔσω δὲ ψυχρότερος· καθεύδων τἀναντία. ἐνθέρμῳ φύσει, ψύξις· ποτὸν ὕδωρ, ἐλινύειν. ὕπνος ἐν ψύχει ἐπιβεβλημένῳ. ὕπνος ἑδραῖος, ὀρθῷ νυσταγμός. αἱ ἀσθενεῖς δίαιται ψυχραί· αἱ δ' ἰσχυραὶ θερμαί. For the doctrinal context, see also above, p. 89—91.

[43] *Epid. VI* 5.338.10—340.1 ὅτι πολλὰ περὶ ἑκάστου ἔστιν ὀρθῶς ἐντείλασθαι, τὰ μὲν ταὐτὰ δυνάμενα, τὰ δὲ οὔ· οἷόν ἐστι τὰ τοιάδε, διαχυθῆναι καὶ πιληθῆναι καὶ ἐξαχθῆναι καὶ σκληρυνθῆναι καὶ πεπανθῆναι † ... †.

[44] *Epid. VI* 5.352.14—15 αἱ δίαιται· ὅσον γνῶναι — μὴ ἐξειδῆσαι —· ξύμφοροι (-φοροι scripsi Johannem Alex. secutus qui habet *congrue* in lemm. [sed *conferentie* in explic.]: -φοραὶ MV, Gal., Pall.) γὰρ πολλαί.

[45] *Loc. Hom.* 6.330.20—338.5 Li. = 70.6—74.2 Joly. The examples are, however, different from those in *Epidemics*.

[46] Syntactically speaking, they are isolated subordinate clauses without main clauses; cf. Langholf, Syntaktische Untersuchungen 47—51.

[47] *Epid. VI* 5.344.17—354.2; cf. Deichgräber, Die Epidemien, p. 35, note 1; Kurt Bardong, Beiträge zur Hippokrates- und Galenforschung, Nachr. der Akad. der Wiss. in Göttingen, Phil.-hist. Kl., 1942, no. 7, 577—603; Manetti/Roselli *ad loc.*

including epidemic diseases which were thought to be brought about by these factors), and on the effects of the seasons on certain age groups. §§ 16 ff. are incoherent in content, but very similar in style. The whole unit bears a kind of title (the opening words of § 7): "From the little writing tablet: to be studied."[48] As Deichgräber rightly observed, paragraphs 7 ff. form a comprehensive medical programme.[49] It is perhaps possible to go a step further. Since their wording is so extremely concise, it seems plausible that this text is a copy from a teacher's note-book (set of several wax-tablets). Whereas one cannot completely rule out that these notes were intended for the composition of a book (although for this purpose they seem, again, to be too summary), it is quite unlikely that they are a record kept by a student listening to his teacher or excerpting literature, because in this case their practical value would have been minimal. Their extreme brevity and their sometimes rather theoretical content make it equally improbable that they were a collection of viewpoints composed to guide the medical practitioner in his daily task of examining patients.[50]

All of the texts mentioned can be compared to Aristotelian texts, some of which are likewise of considerable brevity (e. g. *Poetics*[51]). It would be legitimate to call the *Epidemics* (or part of their text) along with other brachylogical treatises of the Hippocratic Corpus writings for internal use, whereas several more explicit books of the Collection were clearly for public use. Some treatises appear to have an intermediate status, a situation characteristic of a period of transition from oral to written culture,[52] although not unfamiliar to our own experience. Of course, none of these differences in purpose and style permits conclusions as to the identity or non-identity of authors. Unfortunately, it is not possible to locate geo-

---

[48] 344.17 τὰ ἐκ τοῦ σμικροῦ πινακιδίου· σκεπτέα. The punctuation here is Deichgräber's (Die Epidemien p. 35). For the "tablet" see, Langholf, Beobachtungen.

[49] *Loco laud.*

[50] One can never decide whether a passage in the *Epidemics* is a faithful copy of original notes or an excerpt or otherwise modified recast of an original. Some of the material may have been passed on among the authors of the *Epidemics*; cf., for instance, the paragraph *VI* 8.6 immediately preceding the 'tablet' headline (5.344.8–16), which reappears in *Epid. II* 5.116.10–118.1. It is impossible to tell which of the two versions of these notes is a more authentic one, and this is very often the case with the hundreds of other parallel passages in the *Epidemics*.

[51] Very instructive is the discussion of the purpose of the *Poetics* in Alfred Gudeman, Aristoteles, ΠΕΡΙ ΠΟΙΗΤΙΚΗΣ, Berlin/Leipzig, 1934, 1–6. His arguments are similar to the ones adduced above. Ada B. Neschke, Die Poetik des Aristoteles, 2 vols, Frankfurt am Main, 1980. Ingemar Düring, Aristotle's De partibus animalium, Göteborg, 1943, 68–75 (on notebook style and scientific prose). Düring, Aristoteles 34 f.

[52] Cf. generally Lonie, Literacy. On lists of viewpoints generally Smith, Analytical and catalogue structure.

graphically any of the 'internal' instructional texts quoted, whose authors may have been itinerant physicians. These texts can, therefore, not help to elucidate the problem of medical 'schools.'

Although a number of passages of the *Epidemics* were probably notes of one or several teachers who were experts and used their drafts in order to avoid omissions of important topics and/or to memorize the structure of a lesson or of a course of lectures, it would be unsafe to extend this interpretation to the treatises as a whole. Part of them clearly consist of notes taken at, and for, various occasions. Lecturing may have been just one among other purposes. Two examples are particularly revealing.

The first specimen[53] is a description of an anatomical dissection (*Epidemics II* 4.1–2) executed on an animal's carcass[54] and concentrating on (blood-)vessels, 'strands,' and the diaphragm.[55] Before discussing the specific notebook features of this text, it will be useful to comment shortly on its content. The vessels are partly denoted by the substantive *phléps*, partly by the substantive *artēríē*, a distinction which might, at least to some degree, correspond to the one into veins and arteries familiar in later anatomy. The 'strands' have the name *tónos* (plural *tónoi*), literally 'skein,' 'tendon,' 'sinew.' The description makes it obvious that no sinews proper can be meant. Certainly the author makes no systematic distinction between 'strands,' 'nerves,' and other anatomical structures of similar macroscopical appearance. Galen, who held the passage in high esteem and even regarded it as being entirely correct,[56] emphasized that it purposely did not mention some of the major anatomical features, but that it tacitly presupposed them, and he already concluded that the text consists of private notes.[57] Nothing is said explicitly in the text about the goal of the dissection described, but it seems plausible that the anatomist was guided by humoral doctrine[58] commonly accepted among the physicians of his time, namely that at least two body humours are responsible for health and disease of the human organism. The two humours, the pair bile/phlegm, are dis-

---

[53] The second specimen will be discussed in the following section of this chapter, p. 150 ff.

[54] Harris, The heart 62.

[55] *Epid. II* 5.120.12–126.3; cf. generally Lloyd, Magic 156–169. Harris, The heart 61, thought that the passage "seems to represent a state of knowledge intermediate between that of Praxagoras and that of Herophilus." This is hard to prove, even unlikely. Since the text is the record of an actual dissection, it might very well date from much earlier times, namely from around 400 B. C. as does the bulk of the treatise in which it is transmitted. No linguistic features speak against this early date. On the contrary, even according to Harris (*loco cit.*) "the term *liver vein* seems ... to recall an earlier period [than the post-Praxagorean one]." – The parallel version transmitted in *Oss.* 9.178.3–180.23 will be referred to by 'Oss.' in the subsequent footnotes 69 ff.

[56] Gal. *In Hp. Nat. hom. comm.* p. 75 Mewaldt; *In Hp. Epid. II comm.* p. 309 ff. Pfaff.

[57] Gal. *In Hp. Epid. II comm.* p. 314 f. Pfaff.

[58] Cf. generally Lloyd, Magic 162 f.

cussed, or at least mentioned, in numerous Hippocratic treatises.[59] Although this binary scheme was expanded into a quaternary one in some treatises (bile/phlegm/blood/black bile, or: bile/phlegm/blood/water), the pair bile/phlegm still formed a theoretical nucleus in 'physiology' and 'pathology.' Each of the two humours originates in a unique body organ. According to the accepted theory, the source of bile is the liver (with the gall-bladder), and the source of phlegm is the head.[60] According to *Epidemics II* 1.7, the (blood-)vessels and the *tónoi* both have an important function in the disease process: "Segregations (*apóstasis*) occur either through the vessels or the sinews ..."[61] The anatomy of both kinds of ducts was certainly thought to be helpful in the daily task of assessing where the body humours (either harmful or not) wandered in the body, and what would be their effects there. The diaphragm was regarded as being a sort of barrier between the upper and the lower moiety of the body, a sheet separating the thorax cavity from the abdominal one but nevertheless allowing a canalized communication between the two cavities (or body halves) via certain ducts running through it.[62] The expressions 'above the diaphragm' and 'below the diaphragm' found several times in the Hippocratic Collection[63] are not just topographical indications but imply that the upper and the lower body halves form, or contain, rather independent 'sub-systems.' The same doctrine is implied in *Aphorisms IV* 18, "Pains above the diaphragm indicate that purging in upward direction is needed; those below, in downward direction."[64] *On Diseases III*, ch. 14, "*Eileós* [i. e. stoppage of the bowels] occurs when the upper body cavity is warmed and the lower one cooled ... This is the therapy: Purge the upper body cavity ... so that the upper body cavity ceases to be warm. And cool the region above the diaphragm, but not the heart. And warm

---

59 Cf. Jouanna, Archéologie 651 ('Index des notions,' under: 'Humeurs').

60 For the latter doctrine, cf. the following passages (quoted after Littré's edition): *Aer.* 2.46.6–7, *Morb. I* 6.160.9–10, 16–17, 22, 164.13–14, 166.6, 168.12–18 (physical reasons why the phlegm is collected in the head), 174.9–10, *Aff.* 6.212.16–17, 216.14–16, 236.5–7, *Morb. II* 7.8.2–10, 16.23–25, 18.3–4, 12–18 (physical reasons), *Int.* 7.188.26–190.6, *Morb. IV* 7.544.7–9, 548.16–550.16 (physical reasons), 560.7–17, 606.20–21, *Mul. I* 8.32.13, 19, 66.8–10, 72.4–7, 76.11, 13, 18–19.

61 Cf. above p. 80, where the Greek text is quoted.

62 For further details, see below p. 182–184.

63 In the following passages quoted after Littré's edition: *Prog.* 2.122.12, 142.6, *Acut.* 2.272.8, 274.1–2, *Acut. (Sp.)* 2.400.6, 510.8, 12, *Art.* 4.176.7, 178.6, 180.7, *Mochl.* 4.380.15, *Coac.* 5.638.16 (ὑπὲρ τῶν φρενῶν A: καιρίοισι IR, Li.), 680.8, 716.7, *Salubr.* 6.78.6, *Mul. II* 8.384.12, *Judic.* 9.284.17.

64 *Aph.* 4.506.14–15 Li. = 4.138 Jones τὰ ὑπὲρ τῶν φρενῶν ὀδυνήματα ἄνω φαρμακείης δεῖσθαι (φ. δ. C′V: φαρμακίην M) σημαίνει· ὁκόσα (ὁκόσα MV: ὅσα C′) δὲ κάτω, κάτω.

the region below it by having the patient sit in a tub with warm water."[65] Also the numerous passages mentioning the 'upper cavity' or 'lower cavity'[66] reflect this doctrine, as does the famous distinction between 'purging (from) above' (by vomiting) and 'purging (from) below' (by using laxatives or clysters), which is so frequently encountered in Hippocratic therapeutic prescriptions and recipes.

It appears that the anatomical dissection of *Epidemics II* 4.1–2 was executed on an animal and recorded afterwards (see below). In the initial chapter, the liver is the first organ to be laid open,[67] and then the course of the 'liver vein' (*phléps hēpatītis*) is pursued from the loin through the liver and the diaphragm to the heart, the clavicles, the neck, the shoulder-blade and again downward back to the vertebrae and the ribs. One of the main subjects of the chapter seems to be the description of the way in which the two kinds of vessels (*phléps* and *artēríē*) penetrate through the diaphragm. Perhaps these vessels were considered important for the transport of bile from its origin, the liver, through the body.

In the second chapter, the anatomist follows the course of 'strands' (*tónoi*) starting from the brain. One might assume that he regarded them

---

[65] *Morb. III* 7.134.8–20 Li. = 80.29–82.8 Potter εἰλεοὶ δὲ γίνονται τῆς ἄνω κοιλίης θερμαινομένης καὶ τῆς κάτω ψυχομένης ... τοῦτον ὧδε θεραπεύειν· καθῆραι τὴν ἄνω κοιλίην ..., ἵνα παύσηται ἡ ἄνω κοιλίη θερμαινομένη· καὶ ψύχειν τὰ ἄνω τῶν φρενῶν πλὴν τῆς καρδίης· τὰ δὲ κάτω θερμαίνειν ἐν σκάφῃ ὕδατος θερμοῦ καθίζων. *On Hebdomads*, ch. 52 (*Hebd.* p. 79 Roscher = 8.672.23–28 Li. = 4.218–220 Jones) "Boundary of death: When the warmth of the soul has risen above the navel into the place above the diaphragm, and the entire moisture is burnt up ... [Then] ... he exhales all at once the breath of the warmth (out of which the whole was composed) into the whole again." ὅρος δὲ θανάτου, ἐὰν τὸ τῆς ψυχῆς θερμὸν ἐπανέλθῃ ὑπὲρ τοῦ ὀμφαλοῦ εἰς τὸν ἄνω τῶν φρενῶν τόπον καὶ συγκαυθῇ τὸ ὑγρὸν ἅπαν· ... ἀποπνέει ἀθρόον τὸ πνεῦμα τοῦ θερμοῦ, ὅθεν περ ξυνέστη τὸ ὅλον, εἰς τὸ ὅλον πάλιν. The word ὅρος does not seem to mean 'definition' here.

[66] ἄνω or κάτω κοιλίη.

[67] In sacrifices the very first organ to be inspected by the priest immediately after killing the animal, sometimes even before doing so, was the liver (hepatoscopy); for references, see Pease (ed.), Cic., *De div.*, Book I, p. 252–256 (= repr., p. 94–98). Since the dissection described in *Epid. II* was executed on an animal's carcass (Harris, The heart 62) and not on a human body, it would not be surprising if the person slaughtering the animal proceeded according to the normal way. Most of the (relatively little) meat consumed in classical Greece was sacrificial meat (Johannes Haussleiter, Der Vegetarismus in der Antike [Religionsgeschichtl. Versuche und Vorarbeiten, 24], Berlin, 1935, 3 f.), and ritual slaughtering was, therefore, the normal way. Although, however, the procedure in *Epid. II* of laying open the liver first *may* reflect everyday slaughtering rites, it should not be concluded that the dissection as such was in any way a ritual act. It is significant in this respect that at *Nat. Puer.* 7.502.6–7 Li. = 62.6 Joly and at *Mul. I* 8.30.16–17 the fresh, healthy blood of women in childbed is compared not to the blood of butchered animals, but of ritually slaughtered sacrifices. Similarly *Carn.* 8.594.14–16 Li. = 193.20–22 Joly, where the formation of the liver is explained.

as ducts of phlegm. 'Strands' and other anatomic structures such as nerves have a white or light grey colour, as has phlegm.[68] Perhaps the ancient anatomist, in pursuing the *tónoi*, wanted to explore the course taken by the phlegm as it descends from its 'source,' the head. The *tónoi* run from the brain through the neck, and the author of the report was able to follow them to the diaphragm, and partly beyond. Part of them ended there, others sent branches to the abdomen, which were difficult to recognize. The lowest point to be mentioned in the description of the *tónoi* is the *os sacrum*.

These 'minutes' were taken down *after* the dissection (not written or dictated simultaneously), as can be concluded from the numerous verbal forms in the imperfect or pluperfect tenses: vessels "*went* straight to the clavicles," "*had* started somewhat below the diaphragm," "*had* started from the vertebra," "*ceased*;" *tónoi* "*ceased*," "*seemed* to extend," "*extended* along the spine," "*communicated* with the ribs," "*had* started," "*communicated* with the vertebrae."[69] Another expression typical of notes is: "Two veins run from the clavicles ... into the abdomen; where they go on from there *I do not know yet*."[70] The imperfect verbal forms are used in the report together with present tense forms, mostly indiscriminately (e. g., the vessel(s) also "communicates," "turn away," "runs downwards," etc.).[71] For

[68] For the brain as the origin of phlegm, see above note 60. That phlegm is white can be concluded from these passages quoted after Littré's edition: *Aer.* 2.88.3–4, *Epid. III* 3.44.6–7, *VI* 5.318.8, *VII* 5.378.3, *Nat. Hom.* 6.46.19, *Aff.* 6.228.11–17, *Int.* 7.206.17–22, 218.7–8, 260.7–11, *Nat. Mul.* 7.326.1, *Nat. Puer.* 7.510.1–16, *Mul. I* 8.38.6–9, 72.4–9, 114.9–10, *Gland.* 8.556.5–6.

[69] *Epid. II* 5.120.15 ᾖει (Littré: 'sie geht' Gal.: εἴη V: ἡ HIR, Oss. [locus geminus]). 122.16 ἀφωρμήκει. 124.4 ἐξεπεφύκεσαν (sic fortasse legendum: ἐξεπεφύκασιν HIR: πεφύκασιν V: ἐκπεφύκασιν Oss., Littré). 124.5 ἔληγεν. 124.12 ἐτελεύτων. 124.13–14 ἐδόκεον τείνειν. 124.15 παρέτεινεν. 124.16 ἀπένεμεν. 124.18 ἐξεπεφύκεσαν (VHIR, Oss.: ἐξεπεφύκεισαν Littré, falso). 126.1 ἀπεδίδουν (HIR, Littré: ἀπεδίδου Oss.: ἀποδιδοῦν V). Note that in ancient Greek, unlike Latin and modern languages, the pluperfect largely represents an imperfect. – The first scholar to point to the imperfect forms and to interpret them as features typical of 'minutes' kept about a project was Deichgräber, Die Epidemien, p. 104. – Aorist forms have not been mentioned above because aorists may be gnomic (in the Collection, 'general truths' are sometimes expressed in this tense); in the context of the imperfect and pluperfect forms, however, the aorists should have a past tense meaning: 122.3 ἀπέλιπε, προσέδωκε. 122.6 ἤρξατο. 122.10 ἐμετεωρίσθη. 122.11 ἐδιχώθη (Oss.: ἐδιώχθη V: ἐδιαιρέθη HIR, cf. Littré *ad loc.* et E. Nachmanson, Erotianstudien, Uppsala, 1917, p. 355). 122.12 κατηναλώθη (Littré: καταναλώθη VH, Oss.: καταναλωθῇ IR). 124.11 ἦλθεν (VHIR, Littré: ἦλθον Oss.). 124.17 ἐξέλιπον. 126.2 κατηναλώθησαν (Littré: καταν- VHIR, Oss.). – For the abbreviation 'Oss.' see above note 55.

[70] *Epid. II* 5.122.17–124.2 δισσαὶ δὲ ἀπὸ κληῖδων ... ἐς ἦτρον· ὅπη (ὅπη VHIR, Oss.: ὅποι Littré falso) δὲ ἐντεῦθεν, οὔπω οἶδα.

[71] *Epid. II* 5.120.14 προσδιδοῖ (VHIR, Littré: προσδίδοιεν Oss.). 120.17 ἀποκλίνουσιν. 122.5 καταβαίνει. There are also some perfect forms with present tense meaning, e. g. 122.17 προσπεφύκασι. 124.8, 12 πεφύκασιν.

the historian of medicine it is tempting to assume that the 'minutes' reflect a process of generalization. Something "*was*" so and so in the one individual organism dissected, hence it "*is*" always the case. According to modern standards, this generalization by the ancient physician is precipitate, and even in the Hippocratic Collection there are strong tendencies towards taking account of individual variations. One may note here *On Places in Man*, ch. 6: "Some individuals have more, others fewer vertebrae; those who have more have 18 (but with the inclusion of the [two] extreme ones there are [in this case] 20; of these [two], one is above at the head, one below at the seat)." ... "There are many little joints in the body, not the same way in everyone but different ones in the individuals ... The vessels described are the same in everyone, but there are other vessels varying in the individuals; they are, however, not worth mentioning."[72] The opposite tendency of rash generalization from what has been found in one or a few cases is also noticeable in the Collection.[73] In one passage of the record, the anatomist interprets, in an afterthought (and in the present tense), what he has seen during the dissection: there "*came*" two *tónoi* down from the brain, and some branches of them "*seemed* to extend" through the diaphragm to the liver and the spleen. Another *tónos* "*extended*" along the spine. "*I think*," adds the author, "that they *extend* through the diaphragm into the *mesentérion* as the vessels do."[74] Since this was the case with the vessels,[75] it had, according to this physician, to be analogous with the *tónoi*.

This dissection report is characteristic of a large part of the material contained in the *Epidemics*. The two chapters were not composed for publication but as an informal ('esoteric') text intended for personal use or for circulation within a small group of colleagues and/or students. Like many other passages of the *Epidemics*, this record of a dissection is not just a description of facts but starts from a doctrinal basis and interprets the facts.

---

[72] *Loc. Hom.* 6.286.1–4, 290.3–7 Li. = 44.7–11, 46.18–22 Joly. The translation is according to Joly's text. For the problem of general and individual features and the method of generalization cf. Kudlien, Beginn 99 f., 140–145.

[73] Particularly in prognostic aphorisms, e. g. in *Prorrh. I, Coac., Aph.* Rash generalization in medicine is criticized by Aristotle, *Part. anim. IV* 2 (676 b 31–35), cf. Ingemar Düring, Aristotle's De partibus animalium, Göteborg, 1943, 174.

[74] *Epid. II* 5.124.9–17 ὥσπερ αἱ φλέβες (οὕτως add. Li.: om. VHIR, Oss.), οὗτοι διὰ φρενῶν ἐς μεσεντέριόν μοι δοκέουσι τείνειν.

[75] Cf. *Epid. II* 5.124.4 ἀρτηρίαι ... τόνον ἔχουσαι. 126.2 ὥσπερ αἱ φλέβες.

Nosology in the *Epidemics*

Yet another specimen of such notes that deserves examination here as representative of a much larger number of possible examples is a description (*Epidemics II* 2.24) of an historical epidemic of *kynágkhē*, a disease which appeared in two distinct variations, one of them deadly, the other not. Although nosological textbooks of the Hippocratic Collection (*On Diseases II* and *III*) describe several forms of *kynágkhē*, neither of the two variations of *Epidemics II* is mentioned there, and the author of the *Epidemics* passage does not try to harmonize his observations with any of the extant earlier descriptions. He adopts, however, the name of the disease, whose main feature was an affection of the throat or neck similar to angina, and refers to some of its traditional features.[76] One such traditional symptom is difficulty in swallowing (*On Diseases II*, ch. 26; 27; 28; in the younger part of the treatise, ch. 9; *On Diseases III*, ch. 10), which is mentioned in the *Epidemics* report: "They could not swallow, or with considerable difficulty."[77] One nosological description has it that "if he is forced [to swallow], it flows through his nose" (*On Diseases II*, ch. 28), and the same symptom occurred in the historical epidemic: "It flowed into their noses when they tried very hard [to swallow]."[78] *On Diseases III*, ch. 10 states that "he is lying down with his mouth open and lets his saliva flow;" similarly in the historical report: "... they let their saliva flow," however with the restriction, "when they were talking."[79] (Both texts feature the same rare Greek word stem for 'to slaver.'[80]) According to *On Diseases III*, ch. 10, part of the treatment to be prescribed is bloodletting, in particular "to open the veins below the tongue;" in the report, "the veins below the tongue were prominent."[81] The report continues: "... In several individuals, the veins in the forehead and in the head and in the neck were swollen,"[82] which corresponds to the therapeutical prescription of *On Diseases II*, ch. 26 (cf. 27), namely bloodletting at the first vertebra of the neck and near both ears.

---

76 In the nosological books, the chapters describing *kynágkhē* are *On Diseases II*, ch. 26–28 (7.40.9–46.15 Li. = 159.9–164.14 Jouanna); ch. 9 (7.16.23–18.2 Li. = 140.7–13 Jouanna); *On Diseases III*, ch. 10 (7.128.16–130.16 Li. = 76.30–78.20 Potter). Cf. Grmek, Les maladies 479–481.

77 *Epid. II* 5.96.9.

78 *Epid. II* 5.96.9–10.

79 *Epid. II* 5.98.15.

80 σιαλοχοέω and σιαλοχόος respectively; the latter is unique in the Collection, the former found in only one other passage, *Vict. II* 6.548.1, 3 Li. = 168.29, 31 Joly = 4.320 Jones, on the physiology of birds.

81 *Epid. II* 5.96.8–9, *VI* 5.336.8 ἔταμον δὲ καὶ ὑπὸ γλῶσσαν.

82 *Epid. II* 5.96.11–12.

Whereas not all of the traditional *kynágkhē* symptoms are mentioned in the report, a number of symptoms which, according to the nosological descriptions, were to be expected in *kynágkhē* or in certain varieties of it, are explicitly said to have been absent from the historical epidemic. "The throat is inflamed," says *On Diseases II*, ch. 27, and in the same words the report notes that "the throat was *not* inflamed."[83] *On Diseases II*, ch. 9 states that "he breathes with effort;" but as to the patients of the epidemic, "their respiration was *not* raised [or: troubled] very much."[84] Suffocation as a typical occurrence in *kynágkhē* is mentioned at *On Diseases II*, ch. 26, and *III*, ch. 10; the report, however, mentions that "most of them did not experience suffocation unless they wanted to swallow saliva or something else."[85] Fever, finally, is a symptom characteristic of *kynágkhē* according to *On Diseases II*, ch. 26 and 27; in the more recent ch. 9 it is mentioned as a symptom which may or may not be present. In the report of *Epidemics II*, the patients are mostly without fever; only in some cases just the temples have some slight temperature.[86]

A comparison of the historical report with the descriptions of *kynágkhē* contained in the nosological handbooks shows that the authors of the *Epidemics* presupposed a solid professional knowledge on the part of the reader. In the particular case of the *kynágkhē* report, there is even a hint that the intended reader(s) and the author (if they were not identical as in the case of personal notes) stood in a close relationship of permanent communication: "If I catch sight of somebody who has died [viz. of the first, less harmful variety], *I shall mention it*; but all patients, of whom I know *at present*, survived."[87] The report would appear to have been an informal or preliminary ('esoteric') one and written during the epidemic.

As this description of the epidemic *kynágkhē* cases exemplifies, the inexplicitness of the *Epidemics* treatises is particularly evident in one important field of medical knowledge: nosology. When comparing *Epidemics I* and *III* to early nosological texts such as *On Diseases II*, ch. 12–75, one immediately recognizes a difference in perspective. The older approach started from disease units which had a name (e. g. "mortification of the brain," "consumption of the back") or a descriptive label to identify it (e. g. "If water gets to the brain ...," "If he gets struck ...").[88] The physician who read the text was quite obviously expected to identify the

---

83 *Morb. II* 7.42.22 Li. = 161.15 Jouanna ἡ φάρυγξ φλεγμαίνει. *Epid. II* 5.96.4–5 φάρυγξ οὐ φλεγμαίνουσα.

84 *Epid. II* 5.96.10–11.

85 *Epid. II* 5.96.14–15.

86 *Epid. II* 5.96.12–14, 98.3.

87 *Epid. II* 5.96.17–98.1 ἀπολ{λ}όμενον δὲ (δὲ HIR: τε V) εἴ τινα εἶδον, ἀναμνήσομαι· οὓς δὲ οἶδα νῦν, περιεγένοντο.

88 For references and more examples, see above p. 55 f.

disease unit manifested in his own patient as one of the disease units described in the treatise. With regard to this method, modern critics have mistakenly objected that the physician of *On Diseases II*, ch. 12–75 dealt with the disease more than with the patient. It may suffice here to recall what has been said (p. 57 ff.) about the various diagnostic and therapeutic instructions of the treatise which imply a close cooperation, and sometimes even a high degree of communication, between the doctor and the patient: thorough examination of the patient, partly directly (e. g. through auscultation), partly through anamnesis (p. 58 f.); prognoses about the specific turn an individual case may take after certain disease signs have appeared (p. 60 f.); a rather flexible treatment depending on the particular conditions of the individual patient (cf. the types of therapeutic cases outlined p. 68 f.). In fact, the maxim of *Epidemics I* and *III* can be applied also to the procedures prescribed in *On Diseases II*, ch. 12–75: "Medical science and practice [*tékhnē*] have three [aspects]: the disease, the patient, and the physician."[89] Perhaps it is not mere coincidence that the disease and not the patient is mentioned here in the first place; it is the disease that occasions the patient – physician relationship. In the approach of *Epidemics I* and *III* and of the other *Epidemics* treatises, the disease units so prominent in the nosological treatises like *On Diseases II*, ch. 12–75 are not discarded. They are only less conspicuous because the perspective has shifted, but they continue to be important.[90] They are presupposed by the

[89] Cf. above, 'Introduction' p. 1.

[90] Grmek, Les maladies 420–423. The *Epidemics* depend on the nosological approach not only so far as parts of their content are concerned; there is also some affinity in style. This does not indicate that the authors of the *Epidemics* knew any of the *extant* nosological works, but it shows that they perpetuated an older professional language. Typical expressions of the *Epidemics* are ὀδύνη ἐς and similar adverbial phrases without a verb (Langholf, Syntaktische Untersuchungen 78–81) and substantives used 'absolutely,' i. e. without being a formal part of a larger sentence (*ibid.* 30–58). For both features, cf. *Morb. II* 7.62.1–4 Li. = 175.9–13 Jouanna πλευρῖτις ὅταν λάβῃ, πυρετὸς καὶ ῥῖγος ἔχει, καὶ ὀδύνη διὰ τῆς ῥάχιος ἐς τὸ στῆθος. καὶ ὀρθόπνοια, καὶ βήξ, καὶ τὸ σίελον λευκὸν καὶ ὑπόχολον, καὶ ἀποβήσσεται οὐ ῥηϊδίως, καὶ διὰ τῶν βουβώνων ὀδύνη, καὶ οὐρεῖ αἱματῶδες. Another expression typical of the *Epidemics* is an ambiguous ἐκ, which admits of a temporal as well as of a causal interpretation; Diller, Ausdrucksformen 139 (= Kleine Schriften Medizin 112); cf. *Morb. II* 7.60.13 Li. = 174.14 Jouanna ἐκ κόπου ἢ ἐξ ὁδοιπορίης πυρετήνας. More examples of the grammatical features mentioned could be quoted. A further parallel is the use of cardinal instead of ordinal numbers, cf. above p. 61–67, 133 f. As to the vocabulary, a comparison of, for instance, *Morb. II*, ch. 12–75 and the *Epidemics* is a difficult undertaking because both texts are not only of unequal length but also of different scope. It is hard to say how a comparison should be done systematically (e. g. on a statistical basis). A lot of trivial colloquial words would have to be excluded to begin with. However, even a superficial glimpse makes it evident that *Morb. II*, ch. 12–75 has only a few words which do not occur in the *Epidemics*, and that the *Epidemics* have many words not to be found in *Morb. II*, ch. 12–75. This cannot be explained only by the larger compass of the *Epidemics* but may also be necessarily due to innovations.

authors of the *Epidemics*, whose main interest is the influence of internal and external forces (e. g. humours, weather) on the course of the diseases in the patients. In the earlier nosological texts, the diseases, although well-defined units, do not exhibit inflexible, rigid patterns. Some of the symptoms described in *On Diseases II*, ch. 12–75 are considered obligatory, while of others it is said that they may or may not be present (p. 60). Some symptoms have a prognostic value only "generally" or "with most patients" (p. 61). The chronology for many of the nosological disease units is rather flexible (p. 61 ff.).

This fundamental flexibility of the nosological approach is the basis for the method applied by the authors of the *Epidemics* who started from a traditional nosology which they had taken over as a common heritage of the profession, and without which the *Epidemics* cannot be adequately understood. What is written in the *Epidemics* about diseases identifiable by a disease name is largely compatible with the nosological descriptions extant in *On Diseases II*, ch. 12–75 and kindred nosological treatises which, as Jouanna and Grensemann have proved,[91] derive from a common source.[92]

Compatibility does not mean that all the details contained in the disease descriptions of the nosological treatises reappear in the *Epidemics*. Often the *Epidemics* refer to traditional diseases only by their name (never with numbers added[93]), or with very few further indications, presupposing on the part of the reader a professional acquaintance with what the name designates. This procedure is familiar in modern medicine, too. For instance, a *parotitis epidemica*, or mumps, is today such a well-defined entity that in many contexts the very name is sufficient. The following examples are taken from books *I* and *III* of the *Epidemics*; the material could be multiplied by quoting from the other books, but the picture would not change.

A 'term-like' disease name is "long *diárrhoia*" in *Epidemics III*, ch. 14.[94] It finds its explanation in the description *On Affections*, ch. 25.[95] The disease *dysenteríē* (and the adjectives derived from it, *dysenterikós* and *dysenteriṓdēs*) is rather frequent in *Epidemics I* and *III*. A description of it is given in *On Affections*, ch. 23.[96] *Hýdrōps* (dropsy) is mentioned in *Epidemics*

91 Jouanna, Archéologie *passim*, and Grensemann, Knidische Medizin *passim*.

92 A Knidian source (Κνίδιαι γνῶμαι) according to these two authors, but this in particular cannot be proved; cf. above p. 25, 52.

93 On numbering disease types in the nosological books cf. above p. 20; 25, note 46.

94 *Epid. III* 3.98.3–4 Li. = 1.231.17 Kw. = 1.254 Jones; cf. διάρροια without the qualification μακρή in *Epid. I* 2.616.13 Li. = 1.185.2 Kw. = 1.154 Jones; 660.4 Li. = 196.21 Kw. = 176 Jones; 708.2 Li. = 211.11 Kw. = 204 Jones.

95 *Aff.* 6.236.12–25; cf. *Vict. III* 6.616.4–5 Li. = 206.19–20 Joly = 4.394–396 Jones.

96 *Aff.* 6.234.15–236.2; cf. *Vict. III* 6.616.5–8 Li. = 206.20–23 Joly = 4.396 Jones.

I, ch. 4 Li. (= ch. 9 Kw., Jones), and *III*, ch. 3, 12, 13.[97] This disease is described in the nosological treatises *On Affections*, ch. 22, *On Diseases II*, ch. 61, *On Internal Diseases*, ch. 22–26.[98] An ailment bearing the name *íkteros* (jaundice) occurs in *Epidemics I*, ch. 8 Li. (= ch. 15 Kw., Jones);[99] detailed descriptions of it can be found in *On Diseases II*, ch. 38–39, *On Diseases III*, ch. 11, *On Internal Affections*, ch. 35–38.[100] Two adjectives, *leienterikós* and *leienteriṓdēs*, which are formed out of the disease name *leienteríē*, are used in *Epidemics I*, ch. 4 Li. (twice) (= ch. 5 and 9 Kw., Jones); *III*, ch. 8.[101] The disease is described in *On Affections*, ch. 24.[102] A group of patients is called *leukophlegmatíai*, "suffering from white phlegm," *Epidemics III*, ch. 14.[103] This term is elucidated by comparing the description of the white phlegm disease in *On Diseases II*, ch. 71, *On Affections*, ch. 19, and *On Internal Affections*, ch. 21.[104] An adjective *nephrītikós*, 'suffering from the kidneys,' derived from *nephrī́tis* 'disease of the kidneys,' is used in *Epidemics I*, ch. 4 Li. (= ch. 5 Kw., Jones).[105] Descriptions of kidney diseases[106] are given in *On Internal Affections*, ch. 14–17.[107] In *Epidemics III*, ch. 5 *phȳ́mata* of the throat occur.[108] These "growths" are described in *On Diseases II*, ch. 30 and 32.[109] The disease *straggūríē* is mentioned in *Epidemics I*, ch. 4 Li. (= ch. 10 Kw., Jones).[110] Its main symptoms and some general remarks about it can be found in

---

97 *Epid. I* 2.628.9 Li. = 1.188.15 Kw. = 1.160 Jones; *III* 3.70.10 Li. = 1.225.6 Kw. = 1.240 Jones; 92.15 Li. = 230.6 Kw. = 252 Jones; 96.2 Li. = 231.10 Kw. = 254 Jones.

98 *Aff.* 6.232.14–234.14; *Morb. II* 7.94.11–96.8 Li. = 200.8–201.13 Jouanna; *Int.* 7.220.19–236.7 Li. = p. 208–216 Jouanna, Archéologie (ch. 23).

99 *Epid. I* 2.642.12, 644.10 Li. = 1.192.4, 13 Kw. = 1.168 Jones.

100 *Morb. II* 7.54.1–56.2 Li. = 169.18–171.8 Jouanna; *Morb. III* 7.130.17–132.4 Li. = 78.21–80.2 Potter; *Int.* 7.252.17–260.21 Li. = p. 218–219, 382–390 Jouanna, Archéologie (ch. 35 and 37).

101 *Epid. I* 2.616.13 Li. = 1.185.2 Kw. = 1.154 Jones; 628.9 Li. = 188.14 Kw. = 160 Jones; *III* 3.84.13 Li. = 1.228.11 Kw. = 1.246 Jones.

102 *Aff.* 6.236.3–11.

103 *Epid. III* 3.96.5 Li. = 1.231.14 Kw. = 1.254 Jones.

104 *Morb. II* 7.108.4–24 Li. = 210.9–211.14 Jouanna; *Aff.* 6.228.6–19 Li. = p. 100–102 Jouanna, Archéologie; *Int.* 7.218.7–220.18 Li. = p. 206–208 Jouanna, Archéologie.

105 *Epid. I* 2.618.1 Li. = 1.185.6 Kw. = 1.154 Jones.

106 The name νεφρῖτις occurs *Int.* 7.210.7, *Morb. I* 6.144.10, 19 Li. = 8.9, 10.5 Wittern. For a thorough discussion of kidney diseases in the fifth and fourth centuries, see Grmek/Wittern, Krankheit des Nikias.

107 *Int.* 7.202.1–210.6.

108 *Epid. III* 3.76.5 Li. = 1.226.20–21 Kw. = 1.244 Jones.

109 *Morb. II* 7.48.3–11 (especially line 9) Li. = 165.7–16 (14) Jouanna; 48.20 (especially line 22) – 50.3 Li. = 166.10–17 (12) Jouanna.

110 *Epid. I* 2.632.8 Li. = 1.189.14 Kw. = 1.162 Jones; cf. στραγγουριώδης *Epid. I* 2.616.16 Li. = 1.185.5–6 Kw. = 1.154 Jones; 630.10, 632.1 Li. = 189.5, 7 Kw. = 162 Jones; *III* 3.28.6 Li. = 1.215.13 Kw. = 1.218 Jones.

On Affections, ch. 28.[111] The disease name *teinesmós* is used in *Epidemics I*, ch. 4 Li. (twice) (= ch. 5 and 9 Kw., Jones); *III*, ch. 8, 14.[112] This disease is described in *On Affections*, ch. 26.[113]

It is not necessary to assume that the authors of the *Epidemics* used any of the extant nosological treatises of the Hippocratic Collection. Considerable medical literature must have been available in the fifth and fourth centuries. For example, only two meagre quotations and some doxographical notes of the famous *Knídiai gnõmai* are left (cf. *supra* p. 13 ff.); the authors of the *Epidemics* may have used this work or a revised version of it, or any other nosological treatise. Moreover, they must have tapped the profession's store of non-literary common knowledge, which is even likely to have been their main 'source.' There may have existed a commonly accepted nosology.[114]

Two texts are particularly instructive because they show the extent to which nosological knowledge is presupposed in *Epidemics I* and *III*. They form part of the third *katástasis* report of *Epidemics I* (ch. 9 Li. = ch. 18 Kw., Jones)[115] and of the *katástasis* report of *Epidemics III* (ch. 6) respectively.[116] In each of them, the following symptoms in the historical epidemic of a feverish disease, *kaúsos*, are recorded in varying order: fever, rigor, thirst (or absence of thirst), sleeplessness, nausea, disorder of consciousness, coldness of the extremities, quality of urine and stool, nosebleeding (or absence of it). Further symptoms mentioned in only one of the two reports are perspiration (*Epidemics I*) and coma (*Epidemics III*).

Kaúsos is also described in the nosological treatises. The main passages about it are *On Diseases II*, ch. 63; *On Affections*, ch. 11; *On Diseases I*, ch. 29; *On Diseases III*, ch. 6.[117] Several symptoms mentioned in *Epidemics I* and *III* as having occurred in the historical cases of *kaúsos* are not listed in these nosological passages. The symptoms found exclusively in the *katástasis* accounts are rigor, sleeplessness, nosebleeding, perspiration, and coma. It is obvious that they are all quite unspecific, for they are likely to appear in the course of various diseases with high fever.

---

[111] *Aff.* 6.240.5–14.

[112] *Epid. I* 2.616.12–13 Li. = 1.185.1 Kw. = 1.154 Jones; 628.8 Li. = 188.14 Kw. = 160 Jones; *III* 3.84.11 Li. = 1.228.9 Kw. = 1.246 Jones; 98.3 Li. = 231.16 Kw. = 254 Jones. Cf. τεινεσμώδης *Epid. I* 2.688.10–11 Li. = 1.204.21 Kw. = 1.190 Jones.

[113] *Aff.* 6.238.1–9.

[114] Lonie, Literacy.

[115] *Epid. I* 2.650.9–656.1 Li. = 1.194.13–195.14 Kw. = 1.172–174 Jones. On the word *katástasis* see below p. 169 f.

[116] *Epid. III* 3.80.3–82.17 Li. = 1.226.26–227.24 Kw. = 1.244–246 Jones.

[117] *Morb. II* 7.96.17–98.6 Li. = 202.3–17 Jouanna; *Aff.* 6.218.13–220.4 Li. = p. 274–276 Jouanna, Archéologie; *Morb. I* 6.198.6–200.10 Li. = 84.6–86.18 Wittern; *Morb. III* 7.122.23–124.17 Li. = 74.5–21 Potter. Cf. also *Acut. (Sp.)* 2.394.3–398.6 Li. = 1.146.2–147.16 Kw. = 68.2–69.11 Joly. Grmek, Les maladies 416–420.

On the other hand, the four nosological descriptions in *On Diseases I–III* and *On Affections* contain a combination of several specific symptoms not referred to in *Epidemics I* or *III*. All four agree that the tongue of the *kaúsos* patient is rough;[118] three, furthermore, agree that it becomes dark[119] and dry.[120] Another characteristic symptom of *kaúsos* according to the nosological treatises is expectoration,[121] which is described as being viscous[122] (i. e. 'unripe').[123] None of these signs characteristic of *kaúsos* is mentioned in the *katástasis* descriptions of *Epidemics I* and *III*, an omission which cannot be due to an absence of these essential symptoms in the historical cases, and which makes it evident that these historical reports presuppose, on the part of the reader, a professional knowledge of what characterizes *kaúsos*.

The same two *katástasis* reports of *Epidemics I* and *III*, which describe the historical epidemic of *kaúsos*, mention yet another disease, *phrenī́tis*, which is also described several times in the nosological treatises of the Hippocratic Collection, particularly in *On Affections*, ch. 10, *On Diseases I*, ch. 30 and 34, and *On Diseases III*, ch. 9.[124] Typical signs of *phrenī́tis*, according to these descriptions, are fever, disorder of consciousness,[125] and pain localized at the *phrénes* (i. e. the diaphragm[126]) according to *On Diseases III*, in the abdomen according to *On Affections*. Whereas the former two symptoms are listed in the *katástasis* reports, the typical pain is not mentioned there, although it must have been present. The very disease name, *phrenī́tis*, implied that pain at, or near, the *phrénes* must have occurred.

It is particularly revealing that in both *katástasis* accounts *phrenī́tis* and *kaúsos* are described jointly: "... There were cases of *kaúsos*, and also cases of *phrenī́tis* became numerous at that time ... [The description of the *kaúsos* cases follows.] ... In the cases of *phrenī́tis* there occurred all symptoms

---

118 τρηχέα *Morb. II*, *Aff.*; τρηχύνεται *Morb. I*; πέφρικε *Morb. III*.

119 μέλαινα *Morb. II*, *Aff.*; μελαίνεται *Morb. III; Morb. I*, which stresses aetiology, gives an abridged list of the symptoms and omits this feature.

120 ξηρή *Morb. II*, *III*; αὐαίνεται *Morb. I; Aff.* states that the tongue is affected by the hot breath, this implies exsiccation.

121 *Morb. I, II, III.*

122 *Morb. III.*

123 *Morb. I*; according to a theory underlying various treatises of the Hippocratic Collection, 'coction' or 'ripening' of humours consists in their becoming thinner; cf., e. g., above p. 120. All four nosological works moreover agree that *kaúsos* can easily develop into *peripneumoníē* (pneumonia).

124 *Aff.* 6.216.21–218.12 Li. = p. 326–328 Jouanna, Archéologie; *Morb. I* 6.200.11–23 Li. = 86.19–88.13 Wittern; 204.5–14 Li. = 92.7–18 Wittern; *Morb. III* 7.128.5–15 Li. = 76.20–29 Potter.

125 Not necessarily delirium (μανίη): cf. *Morb. I*, ch. 30.

126 Cf. above p. 44–46.

mentioned above [i. e. for *kaúsos*]" (*Epidemics I*). "Cases of *kaúsos* and *phrenĩtis* began early in spring ... This was the condition (*katástasis*) of the *kaúsos* cases: ... In the *phrenĩtis* cases, the symptoms were very similar" (*Epidemics III*). This does not mean that the author(s) did not see, or did not make, any difference between *kaúsos* and *phrenĩtis*, but it illustrates that the physician's perspective had shifted from traditional nosology, which was presupposed, towards an interest in the influence of internal and external forces on the disease cases.

A particularly clear example to illustrate the presupposition of nosology and the shift of interest is that of two descriptions of a disease called *phthísis* (in *Epidemics I* and *III* most often called *tó phthinõdes*), which infested the population twice, once in the period covered by the first *katástasis* account of *Epidemics I* (ch. 2 Li. = ch. 2 Kw., Jones)[127] and once during the time of the *katástasis* account of *Epidemics III* (ch. 13–14).[128]

In the nosological treatises, *phthísis* is described repeatedly; the most important passages are *On Diseases II*, ch. 48 and *On Internal Affections*, ch. 10.[129] The typical symptoms, according to these chapters, which are unanimous in that respect, are: *phthísis* is a disease of the lungs with fever and rigor; there is pain in the chest and in the back; the windpipe yields a whistling noise and is rough or dry; the patient coughs and has expectoration; the upper part of his body is emaciated, but his feet and legs get dropsical; his nails get contorted.

Some of these disease signs reoccur in the reports of *phthísis* in *Epidemics I* and *III*. Both mention fever, rigor, cough, expectoration, emaciation; in *Epidemics III*, furthermore, dropsy is mentioned. Neither of them, however, says a word about the most typical symptoms, namely pain in the chest and in the back, whistling noise and roughness or dryness of the windpipe. Although emaciation is mentioned,[130] nothing is said about its being confined to the upper part of the body; similarly, dropsy is referred to only generally without any details. The specific nail symptom is not mentioned at all. These symptoms cannot all have been absent from the

---

[127] *Epid. I* 2.604.3–610.2 Li. = 1.181.13–182.19 Kw. = 1.148–150 Jones.

[128] *Epid. III* 3.92.18–98.5 Li. = 1.230.9–231.18 Kw. = 1.252–254 Jones.

[129] *Morb. II* 7.72.6–74.21 Li. = 183.5–185.19 Jouanna; in this passage, the name φθίσις does not occur; instead, the description begins Ὅταν πλευμῷ. That it is a φθίσις becomes obvious from the name of the following description, ch. 49 (7.74.22 Li.), which begins Ἄλλη φθόη, "Another *phthísis*" (φθόη is synonymous to φθίσις; in Littré's edition, the description begins Ἑτέρη νοῦσος ἥτις καλέεται φθόη, a wording which is not supported by the only relevant manuscripts θM). In the parallel version, *Int.* ch. 10 (7.188.26–192.7 Li.), the same disease is expressly called φθίσις. — Generally, cf. Grmek, Les maladies 269–283.

[130] In *Epid. I* directly, in *Epid. III* in the description of the urine, cf. below p. 158, note 138.

historical cases if the disease name *phthísis* is supposed to have had any specific meaning. Quite clearly the author(s) of *Epidemics I* and *III* assumed a nosological training on the part of the reader.

The interest of the author(s) who describe(s) these historical cases of *phthísis* is not to test the nosological passages through observation but rather to explore the influence of internal and external conditions (humours, weather changes, seasons) on the disease process. Hence some symptoms of *phthísis* which were left out of account in the nosological chapters are studied in *Epidemics I* and *III*. Both reports describe, among other features, perspiration, coldness, quality of stool and urine, coma, and delirium, and both present these symptomatic features in the same order, often even in the same wording.[131]

The disease manifested itself slowly in the individuals; after some time of feeling unwell they were forced to stay in bed,[132] and many of them succumbed. The symptoms were rigor,[133] continuous, acute fever,[134] perspiration,[135] coldness,[136] stool of certain consistencies,[137] urine of certain qualities,[138] cough and expectoration,[139] symptoms in the windpipe,[140] aversion to food,[141] lack of thirst,[142] and delirium shortly before death.[143]

The congruence in content and arrangement allows the conclusion that the author(s) aimed at a systematic comparison between the two *phthísis* epidemics. He, or they, applied a preconceived set of categories (perhaps some sort of check-list) when writing the two accounts. Two more reports on other epidemic diseases show the same structure, namely the description

---

131 Lichtenthaeler, Le troisième Épidémique 60. — For the following observations cf. Langholf, Symptombeschreibungen.

132 κατεκλίνησαν *Epid. I, III.*

133 φρικώδεες *Epid. I, III.*

134 πυρετοὶ συνεχέες ὀξέες *Epid. I, III.*

135 ἱδρῶτες *Epid. I, III.*

136 ψύξις ἀκραίων πολλή, καὶ μόγις ἀναθερμαινόμενα *Epid. I*; πολλὴ ψύξις, καὶ μόγις πάλιν ἀναθερμαινόμενοι *Epid. III.*

137 κοιλίαι *Epid. I, III.*

138 οὖρα *Epid. I, III*; stool and urine are different in the two *phthísis* reports. In *Epid. III*, the description of the urine contains the formulation συντήξιες κακαί. This must be understood as a sign of emaciation, cf. the urine description of ch. 10 (*Epid. III* 3.90.7–13 Li. = 1.229.6–13 Kw. = 1.250 Jones), οὖρα ... ἐσήμαινεν ... σύντηξιν, and of *Prog.* 2.142.6–8 Li. = 1.90.21–91.1 Kw. = 2.26 Jones καὶ τὰς λιπαρότητας δὲ τὰς ἄνω ἐφισταμένας ἀραχνοειδέας μέμφεσθαι· συντήξιος γὰρ σημεῖα, which is similarly attested for the *Knídiai gnṓmai*, cf. *supra* p. 18 f.

139 ἔβησσον *Epid. I*; βῆχες *Epid. III.*

140 φάρυγξ; different symptoms in *Epid. I* and *III.*

141 ἀπόσιτοι *Epid. I*; ἀποσιτίη *Epid. III.*

142 ἄδιψοι *Epid. I*; διῆγον ἀδίψως *Epid. III.*

143 παράληροι περὶ θάνατον *Epid. I, III.*

of "fevers" in *Epidemics I*, ch. 3 Li. (= ch. 3 Kw., Jones)[144] and the one of "continuous fevers" in *Epidemics I*, ch. 4 Li. (= ch. 7–8 Kw., Jones).[145] Moreover, a large part of the treatise *Prognostics* is composed according to this scheme. The following list (see after p. 160) is designed to demonstrate the congruences in the order of the topics.

It is obvious that these congruences cannot be due to mere chance, but that a model underlies them. Is any of the five texts likely to have been the prototype of the other four? Unfortunately, nothing reliable is known about the chronological relationship of *Epidemics I*, *Epidemics III*, and *Prognostics*.[146] Although it might seem possible that one of the *Epidemics* reports served as a model for the other three *Epidemics* reports, the similarity with the disposition of the material of *Prognostics* precludes this assumption. It is quite unlikely that the disposition of extensive parts of *Prognostics* was modelled on one short report in the *Epidemics*, or on a mode of disposition discernible there only with difficulty. In fact, when one reads the reports in *Epidemics I* and *III*, the congruences are not striking at all. Can the author of *Prognostics* be expected to have noticed them?

Another possible assumption to account for the conformity of arrangement in the five texts would be to regard *Prognostics* as the source of the scheme. This option cannot be discarded completely, but the following considerations make it at least doubtful. The list shows that the scheme of exposition in the *Epidemics* texts comprises additional elements as compared to the one underlying *Prognostics*: shivering, lack of appetite, and lack of thirst. On the other hand, *Prognostics*, too, has elements absent from all of the *Epidemics* reports: in the list, only respiration, the state of the *hypokhóndrion*, dropsies,[147] and vomit have been quoted, but in the text there are more such elements, which shall be examined shortly. The extra elements in both *Epidemics* and in *Prognostics* could, of course, be explained by postulating that *Epidemics* took over the scheme from *Prognostics* via

[144] *Epid. I* 2.610.3–614.1 Li. = 1.182.20–183.18 Kw. = 1.150–152 Jones.

[145] *Epid. I* 2.622.9–628.7 Li. = 1.186.19–188.12 Kw. = 1.156–160 Jones.

[146] On *Epid. I* and *III* cf. Lichtenthaeler, Le troisième Épidémique (*passim*), who contends that book *III* is older than book *I*; there is, however, no proof for this assumption, and the question remains unsolved. Perhaps it is even asked inadequately because it presupposes that both works are homogeneous 'books,' whereas they may be more or less systematic secondary collections of more or less heterogeneous, though doctrinally congruous, materials written by several members of a group of physicians within a period of some years. As concerns the date of *Prog.* in relation to *Epid. I* and *III*, Deichgräber (Die Epidemien 17 ff.) thinks that *Prog.* is older; Lichtenthaeler, Quatrième série 53, 106 is of the opposite opinion, which was also held by Galen. This too remains a moot question. Part of the *doctrine* of *Prog.* should be older than *Prog.*

[147] In *Epid. III*, ch. 13 dropsy is mentioned at another place of the description, namely at its extreme end.

an intermediate source. This source would then have to be regarded as responsible for all the additions and omissions of the *Epidemics* reports. A closer look at the disposition of *Prognostics* in its entirety, however, makes this hypothetical construction improbable. After the chapters 3 to 14 (cf. the list) dealing (almost) exclusively with general or unspecific symptoms, there follow, quite unexpectedly, several chapters which have no counterparts at all in the *Epidemics* reports. It is not very plausible that an intermediate source should have omitted them *en bloc*: a very detailed description of a *specific* disease, *empýēma* (suppuration in the chest), ch. 15 to 17; a description of segregations (*apóstasis*) in another particular disease, *peripneumoníē* (pneumonia), ch. 18; a passage on certain pains, ch. 19 (first half); and some remarks on troubles of the bladder, ch. 19 (second half). *Prognostics* resumes only then the description of general or unspecific symptoms: ch. 20, critical days; ch. 21, headache; ch. 22, ear pain; ch. 23, troubles of the throat;[148] ch. 24, general remarks on relapses, segregations (*apóstasis,* first half of the chapter) and on various symptoms (second half);[149] ch. 25 is an epilogue.

The chapters 15—19 (or at least 15—18, on *empýēma* and *peripneumoníē*) are clearly a 'foreign body' in *Prognostics*, although they in no way differ stylistically or linguistically from the rest of the work, and hence cannot be a later intrusion; they must be supposed to have been written by the same author. There are other compositional "mysteries"[150] in Prognostics, for example the position of chapters 9 and 10 is illogical[151] but, as the comparative list shows, appears also in the reports of the *Epidemics*. These shortcomings in the arrangement of the chapters in *Prognostics* are in marked contrast to the internal elaborateness manifested by most of the same chapters.[152] Moreover, *Prognostics* is far from exhaustive on its subject; important topics are missing.[153] One should, however, not prematurely conclude that *Prognostics* is a book in an unrealized state — namely, that its author had written single chapters and provisionally arranged them,

---

[148] There is an order *a capite ad calcem* in ch. 21—23; generally about this order below p. 249, note 96.

[149] The chapters 21 to 23 also mention, or contain hints to, specific diseases such as *otitis media* and *kynágkhē* (angina), but their main purpose is to give generally applicable prognostic information. Lichtenthaeler, Quatrième série 71, speaks of "nosologie régionale."

[150] The expression is Lichtenthaeler's, *op. laud.*, p. 73.

[151] Lichtenthaeler, *op. laud.*, p. 69, 72—73, 79.

[152] On the elaborate internal structure of the chapters, cf. Lichtenthaeler, *op. laud., passim.* He remarks (p. 73): "Curieux *contraste*! D'un côté, une composition très travaillée, et de l'autre ces 'irrégularités' ... Qu'en penser?" His interpretation of the irregularities in the order of the chapters by using the "principe de congruence" as a "fil conducteur" (p. 71 ff.) explains some, but not all of them.

[153] Lichtenthaeler, *op. laud.*, p. 46 f.

Consumption (φθινῶδες) *Epidemics I*, ch. 2 Li. (= ch. 2 Kw., Jones)	Fevers (πυρετοί) *Epidemics I*, ch. 3 Li. (= ch. 3 Kw., Jones)	Continuous Fevers (συνεχέες πυρετοί) *Epidemics I*, ch. 4 Li. (= ch. 7–8 Kw., Jones)	Consumption (φθινῶδες) *Epidemics III*, ch. 13	*Prognostics*, content of the chapters
"Many of those who had been ailing ... took to their beds," πολλοὶ τῶν ... ὑποφερομένων ... κατεκλίνησαν.			"Many took to their beds ..., ailing," πολλοὶ ... κατεκλίνησαν ..., ὑπεφέροντο.	Ch. 3–4 "Reclining," κεκλιμένον.
				Ch. 5 "Respiration," πνεῦμα.
"Fevers with shivering," φρικώδεες πυρετοί.			"Shivering," φρικώδεες.	
"Continuous, acute fevers," πυρετοὶ συνεχέες, ὀξέες.	"Continuous fevers," πυρετοὶ ... συνεχέες.	"Continuous [fevers]," συνεχέες.	"Continuous, acute fevers," πυρετοὶ συνεχέες, ὀξέες.	
		"Rigors," ῥίγεα.		
"Perspirations," ἱδρῶτες.		"Perspirations," ἱδρῶτες.	"Perspirations," ἱδρῶτες.	Ch. 6 "Perspirations," ἱδρῶτες.
				Ch. 7 "*Hypokhóndrion*," ὑποχόνδριον.
				Ch. 8 "Dropsies," ὕδρωπες.
"Severe chill in the extremities, which with difficulty recovered their warmth," ψύξις ἀκραίων πολλή, καὶ μόγις ἀναθερμαινόμενα.		"Severe chill in the extremities, which with difficulty recovered their warmth," ψύξις δὲ πολλὴ ... ἀκραίων καὶ μόγις ἀναθερμαινόμενα.	"Great chill, with difficulty they recovered their warmth," πολλὴ ψύξις, καὶ μόγις πάλιν ἀναθερμαινόμενοι.	Ch. 9 "Head, hands, and feet being cold," κεφαλὴ ... καὶ χεῖρες καὶ πόδες ψυχρά.

		"Not sleepless," οὐδ' ἄγρυπνοι.		Ch. 10 "As for sleep ...," περὶ δὲ ὕπνου ...
"Stools," κοιλίαι.	"Stools," κοιλίαι.	"Stools," κοιλίαι.	"Stools," κοιλίαι.	Ch. 11 "Stool," διαχώρημα.
"Urines," οὖρα.	"Urines," οὖρα.	"Urines," οὖρα.	"Urines," οὔρων.	Ch. 12 "Urine," οὖρον.
				Ch. 13 "Vomit," ἔμετος.
"They coughed," ἔβησσον.	"Coughing," βηχώδεες.	"Coughs," βῆχες.	"Coughs," βῆχες.	Ch. 14 "Expectoration," πτύελον.
"Expectorating," ἀνάγοντες.	"Expectoration," τὰ βησσόμενα.		"Expectorating," ἀνάγουσαι (βῆχες).	
		"*Krísis* ..., it relapsed," ἔκρινεν ..., ὑπέστρεφεν.		Ch. 20 "Fevers get to a *krísis*," οἱ δὲ πυρετοὶ κρίνονται.
"Throats," φάρυγγες.			"Throats," φάρυγγες.	Ch. 23 "Throat," φάρυγξ.
"Without appetite," ἀπόσιτοι.	"Not without appetite," οὐδ' ἀπόσιτοι.	"Without appetite," ἀποσίτοις.	"Lack of appetite," ἀποσιτίην.	
"Without thirst," ἄδιψοι.		"Not very thirsty," διψώδεες οὐ λίην.	"Without thirst," ἀδίψως.	
	"*Krísis*, ... they relapsed," ἔκρινε, ... ὑπέστρεψαν.	"Segregations," ἀποστάσιες.		Ch. 24 "Relapse ..., segregation," ὑποστροφήν ..., ἀπόστασιν.
"Delirium near death," παράληροι ... περὶ θάνατον.			(Various symptoms follow,) "Delirium near death," παράληροι περὶ θάνατον.	

partly after a traditional scheme of disposition, partly without any scheme, and had also written a preface and an epilogue, when his work was interrupted. Perhaps he just lacked the literary interest or/and energy to undertake the decisive step from catalogue structure[154] to systematic arrangement of his material. The style within his single chapters reveals that he had a rhetorical training. But where could one have learned, by the end of the fifth century B. C., the technique of composing whole medical treatises? This was *terra nova* and possibly beyond the author's more practical interest. So he may have been content to elaborate the chapters as such, not the structure of his treatise. This situation is familiar from other works of the Hippocratic Collection; even the structure of *Epidemics I* and *III* can be explained similarly.

If the conclusion is correct that the author(s) of *Epidemics I* and *III* did not simply follow *Prognostics* in enumerating the symptoms but followed a tradition shared also by *Prognostics*, one might make further cautious inferences about the nature of this tradition. First, the scheme can scarcely have arisen out of systematic (or 'theoretical') reflexion, because the arrangement of the symptoms is not logical and cannot be explained by any of the medical theories transmitted within or without the Hippocratic Collection. How the scheme was first formed cannot be surmised, but it seems likely that it was conceived within the framework of professional, practical activity.

Second, the tradition of the scheme does not seem to have been very wide-spread because it is found[155] only in *Epidemics I* and *III* and *Prognostics*. This is yet further confirmation of the opinion generally accepted among modern historians that these three books have a 'special relationship' with each other.[156]

Third, the scheme comprises, besides 'symptoms,' two doctrinal concepts which have to do with symptoms but are no symptoms themselves, namely *krísis* and *apóstasis*. This doctrine characteristic of the *Epidemics* and kindred treatises is presupposed in the scheme, which must, therefore, be more recent than the doctrine.

---

[154] Smith, Analytical and catalogue structure.

[155] So far as I know.

[156] Deichgräber, Die Epidemien, p. 17–23. Nothing new can be said about the authorship problem. "Ich glaube," says Deichgräber (p. 23), "... daß der Verfasser des Prognostikon in nächster Nähe des Verfassers der Epidd. I und III zu suchen ist, d. h. daß beide zumindest ein und derselben Schule und sicher auch derselben Generation angehören." He favours identity of authorship. Even *Epid. I* and *III* may, however, have been written by several authors, perhaps persons in a teacher – student relationship. Also, the differences in the systems of critical days in *Epid. I, III* and in *Prog.* speak against Deichgräber's opinion (Lloyd, Hippocratic question 185). Generally on problems of authorship Langholf, Kallimachos 21–30.

Fourth, neither concepts of meteorological medicine nor special humours such as bile or phlegm are mentioned in the scheme. This does not prove that these doctrines were not presupposed.

Fifth, the scheme occurs only in connexion with *general* case descriptions (i. e. with historical descriptions of groups in the *Epidemics*, with prognostic descriptions in *Prognostics*). In the *individual* descriptions of historical cases in the *Epidemics*, the method applied is different (day-to-day reports about selected symptoms). This does not prove that the scheme was unknown when the individual case reports were written.[157]

The scheme is clearly an analytic tool. The original nosological approach (e. g. in *On Diseases II*, ch. 12–75) dealt with autonomous disease units (A, B, C, ... N) and tried to adjust the doctrine to 'reality' by increasing the number of disease units (A_1, $A_{2...n}$, B_1 ... N_n), e. g. *On Internal Affections*, ch. 10–12 "There are three kinds of *phthísis*: This one ... (follows description, ch. 10). Another *phthísis*... (ch. 11). Another *phthísis* ... (ch. 12)."[158]

In *Epidemics I* and *III* and *Prognostics*, one can see how the firm units were broken into universally applicable sub-units. A kind of 'questionnaire' was used in *Epidemics I* and *III* in order to control the multitude of 'data' relating to patients in an epidemic disease. 'Questionnaire' and 'data' should not be taken in the modern sense. There was certainly no flood of paper, nor was there much *numerical* data except for the numbers of the days with paroxysm and *krísis*. With this reservation, the two words denote quite well the method utilized. A physician who relied solely on traditional nosology must have felt helpless vis-à-vis some forms of epidemic diseases whenever an individual case diverged from the 'norm,' or the standard of the handbooks. The most natural question asked by a patient is: "What is my disease called?" The answer which a traditional nosologist would give in numerous cases was: "It is a new variety of disease A." Quite often the only possible answer was: "I don't know." This must have been a delicate situation for the physician who worked in a small Greek city state without the protection of any public certificate or diploma. A doctor was dependent exclusively on his reputation – and this in communities where (unlike modern cities) everybody knew everybody and direct communication was much more widespread than in modern states.[159]

---

[157] On the relationship between individual and summary (collective) case descriptions, see Grmek, Les maladies 423–425 ("Le passage du cas concret à la règle générale").

[158] *Int.* 7.188.26–198.24 φθίσιες τρεῖς· αὕτη μὲν γίνεται ἀπὸ φλέγματος ... ἄλλη φθίσις· γίνεται μὲν ἀπὸ ταλαιπωρίης ... ἑτέρη φθίσις· ὑπὸ ταύτης τάδε πάσχει· ... (textus secundum M: deest θ). Cf. above p. 20; 25, note 46.

[159] Cohn-Haft, Public physicians 12 ff.

Splitting the traditional disease units into smaller secondary units of disease signs ('symptoms') was a less problematic procedure, particularly so because many of the 'symptoms' had already had some significance within the framework of traditional nosology. The scheme of exposition underlying some of the descriptions in *Epidemics I* and *III* gives a good idea of how the physicians proceeded when trying to master the variety of pathological phenomena present in the many individual cases of an epidemic. The method made it also possible to recognize whether any 'symptoms' were lacking. The texts excerpted in the list contain examples of such negative indications: "Not sleepless," "not without appetite," "not very thirsty." The scheme did not contradict the earlier approach and was easily comprehended by the layman on whose appreciation the physician depended so much. It permitted furthermore the comparison not only of different cases of one sort of disease (by forming 'groups' of patients, cf. below, p. 194 ff.), but even of diseases with different names,[160] and the application of generally valid rules. For instance, the *krísis*, *pépsis*, and *apóstasis* doctrine including the doctrine on critical days could be applied quite easily on the basis of such analyses. All this did not make it necessary to abolish the disease units denoted by the traditional disease-names, which had been current among the lay public as well as the physicians, and which continued to be another useful tool.

It seems as though *Prognostics* is an essay to evaluate the prognostic relevance of the 'symptoms' of acute diseases on the basis of an inherited 'questionnaire'-scheme, independently of the traditional denominations of any specific diseases. Irrespective of the chronological relationship between *Epidemics I* and *III* and *Prognostics* – books that might be but literary samples of a more wide-spread approach –, it is legitimate to ask which of the two *stages as such*, namely description (represented by *Epidemics I* and *III*) and prognostic evaluation (represented by *Prognostics*), is the older one. At first sight one should say that observation (and description) must have preceded evaluation. However, when taking into account how closely 'investigation' or 'research'[161] was connected with the everyday

---

160 According to the author of *Acut.*, diseases may be identical even if they do not have the same name: the revisors of the *Knídiai gnṓmai* were mistaken because they considered rather the differences between diseases than the features common to them, and because they assumed "that two diseases are not identical unless they have the same name" (cf. above p. 14 f.). The idea is similarly expressed in the very last sentence of *Prog.* (2.190.6–9 Li. = 1.108.8–11 Kw. = 2.54 Jones), "You should not regard relevant the name of any disease unless it has been mentioned above ..." The scheme of the 'questionnaire' and its application are illustrative of these two statements, which appear to criticize a habit of correlating directly and unequivocally a thing and its name; Manfred Kraus, Name und Sache. Ein Problem im frühgriechischen Denken (Studien zur antiken Philosophie, 14), Amsterdam, 1987 (1988).

161 On both words cf. below p. 179 f.; 211.

practical work of the physician, one comes to realize that the question in this alternative form implies too strict a schematism. It is not out of place for the historian of medicine to start from logical considerations and subsequently to try to distill his logical procedures, such as induction or deduction, out of a complex pre-Aristotelian historical reality. Such logical procedures can in fact easily be read *into* the extant medical texts of the fifth and fourth centuries B. C., and the Hippocratic authors must, therefore, to some extent have been aware of the existence of logical rules.[162] Since, however, these writers are never specific with regard to this point, we do not know how far they were guided by anything like abstract logic.[163] An historically more plausible assumption would be that observation and prognostic evaluation went hand in hand in the professional practice of these Greek physicians; that in their very acts concerning the single patient, evaluation influenced and biased observation, and *vice versa*. Apart from abstract logic, there must have been a rather high methodological awareness in the authors of the *Epidemics, Prognostics,* and of kindred treatises. This can be inferred not only from their explicit methodological remarks, but also from the fact that they presupposed an older approach (nosology) while following a new one, and that they obviously felt free to emphasize the new or the old approach according to circumstances in their practical activity.

Meteorological Doctrines Amalgamated with the Doctrinal System of *krísis*, *pépsis*, and *apóstasis*

The *krísis*, *pépsis*, and *apóstasis* doctrine forms the core of the medical theories of the *Epidemics*. The doctrine was not created *ex nihilo* by the authors of the *Epidemics* or by their forerunners; primitive features of it are 'foreshadowed' in the oldest nosological texts and could be re-interpreted in the light of the developed *krísis*, *pépsis*, and *apóstasis* doctrine.[164] This latter doctrine contains itself doctrinal elements taken over from older stages of Greek medicine. Such elements could be combined with the *krísis*, *pépsis*, and *apóstasis* concept because it was universal and vague enough, and because it did not affect the content of the other medical traditions. Indeed, it concerned other aspects of medicine than the nosology represented by *On Diseases II*, ch. 12–75 and by kindred treatises, also other aspects than the various concepts of elementary qualities (warm/

---

[162] For details, see below on 'types' and 'groups' in the *Epidemics*, p. 194 ff.

[163] For 'induction,' see above p. 113, and below p. 213–224.

[164] Cf. above p. 67 f.; 123–126.

cold, moist/dry) and of humours (the best-known humoral doctrine being the one featuring blood, phlegm, bile, and black bile). All of these doctrines, which were mutually compatible (at least in principle), could easily be amalgamated with the doctrinal system of *krísis*, *pépsis*, and *apóstasis*.

This holds true also of the meteorological approach, which tried to establish correlations between the astronomical events, the weather, and the diseases attendant upon the changes of the seasons. Traces of a medical interest in meteorology are found in some of the nosological treatises (*On Internal Diseases, On Affections, On Diseases I*).[165] The idea that diseases are influenced by the weather and its changes must have been old.[166] Herodotus, for example, contends that the Egyptians are healthy because their seasons do not change. "For people are most likely to be seized with maladies during changes; changes of anything, but in particular of the seasons."[167] The author of *On Airs, Waters, Places*, ch. 2, states about the physician: "If he knows the changes of the seasons, the risings and settings of the stars, and how each of these happen, he will know beforehand how the year is going to be."[168]

The method advocated consisted in observing the weather during certain astronomical events: the differentiation between astronomical and meteorological phenomena was not yet made around 400 B.C.[169] In ch. 10 it is stated: "As to the seasons, one may in the following way assess whether the year will be unhealthy or healthy: If the signs (viz. of the weather and in heaven) are normal during the settings and risings of the stars, then the year is likely to be very healthy."[170] "If during the rising of Sirius there is rain and storm and the Etesian winds blow, one may

---

165 For references, see Jouanna, Archéologie 248–250, 302, and 355 respectively; also his 'Index des notions' s. v. 'saisons' (p. 652). His assumption (p. 250, note 4; 511) that the doctrine of the influence of the climate is a Koan achievement taken over by the 'Knidian' nosological authors is unlikely, cf. above generally about Kos and Knidos (p. 12–36).

166 Kudlien, Beginn 57–59, 128–132.

167 Hdt. *II* 77.3 ... ὅτι οὐ μεταλλάσσουσι αἱ ὧραι· ἐν γὰρ τῇσι μεταβολῇσι τοῖσι ἀνθρώποισι αἱ νοῦσοι μάλιστα γίνονται, τῶν τε ἄλλων πάντων καὶ δὴ καὶ τῶν ὡρέων μάλιστα.

168 *Aer.* 2.14.10–12 Li. = 1.34.18–21 Kw. = 1.72 Jones εἰδὼς γὰρ τῶν ὡρέων τὰς μεταβολὰς καὶ τῶν ἄστρων ἐπιτολάς τε καὶ δύσιας κατότι ἕκαστον τούτων γίγνεται προειδείη ἂν τὸ ἔτος ὁκοῖόν τι μέλλει γίγνεσθαι. (Text quoted after Diller's edition.)

169 See, e. g., Der Kleine Pauly III 1266 s. v. 'Meteorologie' (Robert Böker); Pauly/Wissowa, Suppl. VI 316 ff. s. v. 'Meteorologie' (W. Capelle). An example from *Morb. Sacr.* will be quoted shortly below p. 171, note 202. Another example is the influence of the air on the heavenly bodies in *Flat.*, cf. below p. 244. Significant in this connection is, for instance, also the belief ascribed to various Pre-Socratics that the solstices are due to the influence of the air on the sun (see, Diels/Kranz, vol. 3, 'Wortindex,' s. v. τροπή). The expression ἄνευ τῆς τοῦ ὅλου φύσεως (Plat. *Phdr.* 270 c; cf. below p. 196 f., note 324) could, therefore, refer both to the entire immediate environment and to the whole universe.

170 *Aer.* 2.42.8–13 Li. = 1.48.17–49.3 Kw. = 1.98 Jones (quoted below, note 208).

expect that [the fevers] cease, and that the autumn will be healthy."[171] Unhealthy years were predicted correspondingly. The treatise mentions in particular the rising of the Dog-Star (Sirius) and Arcturus, and the setting of the Pleiades (ch. 10–11).[172]

A similar method is reported by an author of the fourth century B. C., according to Cicero, *On Divination I* 130: "We possess information that the inhabitants of Keos have the custom of diligently observing the rising of Sirius every year and of assessing, as Herakleides Pontikos writes, whether the year will be healthy or unhealthy: If the star rises darker and as it were covered with mist, he says, the heaven is dense and thick, so that its exhalation will be heavy and unhealthy; but if the star appears bright and shining, this signifies that the heaven is thin and pure and, therefore, healthy."[173] If no other report besides the one by Herakleides was available to us, we would perhaps infer that a group of physicians or meteorologists were executing this annual observation on Keos. In fact, Herakleides could even have known *On Airs, Waters, Places*. That his report, however, attests to activities of a different kind, can easily be inferred.

Two early Alexandrian poets, Apollonius Rhodius and Callimachus, mention the observations made traditionally on Keos, and from the details mentioned by them it becomes obvious that the observations of Sirius were a religious act. Apollonius (*II* 500–527) describes how the rural god Aristaios, son of Apollo and Cyrene, was brought up by the centaur Chiron and was taught "medicine and divination."[174] When Sirius burned the Cyclades and there had been no remedy[175] for a long time, the inhabitants called Aristaios to ward off the pestilence.[176] He came to Keos with people from Arcadia, built a large altar to Zeus Ikmaios and offered sacrifices on the mountains to the star Sirius and to Zeus. "For this reason,

---

171 *Aer.* 2.44.8–10 Li. = 1.49.17–19 Kw. = 1.98 Jones καὶ ἢν μὲν ἐπὶ κυνὸς ἐπιτολῇ ὕδωρ ἐπιγένηται καὶ χειμὼν καὶ οἱ ἐτησίαι πνεύσωσι, ἐλπὶς παύσασθαι καὶ τὸ μετόπωρον ὑγιηρὸν γενέσθαι.

172 Pauly/Wissowa, Suppl. VII 175–198 s. v. 'Episemasiai' (Albert Rehm).

173 Etenim Ceos accepimus ortum Caniculae diligenter quotannis solere servare coniecturamque capere, ut scribit Ponticus Heraclides, salubrisne an pestilens annus futurus sit. nam si obscurior ⟨et⟩ quasi caliginosa stella extiterit, pingue et concretum esse caelum, ut eius adspiratio gravis et pestilens futura sit; sin inlustris et perlucida stella apparuerit, significari caelum esse tenue purumque et propterea salubre. For other ancient weather prognoses from the rising of Sirius, see Pauly/Wissowa III.1 A, 314–351 s. v. 'Sirius' (Gundel), in partic. 346 f. More generally Pauly/Wissowa, Suppl. IX, 1609–1692 s. v. 'Wetterzeichen' (Robert Böker), in partic. 1631–1633.

174 512 ἀκεστορίην τε θεοπροπίας τ' ἐδίδαξαν, sc. Μοῦσαι.

175 817 ἄκος.

176 519 λοιμοῦ ἀλεξητῆρα.

the Etesian winds from Zeus cool the land for forty days."[177] Apollonius tells the story in order to explain the origin of the Etesians and of the religious rite, which was still performed in his day: "Still now, the priests offer sacrifices before the rising of the Dog-Star (= Sirius)."[178] The ancient scholia provide the additional information that Aristaios ordered the islanders of Keos to watch the rising of Sirius every year "with weapons" and to sacrifice.[179]

Callimachus tells virtually the same story, although shorter and with some minor divergences and additions: The priesthood of Zeus Aristaios Ikmios, as he calls the god,[180] had been handed down in a clan for generations. The ritual task was "on mountain heights to appease the violence of the rising Sirius and to pray to Zeus for the Etesians."[181]

The testimonia about the cult on Keos suggest that the observation of a star for the prognosis of weather and health was not an achievement of the author of *On Airs, Waters, Places*, not even of physicians. It had ancient roots. In the case of Sirius, we can observe how a cult[182] still

---

[177] 522–526 καὶ βωμὸν ποίησε μέγαν Διὸς Ἰκμαίοιο, | ἱερά τ' εὖ ἔρρεξεν ἐν οὔρεσιν ἀστέρι κείνῳ | Σειρίῳ αὐτῷ τε Κρονίδῃ Διί. τοῖο δ' ἕκητι | γαῖαν ἐπιψύχουσιν ἐτήσιοι ἐκ Διὸς αὖραι | ἤματα τεσσαράκοντα.

[178] 526–527 Κέῳ δ' ἔτι νῦν ἱερῆες | ἀντολέων προπάροιθε Κυνὸς ῥέζουσι θυηλάς.

[179] Scholia in Apollonium Rhodium vetera, rec. Carolus Wendel, Berlin, 1935, p. 172 ἐνομοθέτησε γὰρ τοῖς Κείοις κατ' ἐνιαυτὸν μεθ' ὅπλων ἐπιτηρεῖν τὴν ἐπιτολὴν τοῦ Κυνὸς καὶ θύειν αὐτῷ. Other ancient attestations of the myth and bibliography in: Martin P. Nilsson, Griechische Feste von religiöser Bedeutung, Leipzig, 1906, 6–8; Nilsson, Geschichte der griechischen Religion, vol. 1. 395 f.; Apollonios de Rhodes, Argonautiques, ed. Francis Vian, trad. Émile Delage, Paris, 1974, *ad loc.* and p. 272 f.; Walter Burkert, Homo necans. Interpretationen altgriechischer Opferriten und Mythen, Berlin/New York, 1972 (Religionsgesch. Versuche und Vorarbeiten, 32), 125–127. The explanation of the name Ζεὺς Ἰκμαῖος given by the scholiast of Apoll. Rhod. and accepted by modern scholars (Διὸς Ἰκμαίοιο· ἕνεκα τῆς ἰκμάδος. ἐν τῇ Κέῳ δέ ἐστιν ἱερὸν Διὸς Ἰκμαίου, τουτέστι διύγρου, ἐπεὶ αἴτιος γέγονε τῆς πνοῆς τῶν ἀνέμων), although linguistically and mythologically possible (Zeus = god of rain), cannot be right, because the Etesians are dry, not wet (cf., e. g., Der Kleine Pauly II 381 s. v. 'Etesien' [Robert Böker]). Moreover, Callimachus' collateral form Ἴκμιος (see below) cannot be explained so linguistically (ἴκμιος 'moist' in Nonnos *II* 490 is glossematic). This Zeus seems rather to be related to Ζεὺς οὔριος and Homer's enigmatic ἴκμιος οὖρος.

[180] On Aristaios and his identification with Zeus see, Lexicon iconographicum II.1, 603–607 s. v. 'Aristaios' (Brian F. Cook), where literature is listed.

[181] Call. *Aet. III*, frg. 75.32–37 Pfeiffer Ἀρισταίου [Ζη]νὸς ἀφ' ἱερέων | Ἰκμίου οἷσι μέμ[η]λεν ἐπ' οὔρεος ἀμβώνεσσιν | πρηΰνειν χαλ[ε]πὴν Μαῖραν ἀνερχομένην, | αἰτεῖσθαι τὸ δ' ἄημα παραὶ Διός. Cf. the commentary in: Callimachus, ed. Rudolfus Pfeiffer, Oxford, 1949–1953. For the passages from Apollonius and Callimachus see also Fraser, Ptolemaic Alexandria, vol. 1. 638 f. 725–727.

[182] A cult for Zeus *and* Sirius, cf. Burkert *loco cit.*; stars were rarely the object of a cult in classical Greece, although the belief in the influence of the stars was popular even before the spread of astrology; cf. Roscher, Lexikon VI 867–1071 (Nachträge) s. v. 'Sternbilder, Sternglaube und Sternsymbolik' (Boll, Gundel), in partic. 867–869 (bibliography), 995–

existing at the time of the Alexandrian poets or of their sources was reinterpreted, or rationalized, by Herakleides Pontikos, who does not make reference to any religious cult.[183] The prognostic doctrine of *On Airs, Waters, Places* can similarly be interpreted without presupposing popular beliefs.

In *On Airs, Waters, Places* it is left ambiguous whether the astronomical events are themselves the cause of changes in the body.[184] Ch. 11 indicates only the simultaneousness: "You must in addition [to solstices and equinoxes] pay attention to the risings of the stars, in particular of the Dog-Star, then of Arcturus, and also to the setting of the Pleiades, because diseases get to their *krísis* mostly on these days: some of the diseases end fatally, others favourably, and all others change their form and state (*katástasis*)."[185] The traditional belief[186] in the direct influence of the stars on human life is neither explicitly expressed nor repudiated in the treatise, whose contemporary reader could interpret the respective passages in either sense, i. e. either in terms of popular tradition or of contemporary rationalization.[187] Explicitly explained is the influence of the climate, the environment, and the weather. In interpreting *On Airs, Waters, Places*, the philologist or medical historian should, therefore, take both aspects into account.

The local cult of Sirius on Keos is of unknown age but cannot have been recent at the time of Herakleides and of the Alexandrian poets. How ancient generally the belief in the influence of Sirius is, can be inferred from its mention in early epic poetry: Hesiod, *Works and Days* 575–588, "... at harvest-time, when the sun parches the skin ... Then the goats are fattest, the wine at its best, the women most lustful, the men most

---

1002 (Sirius), 1055–1058 ('Astrometeorologie,' where additional literature is listed); Pfeiffer, Studien zum Sternglauben 1–16; Lexicon iconographicum II.1, 904 ff. s. v. 'Astra' (Semni Karusu), with bibliography; Burkert, Griechische Religion 271–273.

183 There is 'rationalization' in Herakleides' report, although its general context must have been divination; Fritz Wehrli, Die Schule des Aristoteles, Herakleides Pontikos, 2nd ed., Basel, 1969, frg. 141 (also comm., p. 104–107); H. B. Gottschalk, Heraclides of Pontus, Oxford, 1980, 130.

184 For a similar ambiguity, namely the inexplicitness as to whether certain 'signs' *indicate* or *cause* subsequent phenomena, see above, p. 60, and below note 189; 224, note 450.

185 *Aer.* 2.52.4–8 Li. = 1.52.19–53.4 Kw. = 1.104 Jones δεῖ δὲ καὶ τῶν ἄστρων τὰς ἐπιτολὰς φυλάσσεσθαι, καὶ μάλιστα τοῦ κυνός, ἔπειτα ἀρκτούρου, καὶ ἔτι πληϊάδων δύσιν. τά τε γὰρ νοσεύματα μάλιστα ἐν ταύτῃσι τῇσιν ἡμέρῃσι κρίνεται καὶ τὰ μὲν ἀποφθίνει, τὰ δὲ λήγει, τὰ δὲ ἄλλα πάντα μεθίσταται εἰς ἕτερον εἶδος καὶ ἑτέρην κατάστασιν. On the meaning of *katástasis* see shortly below.

186 The old belief in the influence of stars was only in later (Hellenistic) times amalgamated with the 'Chaldaean' system of astrology; Burkert, Griechische Religion 184, 484; Nilsson, Geschichte der griechischen Religion, vol. 2. 268–281.

187 A popular tradition clearly appearing in *On Airs, Waters, Places* is the belief in a 'privilege' of the east, see below p. 245.

powerless, because Sirius dries up head and knees, and the skin is parched from heat."[188] In Hesiod, the heat of the sun is brought about by Sirius (the text does not explain, how[189]), the star brings about 'pathological' changes in the body, particularly in the head.[190] This is strongly reminiscent of the pathological mechanism explained in *On Airs, Waters, Places* (and *On the Sacred Disease*). The *Iliad*, too, mentions the effect of Sirius, *XXII* 29–31: The Dog-Star "brings much *pyretós* to the miserable mortals."[191] Although the meaning of *pyretós* cannot be determined with certainty here,[192] it seems plausible to understand the word in its normal meaning, 'fever.'[193]

Astronomical and meteorological events are mentioned time and again in the *Epidemics*, above all in the so-called *katástasis* descriptions of books *I* and *III*. The Greek word *katástasis* means 'condition,' 'situation,' 'state' and can be used for the 'state' of a disease[194] as well as for the 'condition' of the weather.[195] In a number of passages one cannot decide which of the two meanings is intended.[196] Both meanings are implied in *Epidemics I*, ch. 10 (= ch. 23 Kw., Jones), "... the whole *katástasis* and particularly

---

188 ὥρῃ ἐν ἀμήτου, ὅτε τ' ἠέλιος χρόα κάρφει. | ... τῆμος πιόταταί τ' αἶγες καὶ οἶνος ἄριστος, | μαχλόταται δὲ γυναῖκες, ἀφαυρότατοι δέ τοι ἄνδρες | εἰσίν, ἐπεὶ κεφαλὴν καὶ γούνατα Σείριος ἄζει, | αὐαλέος δέ τε χρὼς ὑπὸ καύματος. Cf. *Scut.* 397 ὅτε τε χρόα Σείριος ἄζει.

189 "Da mit dem Auf- oder Untergang bestimmter Sterne oder Sternbilder verschiedene Witterungserscheinungen auftraten ..., entstand der Glaube, daß diese Sterne solche Wetteränderung bewirkten, nicht nur andeuteten." (Der Kleine Pauly V 365 s. v. 'Sternglaube' [Emilie Boer]) Cf. above p. 60, 168 and below p. 224, note 450 on indication and causation of symptoms.

190 The changes in the males can partly be explained in terms of doctrines manifest in the Hippocratic Collection and elsewhere: The head, which should be cool, as it contains the cold phlegm ≅ semen (Lonie, Hippocratic treatises 101–103), is warmed and impairs the whole body. Cf. the commentary by Martin L. West (ed.), Hesiod, Works and Days, Oxford, 1978, 305, with some parallels and bibliography; Fridolf Kudlien, Zur Erforschung archaisch-griechischer "Zeugungslehren," Medizinhist. Journ. 16 (1981), 323–339.

191 φέρει πολλὸν πυρετὸν δειλοῖσι βροτοῖσι.

192 'Fever'? Or (as Liddell/Scott/Jones translate) 'burning heat,' 'fiery heat'?

193 But not necessarily in the narrow technical sense as in the Collection: Perhaps the language of the early epic did not yet differentiate between 'heat' generally and 'fever.' Kudlien, Primitive medicine 321. For the more comprehensive meaning of some words in Homeric poetry, see above p. 37–43.

194 E. g., *Epid. I* 2.674.14 Li. = 1.200.22 Kw. = 1.182 Jones; *III* 3.80.5 Li. = 227.2 Kw. = 244 Jones.

195 E. g., *Epid. I* 2.598.11 Li. = 1.180.11 Kw. = 1.146 Jones; 640.8 Li. = 191.9 Kw. = 166 Jones; *III* 3.100.5 Li. = 232.6 Kw. = 256 Jones.

196 E. g., *Epid. I* 2.614.2 Li. = 1.183.19 Kw. = 1.152 Jones; 642.7 Li. = 191.22 Kw. = 166 Jones; 656.7 Li. = 195.21 Kw. = 1.174 Jones; 664.5 Li. = 197.17 Kw. = 176 Jones.

that of the weather and of each (geographic) region."[197] The semantic ambiguity is due to the underlying medical doctrine of a close interrelation between the weather and the diseases, which both form one 'system.' According to the *Epidemics* it is useless to observe or treat a disease without paying attention to the weather. Apart from medicine, the belief in the importance of wind and weather for human life, health and disease was popular lore as expressed in a number of Wind cults (sacrifices, prayers, etc.)[198]

Astronomical events (solstices, equinoxes, risings and settings of stars) are very frequently mentioned[199] in the *Epidemics*, but as in *On Airs, Waters, Places*, it is never said explicitly that these events are themselves responsible for health or disease. It appears that the *Epidemics* use them merely for purposes of dating. Since, however, these treatises are not explicit concerning their respective underlying theories, one cannot rule out the possibility that the events were thought to be responsible either directly or indirectly, namely as agents determining the weather.

The physician, by observing the meteorological phenomena, tried to predict which diseases were likely to appear, and he even thought it feasible to predict the weather from observing the diseases: *On Humours*, ch. 17, "As it is possible to conjecture about the diseases by starting from the weather, it is sometimes also possible to predict rainfalls and winds and droughts on the basis of the diseases, for example northwind, southwind."[200]

Basic constituents of the meteorological approach to medicine are the weather conditions characterized as wet/dry and northern/southern;[201] the

---

[197] *Epid. I* 2.670.4–5 Li. = 1.199.13–14 Kw. = 1.180 Jones ἐκ τῆς καταστάσιος ὅλης καὶ κατὰ μέρεα τῶν οὐρανίων καὶ χώρης ἑκάστης.

[198] Nilsson, Geschichte der griechischen Religion, vol. 1. 116 f.; Roland Hampe, Kult der Winde in Athen und Kreta, Sitzungsber. d. Heidelberger Akad. d. Wiss., Philos.-histor. Kl., 1967, no. 1; Lanata, Medicina magica 65–69; Burkert, Griechische Religion 272, with bibliography; Der Kleine Pauly V 1380 f. s. v. 'Winddämonen, -kult' (Dietrich Wachsmuth).

[199] Phillips, Hippocratic physician.

[200] *Hum.* 5.498.7–9 Li. = 4.90 Jones ὡς (ὡς A: ὥσπερ M) ἐκ τῶν ὡρέων (ὡ- M: ὁ- A) τὰς νούσους ἔστι τεκμήρασθαι, ἔστι ποτὲ καὶ ἐκ τῶν νούσων ὕδατα καὶ ἀνέμους καὶ ἀνυδρίας προγινώσκειν, οἷον (οἷον A: om. M, suppl. supra lin.) βόρεια, νότια. An example taken from Ps.-Theophrastus, *De signis*, will be quoted below p. 251.

[201] Moreover, the physicians tended to amalgamate this "Zweiwindetheorie" (Pauly/Wissowa VIII A.2 [2. Reihe, 16. Halbband], 2332 ff. s. v. 'Winde' [Robert Böker]) and the binary phlegm/bile doctrine. Generally on the amalgamation of medical theories in the Hippocratic Collection Langholf, Kompatibilität. – Perhaps it is no coincidence that one of the supporters of the two-wind theory originated from, or lived on, the island of Thasos, where parts of the *Epidemics* are localized: Thrasyalkes. For the scarce testimonia available about him, see Pauly/Wissowa VI A.1 (2. Reihe, 11. Halbband), 565–567 s. v. (W. Capelle); Der Kleine Pauly V 784 s. v. (François Lasserre).

qualities warm/cold play a less prominent rôle. The most detailed meteorological description comprising these constituents is *On the Sacred Disease*, ch. 13 Li., Gr. (= ch. 16 Jones): "I say that for the following reasons one gets seizures during the changes of the winds, particularly of the southern ones, but also of the northern ones and the others (these two are the strongest as compared to the others, and the ones most strongly opposed to each other in direction as well as in force): The northwind contracts the air and segregates what is turbid and wet in it, and makes it clear and transparent; and it has the same effect on everything else that has its origin in the sea and in the other waters. It segregates the wet and turbid from everything, also from the people. Therefore it is the most healthy wind. The southwind has the exactly opposite effect. It begins by diluting the contracted air and making it thinner, wherefore it does not blow violently at once but begins gently (because it cannot immediately overwhelm the previous air which is thick and contracted, but needs some time to make it thin). Its effect is the same also on the sea, the rivers, the sources, the wells, and whatever lives and contains moisture — which is in everything more or less. It all feels this wind and turns turbid from being clear, warm from being cold, and wet from being dry. Ceramic vessels stored in the houses or below the earth and filled with wine or another liquid all feel the southwind and change the quality [of their contents]. It also renders the sun and the moon and the stars much less clear than normally. Since it has power over these which are so huge and strong, it must of necessity rule also over the human nature[202] and cause[203] the body to feel it and to undergo changes."[204]

A similar doctrine underlies the four *katástasis* accounts of *Epidemics I* and *III*, although one cannot determine with any precision in which details the doctrines are identical, because the *Epidemics* are not explicit enough as to the underlying theory. At any rate, the *Epidemics* seem to represent a later stage of doctrinal evolution.[205]

Each *katástasis* account in *Epidemics I* and *III* begins with a meteorological description of one particular year, followed by a detailed report of the prevailing diseases. Whereas the weather as such is described each time from autumn until summer, the diseases are recorded for another period of time, namely from winter (*katástasis* no. 2, 3, 4) or next year's

---

202 An argument *a fortiori* (cf. above p. 98, note 81). Note the lack of differentiation between meteorological and astronomical phenomena.

203 Legendum ποιεῖ⟨ν⟩.

204 *Morb. Sacr.* 6.384.4—386.14 Li. = 2.170—172 Jones = 80.4—82.34 Grensemann. The translation proposed above is based on the latter edition.

205 See below, and Grensemann, Gynäkologie 35: [To date *Aer.* around 400 B. C., i. e. *after Epid. I* and *III*] "bedeutet eine Abwertung von Aer. Nach den Epidemien brauchte auch niemand für die Übernahme astronomischer Faktoren in die Medizin einzutreten."

spring (*katástasis* 1) until next year's winter (*katástasis* 1, 2, 3) or autumn (*katástasis* 4).[206] The author(s) do(es) not seem to be primarily interested in the relationship between the weather of a certain season and the *simultaneous* diseases but rather in the relationship between the weather of one season and the diseases of another *subsequent* season. The interest seems to be prognostical: what is the future effect of given weather conditions on the occurrence of diseases, or on the health of the people?

The same question is asked, and answered, in the Hippocratic treatises *On Airs, Waters, Places*, ch. 10 and 11, and *Aphorisms III*, ch. 11—14, and in the pseudo-Aristotelian *Problemata I*, ch. 8—11, 19—20. Some striking similarities and specific differences between these texts and the *katástasis* descriptions of *Epidemics I* and *III* allow a tentative interpretation of the texts in terms of a scientific evolution from *a priori* dogmas towards ways of asking questions within the framework of the dogmas.

On Airs, Waters, Places, ch. 10 and 11 present the following doctrine:[207] "With regard to the seasons, one can prognosticate [*diaginṓskō*] in the following way as to how the year will be characterized, whether unhealthy or healthy: If the [meteorological] features are normal [*katá lógon*] when the stars set and rise; and if there is rain in autumn, and the winter is moderate, neither too warm nor excessively cold, and if in spring and summer there is rain appropriate to the season — then the year is likely to be very healthy."[208]

In this description of the ideal year, the northwind and southwind are not mentioned. They are introduced only in the subsequent collection of general cases, which seems to have been taken over from a lost literary source (cf. below): "But if the winter is dry and northerly and the spring rainy and southerly, the summer must of necessity bring about fever and eye-inflammation and dysentery."[209] "And if the winter is southerly and rainy and warm, and the spring northerly and dry and cold, ..." (a

206 *katástasis* 1: *Epid. I* 2.598.3—614.5 Li. = 1.180.2—183.22 Kw. = 1.146—152 Jones; *katástasis* 2: *Epid. I* 2.614.7—632.11 Li. = 1.184.1—189.17 Kw. = 1.152—164 Jones; *katástasis* 3: *Epid. I* 2.638.7—668.14 Li. = 1.190.21—199.7 Kw. = 1.164—180 Jones; *katástasis* 4: *Epid. III* 3.66.13—100.6 Li. = 1.224.6—232.19 Kw. = 1.238—256 Jones.

207 *Aer.* 2.42.7—52.9 Li. = 1.48.16—53.4 Kw. = 1.98—104 Jones.

208 περὶ δὲ τῶν ὡρέων ὧδε ἄν τις ἐνθυμεύμενος διαγινώσκοι, ὁκοῖόν τι μέλλει ἔσεσθαι τὸ ἔτος, εἴτε νοσερὸν εἴτε ὑγιηρόν· ἢν μὲν γὰρ κατὰ λόγον γένηται τὰ σημεῖα ἐπὶ τοῖς ἄστροισι δύνουσί τε καὶ ἐπιτέλλουσι, ἔν τε τῷ μετοπώρῳ ὕδατα γένηται, καὶ ὁ χειμὼν μέτριος καὶ μήτε λίην εὔδιος μήτε ὑπερβάλλων τὸν καιρὸν τῷ ψύχει, ἔν τε τῷ ἦρι ὕδατα γένηται ὡραῖα καὶ ἐν τῷ θέρει, οὕτω τὸ ἔτος ὑγιεινότατον εἰκὸς εἶναι. As in *Epidemics I* and *III*, the year begins in autumn; Deichgräber, Die Epidemien p. 9.

209 ἢν δὲ ὁ μὲν χειμὼν αὐχμηρὸς καὶ βόρειος γένηται, τὸ δὲ ἦρ ἔπομβρον καὶ νότιον, ἀνάγκη τὸ θέρος πυρετῶδες γίνεσθαι καὶ ὀφθαλμίας καὶ δυσεντερίας ἐμποιεῖν.

description of the diseases to be expected follows).[210] "And if the summer is rainy and southerly, and the autumn is so, too ..."[211] "And if the summer is dry and northerly and the autumn rainy and southerly, ... But if it [the autumn] is northerly and dry, ..."[212] After each sequence of weather conditions, a prognostic statement is made about the diseases to be expected in the ensuing third season, namely summer or winter respectively. The focus of the dogmatizing collection of cases is on these two main seasons, for which the predictions are made.

The prognostic signification of the sequences spring – summer and autumn – winter is not considered (in *Epidemics I* and *III* it is, cf. shortly below). It is also remarkable that not all of the possible combinations of the qualities northerly/southerly and dry/rainy are taken into account (see the following diagram, where only the weather conditions are represented and the third season, for which each prognosis is made, has been omitted):

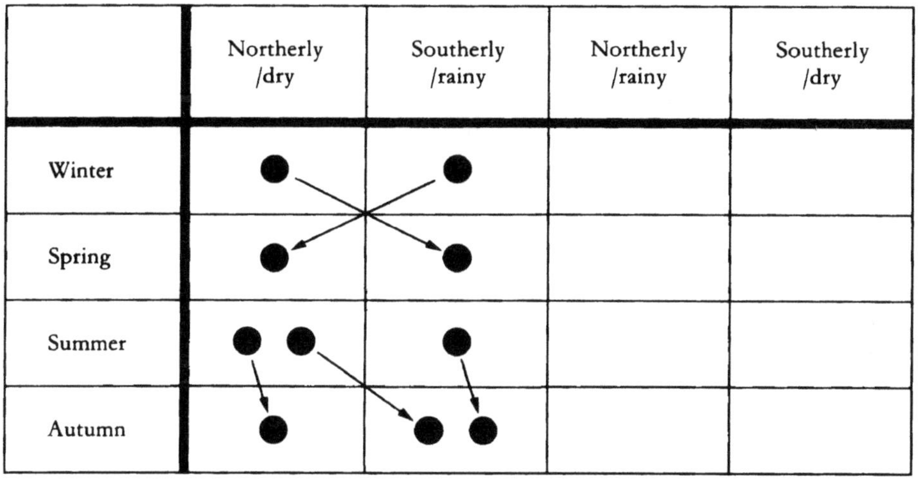

In the columns 'northerly/dry' and 'southerly/rainy' three more combinations are theoretically possible for the sequences considered (two of them are studied in *Epidemics I* and *III*, cf. below). The combinations 'northerly/rainy' and 'southerly/dry' (which are prominent in *Epidemics I* and *III*, cf. below) do not appear at all; and in fact they do not do so in

---

[210] ἢν δ' ὁ μὲν χειμὼν νότιος γένηται καὶ ἔπομβρος καὶ εὔδιος, τὸ δὲ ἦρ βόρειόν τε καὶ αὐχμηρὸν καὶ χειμέριον, ...

[211] ἢν δὲ τὸ θέρος ἔπομβρον γένηται καὶ νότιον καὶ τὸ μετόπωρον, ...

[212] ἢν δὲ τὸ θέρος αὐχμηρὸν γένηται καὶ βόρειον, τὸ δὲ μετόπωρον ἔπομβρον καὶ νότιον, ... ἢν δὲ βόρειόν τε ᾖ καὶ ἄνυδρον, ... (On the variant readings cf. Flashar (transl.), [Aristoteles], Problemata, p. 395 f.)

the whole treatise *On Airs, Waters, Places.*[213] The wind system here is the same as in *On the Sacred Disease*, where the northwind is never wet, and the southwind never dry.[214] This seems to be an ancient folk tradition. Already in Homer, the northwind is dry (*Iliad XXI* 346 f.), it drives away the clouds (*Iliad V* 524–526) and is therefore called *Aithrēgenés* or *Aithrēgenétēs*, 'born in the (or: creating) clear sky' (e. g. *Odyssey V* 296). The southwind, on the other hand, has its origin in the clouds (*Iliad II* 145 f.) and covers the mountaintops with mist (*Iliad III* 10).[215] The very word for southwind, *nótos*, originally means 'wet wind' (*notís* 'moisture'). In *On Airs, Waters, Places*, ch. 6, a region is described whose moisture is not sufficiently "segregated" by the northwind.[216] This is also the doctrine of *On the Sacred Disease.*

As in *On the Sacred Disease*, the northwind and southwind in *On Airs, Waters, Places* have a direct influence on the body by acting on the veins and on their contents. For instance, as a consequence of a southerly and rainy winter followed by a northerly and dry spring,[217] it is stated that in summer certain diseases provoked by harmful fluxes from the brain will occur, "because when during the southerly and warm winter the body is not contracted nor are the veins so, the brain will, when the northerly and dry and cold spring comes, get hard and be contracted, when it ought to be loosened and purged from mucus and coarseness during spring; with the consequence that, when suddenly the summer with its heat arrives, the aforesaid diseases occur." (Ch. 10)[218] This is the same physiological

---

213 With regard to geographic places, however, the elementary qualities are freely combined in *Aer.*: warm/dry, warm/wet, cold/dry, cold/wet. Details in Hermann Grensemann, Das 24. Kapitel von De aeribus, aquis, locis und die Einheit der Schrift, Hermes 107 (1979), 423–441.

214 Cf. what has been quoted shortly above from *Morb. Sacr.*: "The northwind ... segregates what is ... wet in it [in the air] ... The southwind has the exactly opposite effect [and makes everything wet that was dry before]." For the similarities between *Morb. Sacr.* and *Aer.* see Grensemann (ed.), Hippokrates, Heilige Krankheit, p. 7–18 (with bibliography). One author seems to have written both treatises. For the structural unity of *Aer.* see Grensemann's article quoted in the preceding note.

215 It would be a tempting task to try to determine for which parts of Greece and Asia Minor these two combinations are typical. Cf. Pauly/Wissowa XVII.1 (33. Halbband), 1116–1120 s. v. 'Notos' (W. Capelle).

216 *Aer.* 2.26.1–3 Li. = 1.40.1–3 Kw. = 1.82 Jones; instead of νοσώδης (V, Littré), νοτώδης (*austrinus* Latin version, Arabic version, Galen) has to be read, cf. Diller (ed.), Hippokrates, Über die Umwelt, *ad loc.*

217 Cf. above p. 172 f.

218 *Aer.* 2.46.11–48.3 Li. = 1.50.15–22 Kw. = 1.100–102 Jones; the translation is after the text edition by Diller, p. 50, 3–9: ὁκόταν γὰρ τοῦ χειμῶνος ἐόντος νοτίου καὶ θερμοῦ ⟨τὰ⟩ τοῦ σώματος μὴ συνίστηται μηδὲ ⟨αἱ⟩ φλέβες, τοῦ ἦρος ἐπιγινομένου βορείου καὶ αὐχμηροῦ καὶ ψυχροῦ ὁ ἐγκέφαλος, ὁπηνίκα αὐτὸν ἔδει ἅμα τῷ ἦρι διαλύεσθαι καὶ καθαίρεσθαι ὑπό τε κορύζης καὶ βράγχω⟨ν⟩, τηνικαῦτα πήγνυταί τε καὶ ξυνίσταται· ὥστε ἐξαίφνης τοῦ θέρεος ἐπιγενομένου καὶ τοῦ καύματος ... ταῦτα τὰ νοσεύματα ἐπιπίπτειν.

mechanism as in *On the Sacred Disease*, where seizures are explained by it;[219] the northwind or southwind respectively act on the brain, the brain with its fluxes acts on the veins, and the disturbed action of the veins results in diseases.

The general cases of *On Airs, Waters, Places*, ch. 10 and 11 are paralleled in a more recent treatise transmitted among the works of Aristotle, namely, the *Problemata*. The treatise is post-Aristotelian; its composition can be dated in the third century B. C.[220] When comparing the pseudo-Aristotelian version (*Problemata I*, ch. 8–11, 19–20),[221] one is at first sight tempted to believe that the older treatise *On Airs, Waters, Places* was the source of it.[222] But a closer examination reveals that, although the statements about changes in the weather and about the resulting diseases are similar, a third element is different in the two works: the aetiology. In each of the cases of the *Problemata*, an aetiology is given (the whole work is but a collection of problems of various sorts, each introduced by the interrogative "Why ...?"). In *On Airs, Waters, Places*, most cases have an aetiology, but not all. The aetiologies of both works are similar in so far as both treatises operate with the constitutive humours phlegm and bile and have other concepts in common; they diverge in details and also in their wording. Neither of the two versions of the aetiological parts seems to be influenced by, or dependent on, the other. This permits the assumption that *On Airs, Waters, Places* and *Problemata* used a common source for the general weather cases as such (scheme: weather of season 1 + weather of season 2 = diseases of season 3), but that none of the surviving *aetiologies* was contained in this common source. The assumption is supported by the fact that the same weather cases, but without any aetiology, are transmitted in another Hippocratic treatise, *Aphorisms III*, ch. 11–14.[223] The lost common source

---

219 *Morb. Sacr., passim.*

220 K. Abel, Gnomon 38 (1966), 229–236, favours the years 300–285, whereas Flashar (*op. cit.*, p. 356–358) had dated the work around 250 B. C.

221 *Probl.* 859 b 21–860 b 14; 861 b 1–862 a 3.

222 This is the opinion of Flashar, *op. cit.*, p. 385, 392. – Albert Rehm, Parapegmastudien, München, 1941 (Abhandl. der Bayer. Akad. d. Wiss., Philos.-histor. Abteil., N. F. 19, 1941), 37 f., 122–140, was of the same opinion. He assumed, moreover, that the method of indicating correlations between the seasons and typical events originated with the astronomer Euktemon (Pauly/Wissowa, Suppl. VII 175–198 s. v. 'Episemasiai' [Albert Rehm], in partic. 184–191), which would date the common source (see shortly below) of the passages in *Aer., Aph.*, and *Probl.* in the second half of the fifth c. B. C. This is, however, a wide temporal range, and the assumption is not sure; therefore I shall not draw any conclusions from it.

223 *Aph.* 4.490.2–492.6 Li. = 4.124–126 Jones. One can check systematically whether the three versions are likely to be dependent on each other, or whether it is more probable to postulate a lost common source (arguments of absolute date will not be used since

inferable[224] from the three kindred texts was, of course, older than any of these texts,[225] and it must have been authoritative and widely distributed – otherwise its reiteration would be unexplained.[226] Its main features were the opposition of the northwind and the southwind (with the former being always dry, the latter always wet) and the prognosis of the diseases

both *Aph.* and *Probl.* are compilations which might include old material):

(1) *A. W. P.* ↓ *Aph.* ↓ *Probl.*

(2) *A. W. P.* ↓ *Probl.* ↓ *Aph.*

(3) *Aph.* ↓ *A. W. P.* ↓ *Probl.*

(4) *Aph.* ↓ *Probl.* ↓ *A. W. P.*

(5) *Probl.* ↓ *A. W. P.* ↓ *Aph.*

(6) *Probl.* ↓ *Aph.* ↓ *A. W. P.*

(7) *A. W. P.* ↙ ↘ *Aph.* *Probl.*

(8) *Aph.* ↙ ↘ *A. W. P.* *Probl.*

(9) *Probl.* ↙ ↘ *A. W. P.* *Aph.*

A. W. P. has one case (summer and autumn wet and southerly) more than *Aph.*; this excludes (3), (4), (6), (8) unless the case has been omitted in *Aph.* during a later stage of the transmission; but since the same case is missing also in *Probl.* (where it has been supplied in a postscript as ch. 20), this seems unlikely. The different arrangement of the cases in *Probl.* and in *A. W. P.* excludes (5). *A. W. P.* and *Aph.* agree in giving more details in the disease descriptions than does *Probl.*; furthermore, the formulation of *Probl.* in each case, "Why ...?", and the grammatical subordination of the disease descriptions under the aetiology do not reoccur in the other two texts. (2) and (9) are therefore excluded. Both *A. W. P.* and *Probl.* have in common an additional element as compared to *Aph.*, namely a pathology based on the two humours bile and phlegm, which is absent from the *Aph.* chapters (another additional element they share is the formulation at the end of *A. W. P.*, ch. 10, "they reach the winter being not watery," which is also found at the end of *Probl. I*, ch. 11). This excludes (1). There remains (7), and it is unlikely because no trace of the aetiology of *A. W. P.* can be found in either *Aph.* or *Probl.*

224 A strict proof is impossible because the probability of later spontaneous change and of contamination cannot be assessed with any certainty. – For a possible common source of *Morb. II* and parts of *Aph.* see Paul Demont, Rev. Ét. Grecques 98 (1985), 427–429.

225 There may even have been intermediate sources.

226 It underwent the same changes as did some nosological books: addition of an aetiology to a descriptive text fund. On the nosological books, cf. Grensemann, Knidische Medizin, and Jouanna, Archéologie *passim*.

of a third season from the weather of the two preceding ones. The author of *On Airs, Waters, Places* incorporated the doctrine into his treatise because he took it to be useful, and because it was compatible with it. This treatise, which in turn is very similar to *On the Sacred Disease*, reveals, on the part of the physician(s), a fundamental interest in the influence of the weather, more precisely, of the northwind and the southwind, the dry and the wet, on the diseases, which were conceived as being generated by these weather changes. There is no proof for the belief that the author(s) of *Epidemics I* and *III* knew the treatises *On Airs, Waters, Places* or *On the Sacred Disease*; he (or they) may have known them, though, and must certainly have been familiar with the general discussion on the medical effects of the northwind and the southwind, the dry and the wet. This becomes obvious because the author(s) *systematically* collected material with this particular viewpoint in mind. It seems as though he (or they) started from a more or less specific doctrine about these weather features and then gathered observations in order to find out more about the relationship weather – diseases. The passages of *Epidemics I* and *III* in which this material is presented are the above-mentioned *katástasis* descriptions.[227]

There are four of them, each covering one of the four possible combinations of the features northwind/southwind and dry/wet. The free connexion of these constituents contrasts to the two invariable combinations, dry northwind and wet southwind, found in *On Airs, Waters, Places*, in *Aphorisms*, and in the pseudo-Aristotelian *Problemata*. In the 1st *katástasis*, it is stated that "the whole tendency was toward the southwind with dryness."[228] The 2nd *katástasis* says, "the whole year was wet and cold and northerly."[229] The 4th has two statements of this kind: "The year was southerly and wet and mild,"[230] and the headline "Southerly Rainy Year."[231] This title particularly makes clear what the leading principles of the *katástasis* description were. The 3rd *katástasis* is the only one not to contain a general formulaic summary of the year's weather tendency as do the other ones. From the detailed description of the weather of each season[232] it becomes, however, obvious that the year was mainly under the influence

---

[227] Cf. above p. 171 f.

[228] *Epid. I* 2.598.10–11 Li. = 1.180.10–11 Kw. = 1.146 Jones γενομένης δὲ τῆς ἀγωγῆς ὅλης ἐπὶ τὰ νότια καὶ μετ' αὐχμῶν ... The ensuing words, πρωῒ μὲν τοῦ ἦρος ἐκ τῆς πρόσθεν καταστάσιος ὑπεναντίης καὶ βορείου γενομένης, are unclear. Littré (598.11–12) and Jones (146) follow two possible ways of understanding them.

[229] *Epid. I* 2.616.5–6 Li. = 1.184.17–18 Kw. = 1.154 Jones γενομένου δὲ τοῦ ἔτεος ὅλου ὑγροῦ καὶ ψυχροῦ καὶ βορείου ...

[230] *Epid. III* 3.68.9–70.1 Li. = 1.224.18–19 Kw. = 1.240 Jones γενομένου δὲ τοῦ ἔτεος νοτίου καὶ ὑγροῦ καὶ μαλθακοῦ ...

[231] *Epid. III* 3.66.14 Li. = 1.224.7 Kw. = 1.238 Jones Ἔτος νότιον ἔπομβρον.

[232] *Epid. I* 2.638.8–640.7 Li. = 1.190.22–191.8 Kw. = 1.164–166 Jones.

of the northwind, and dry.[233] The four *katástasis* descriptions of *Epidemics I* and *III* thus represent the four possible combinations of the four constituents contained in the two classes northwind/southwind and dry/wet.[234] The combinations northwind/wet and southwind/dry are a new achievement as compared to the treatises *On the Sacred Disease* and *On Airs, Waters, Places* and also to the common source of the above-mentioned collection of general weather cases, a more flexible approach. The fact that the four years exhaust all four possibilities of combination makes it highly unlikely that they formed an immediate historical sequence. The descriptions may represent a selection out of a larger number of *katástasis* descriptions now lost.

Although the author(s) chose four years whose "whole tendency" followed the four patterns, he (or they) nevertheless paid attention to the smaller weather changes within each year, and consequently recorded which effects they had on the health of the people. The following diagram shows the weather conditions in each of the four seasons of the four years:

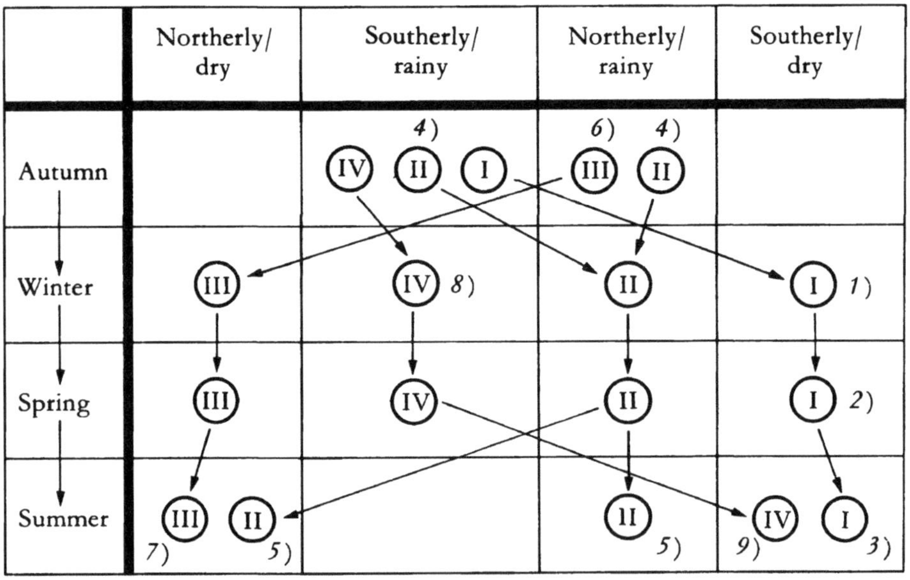

---

233 Northerly and dry from Nov. 8 (apparent cosmical setting of the Pleiades) through Sept. 20 (heliacal rising of Arcturus) of the next year according to our calender. For the dates of the rising and setting of the most important stars in the fifth century B. C., see Pauly/Wissowa VI.2 (12. Halbband), 2427 f. s. v. 'Fixsterne' (Boll). I am following these results. Slightly different dates are found in Lloyd (ed.), Hippocratic Writings, 65–66. On problems involved, see Martin L. West (ed.), Hesiod, Works and Days, Oxford, 1978, 376–381.

234 Similarly already Daremberg, Œuvres choisies d'Hippocrate, p. 401; he identified, however, 'southerly' with 'warm' and 'northerly' with 'cold,' which is a simplification.

The Roman numerals I–IV refer to the four *katástasis* descriptions of *Epidemics I* and *III* (cf. above p. 171 f.), the Arabic to the following notes: *1*) "Southerly winter, little northwind." *2*) "Spring southerly ..., little rain." *3*) "The Etesians blew only seldom, faintly, and with interruptions." *4*) "Wet with northwind and southwind." *5*) "The Etesians blew continuously; but soon around (the heliacal rising of) Arcturus (= September 20) there was again much rain with northwind" (i. e., most of the summer must have been dry; but this is not explicitly said). *6*) "But around the (autumnal) equinox until the (apparent cosmical setting of the) Pleiades (= November 8) there were a few southerly rainfalls." This was only a short interlude. *7*) There was another short interlude: "But around the summer solstice there was a little rain ... until (the heliacal rising of) Sirius (= July 28)." Also "around (the heliacal rising of) Arcturus (= September 20) until the (autumnal) equinox there was southerly rain." *8*) With an exception: "Around the equinox, there was northwind ... for a short time." *9*) "The summer was sunny ..., the Etesians blew only faintly and with interruptions. But around (the heliacal rising of) Arcturus (= September 20, i. e. during the last few days of the year described) there was much rain with northwind." Cf. ch. 15, on the same summer: "The summer ... was southerly and without wind."

When comparing the diagram to the one representing the general cases of weather changes in *On Airs, Waters, Places* and its source (above p. 173), one immediately recognizes that between the earlier dogmatizing approach and the observations of *Epidemics I* and *III* no contradictions occur as to the effects of the changes on health and diseases. They *cannot* occur, because none of the combinations of weather change contained in the older, influential collection of general cases reoccurs in the descriptions of *Epidemics I* and *III*. It looks as though the author(s) of *Epidemics I* and *III*, when collecting or presenting the observation material, had consciously avoided questioning the correctness of the case collection, although such a test would probably have been quite easy.

Theoretical Questions Asked in the *Epidemics*

To speak of research methods traceable in the *Epidemics* is to narrow down the historical perspective considerably. 'Research' is only one aspect of the work undertaken by the physicians who wrote these texts. The word *tékhnē*, by which the medical practitioners of that epoch denoted their professional activity, comprised not only cognition but also professional performance, not only science but also the everyday practical routine.[235] They did not possess a word which unambiguously designated 'medical science.' And just as there was no term for 'theory,'[236] there was

[235] Cf. above p. 18.
[236] Cf. above p. 1 f.

none for 'research' in the field of medicine.[237] The scientific investigation undertaken by the authors of the *Epidemics* and by other writers of the Collection originated directly from practical problems and was supposed to solve them immediately. Questions asked and answers given were never so specialized as not to have immediate bearing on the daily interaction between "the disease, the patient, and the physician," in which "the physician is the servant of [or: has an ancillary function in] the *tékhnē*; together with the physician, the patient must fight the disease."[238] The physician had to determine, if possible, the plan according to which the disease manifested itself in the body. This implied his knowing about *krísis* (including critical days), *pépsis*, and *apóstasis*. For the medical historian who examines these doctrines or 'theories' as a system (as has been done above, ch. III 1) and in their putative historical evolution (ch. III 2), it is instructive to see the multifarious influences that appear to have created them. The historian can single out some of the elements and some of the influences which helped constitute several of the doctrines, but it is not possible, in or through the surviving texts, to observe the very acts by which the central doctrines were formed. It cannot be denied that the authors of at least parts of the *Epidemics* did systematic research work. The investigation by the author(s) of books *I* and *III* into the general importance of the even days (an investigation based on historical case descriptions) is a typical example in so far as the subject of the research was relevant only for a marginal component of the medical theory underlying books *I* and *III*. The scope of that particular investigation was perhaps further limited by the fact that probably some earlier doctrines on critical days, as well as lists of such days, had already included even numbers.[239] We never witness one of the great fundamental doctrines coming into existence. In all instances in which research activity with the aim of doctrinal innovation can be observed, only the margin of a system of central theories is affected.

When trying to reconstruct the research methods applied by the authors of the *Epidemics*, and to determine the scope of their research, it seems useful to consider all the explicit theoretical *questions* they asked.[240] There

---

[237] According to Diller, Ausdrucksformen 142 (= Kleine Schriften Medizin 115), the verb σκέπτεσθαι denoted "das Forschen im weitesten Sinn;" but see below p. 193. The semantic field of ἱστορ- comprises research but is much broader.

[238] Cf. above p. 1.

[239] Cf. above p. 93–103.

[240] On the following pages, *all* explicit questions will be discussed; not included are syntactically isolated dependent clauses (i. e. 'elliptic' subordinates without main clause) introduced by ὅτι, οἷος, ὅτε etc., which Diller, Ausdrucksformen 142f. (= Kleine Schriften Medizin 115f.) interpreted as indirect interrogative clauses. They may, however, be relative clauses, Langholf, Syntaktische Untersuchungen 48f.

are no questions which can be fully understood without taking into account the medical doctrines and theories typical of the Hippocratic Collection. Sometimes the theoretical context can only apparently be dismissed. One such question is formulated in *VI* 8.22: "One must investigate what is inside the joints. Do they not suppurate?"[241] The belief that the articulations do not suppurate must have seemed paradoxical to the Hippocratic physician, because pain in the joints was considered a form of *apóstasis.*[242] Hence the question should probably be taken as meaning: "Is it really true that the joints do not suppurate although, according to the theory, they ought to?" For the sake of the applicability and coherence of his doctrine, the author would have welcomed every observed case of articular suppuration.

Another question appears, at first sight, to be asked independently of any specific doctrine, *VII* 57 (in an individual case history): Ekhekrates the Blind was affected with an *otitis media.* The pain is described at length; he had fever, "during the day it was less, but by night there was pain." Then a question is asked which aims at extending the applicability of a medical doctrine: "Is it towards night that there are the pains in *all* cases of suppuration, also the ones at the eye?"[243] Although the underlying observation could have been made without any reference to a theory, other passages of the *Epidemics* show that there was a more general discussion, in which an analogy was drawn between the four periods of the day and the four seasons. The evening was supposed to correspond to autumn, at both times exacerbations were believed to occur (*II* 1.3–4; *VI* 1.11; *Aphorisms III* 9).[244] If this doctrinal background had any influence on the answer to be given to the question, it should have been "yes." Concepts mentioned in these texts, i. e. presupposed in the discussion, are paroxysm,[245] *katástasis,*[246] periodicity in the course of the diseases, and the doctrine that black bile is prevalent in autumn.[247] As far as the discussion can be reconstructed from the extant texts, it did not aim at questioning any of the principal constituents of the medical doctrine.

---

241 *Epid. VI* 5.352.6–7 Οἷον ἔνεστιν (ἔ. MV: ἔστι τὸ Pall.) ἐν τοῖσιν ἄρθροισι σκεπτέον· ἦρα οὐκ (οὐκ MV: μὴ Pall.) ἐκπυοῦνται (-νται MV: -ται Pall.).

242 The idea is frequently expressed in the Collection; see, for instance, the "Table alphabétique des matières" in Littré, vol. 10, s. v. 'articulation,' 'genoux,' 'hanche.'

243 *Epid. VII* 5.422.23–424.6 ≈ *V* 5.248.12–13 ἦρά γε ἐν πᾶσι τοῖσιν ἐμπυήμασι, καὶ τοῖσι περὶ ὀφθαλμόν, ἐς νύκτα οἱ πόνοι;

244 *Epid. II* 5.72.14–74.5; *VI* 5.272.1–4; *Aph.* 4.488.16–17 Li. = 4.124 Jones; cf. *Epid. IV* 5.158.5–8 Li. = Per. 138–139 La.

245 Cf. above p. 103 f., 113–118.

246 Cf. above p. 169 f., 171 f., 177–179.

247 For the latter two topics, cf. the treatise *On the Nature of Man, passim.*

In *II* 2.9 a group of three patients suffering from kidney affections are mentioned. The short reference is concluded by: "Questions: Whether it is easier always to be filled with drink or with food."[248] The alternative question can very well be understood without the background of any specific doctrine, but again it is evident from other passages that there must have been a medical discussion on the subject. One of the passages mentions phlegm, *VI* 1.5: "And in the kidney there is heavy pain when they [the patients] are filled with food (or drink); they vomit phlegm ... It helps ... not to be filled ..."[249] The words bracketed, "or drink," are missing in an important manuscript and in Galen's commentary, and it is impossible to determine whether they are authentic or a later addition. A similar text is *Aphorisms II* 11, an isolated sentence without any explicit context: "It is easier to be filled with drink than with food."[250] Nothing is known about the chronological relationship of the three passages. The identical wording suggests that they are dependent either on each other or on another lost text. Therefore, the situation in which the research question of *Epidemics II* 2.9 was asked is not clear. Was it a commonly accepted doctrine that it is easier in any disease to be filled with drink than with food (*Aphorisms*)? Was it believed that in the special case of kidney diseases it is harmful to be filled with food alone, or with either food or drink (*Epidemics VI*, depending on how one chooses among the variant readings)? Did the question formulated at the end of *Epidemics II* 2.9 try to find out modifications of any of these two (or of both) doctrines? Or are, on the contrary, both of these assertions answers (perhaps generalized answers) to the question formulated in *Epidemics II*? The medical historian cannot solve that puzzle. One can only outline the possible framework of a fifth and fourth century discussion; despite the lack of further source material, however, it becomes sufficiently clear that the discussion was about marginal constituents of the doctrine.[251]

A kind of research project is sketched in *VI* 2.5. The text is formulated in the usual concise notebook style.[252] Although details of the wording must have undergone changes in the course of the text transmission, all extant text sources agree on the principal points. The main content of the passage is, therefore, clear. The questions asked refer to a phenomenon

---

248 *Epid. II* 5.88.11–12 Li. = Per. 18 La. ἐρωτήματα· εἰ ῥήϊον (εἰ ῥήϊον ci. Nikitas, Untersuchungen 173: 'ob es leichter ist' Gal.: εἴρεον V: ἤρεον γὰρ αὐτοὺς HIR) ἀεὶ πληροῦσθαι ποτοῦ ἢ σίτου. A similar question (?) concerning diet, *Epid. VI* 2.21 (5.288.10–11), has been discussed above p. 31, n. 91 f.; cf. 187 f., n. 273.

249 *Epid. VI* 5.268.3–7 καὶ ἐς νεφρὸν ὀδύνη βαρείη, ὅταν πληρῶνται τοῦ σίτου ἢ ποτοῦ (τ. σ. ἢ π. V: σίτου M, Gal.), ἐμέουσί τε φλέγμα ... ξυμφέρει ... μὴ ἐμπίπλασθαι.

250 *Aph.* 4.472.8 Li. = 4.110 Jones Ῥᾷον πληροῦσθαι ποτοῦ ἢ σίτου.

251 For an extensive interpretation of the passages, see Nikitas, Untersuchungen 161–188.

252 Deichgräber, Die Epidemien p. 38, called the passage a scientific soliloquy.

repeatedly described in individual case descriptions. If certain symptoms or segregations (*apóstasis*) occur together, they tend, according to these case reports, to be confined to one side (left or right) of the body.[253] "On the same side [of the body] are pain in the ribs, tensions of the *hypokhóndrion*, swellings of the spleen, nosebleeding, and ear affections. Most of this occurs on the same side. The same [symptoms, or segregations] affect also the eyes. — Are, therefore, all [symptoms, or segregations, on the same side]? Or [only] the ones above coming from below, e. g. the ones at the jaws or the eye or the ear, whereas the ones below coming from above do not occur on the same side? However, angina-like inflammations and pains in the ribs *do* occur on the same side, as do the [symptoms, or segregations] below the liver that come from above, e. g. the ones going into the testicles and into the varicose veins. — One must investigate to whom this occurs and where and whence and why."[254] The body is traditionally divided not only into a right and a left side, but also into an upper and a lower section, with the diaphragm being the barrier between these two halves. The author does not doubt that an *apóstasis* ascending from the lower part to the upper part of the body stays on the same side; but as to the segregations descending from above the midriff to the places below it, he is not sure, and he formulates the problem as an alternative. (The midriff must have been credited with an important function in the physiology of the humour-ducts such as vessels and 'strands,' *tónoi*, because the anatomical dissection report of *Epidemics II* 4.1—2 concentrates on the diaphragm, in whose region the course of the ducts is described as being particularly complicated and unclear. For more details on the dia-

---

253 For the left side, cf. the examples quoted in Littré's "Table alphabétique" s. v. 'rate' (vol. 10, p. 764 f.); for the right side, cf. *Epid. I*, case 10 ἰσχίου ὀδύνη δεξιοῦ ... ὀφθαλμὸν δεξιὸν ἤλγει. *Epid. III*, 1st series, case 3 ἰσχίου δεξιοῦ ὀδύνη ... ὀφθαλμοῦ δεξιοῦ ὀδύνη. *Epid. II* 5.90.15—92.2 Li. = Per. 25—26 La. ἐν κνήμῃ κάτω δεξιῇ ... καὶ ἐν χειρὶ δεξιῇ. Cf. *Epid. II* 5.136.5—7. The passages concerning the left side are by far more numerous.

254 *Epid. VI* 5.278.12—280.3 κατ' ἴξιν καὶ πλευρέων ὀδύνη καὶ ξυντάσιες ὑποχονδρίων (-ων MV, Gal.: -ου Pall.) καὶ σπληνὸς ἐπάρσιες καὶ ἐκ ῥινῶν ῥήξιες καὶ ἐς (ἐς Galeni interpr. Arab.: om. cetera memoria) ὦτα. κατ' ἴξιν τούτων τὰ πλεῖστα, ταὐτὰ (ταὐτὰ Galeni interpr. Arab.: ταῦτα cetera memoria) καὶ ἐς ὀφθαλμούς. — πότερον ἦρα (ἦρα MV, Pall.: μὴν ἄρα Gal.) πάντα (scil. κατ' ἴξιν); ἢ τὰ μὲν κάτωθεν ἄνω (scil. κατ' ἴξιν), οἷα τὰ παρὰ γνάθους (-ους MV, Gal.: -ον Pall. ed. Dietz: -ον καὶ ῥῖνα Pall. codex Urbinas Gr. 64) ἢ παρ' ὀφθαλμὸν ἢ (ἢ Gal.: καὶ MV, Pall.) οὖς, τὰ δὲ ἄνωθεν κάτω οὐ κατ' ἴξιν; καίτοι καὶ τὰ συναγχικὰ (καὶ τὰ συν- Gal.: τὰ κυν- Pall.) ἐρυθήματα καὶ πλευρέων ὀδυνήματα κατ' ἴξιν (καίτοι ... ἴξιν Gal., Pall.: om. MV), ᾗ (ᾗ scripsi: ἢ MV, Gal., Pall.) καὶ τὰ κάτω τοῦ (τοῦ Gal., Pall.: om. MV) ἥπατος ἄνωθεν διαδιδόντα, οἷον τὰ ἐς ὄρχιας καὶ κιρσούς. — σκεπτέα (-έα M, Gal., Pall.: -έον V) ταῦτα, οἷσι καὶ (οἷσι καὶ Pall.: om. MV, Gal.) ὅπῃ καὶ ὅθεν καὶ διότι (διότι MV: διὰ τί Gal., Pall.).

phragm, cf. above p. 145 ff.)[255] Subsequently, the author mentions those segregations which do not cross the barrier formed by the diaphragm but stay above or below it, and again he does not express any doubt at the assumption that in these cases the 'harmful matter' stays on its left or right side respectively. Finally, he formulates another question, or rather a series of questions, not to test the assumptions, but to determine some more specific conditions under which the *materia peccans* stays on its body side or changes it: In which patients? In which parts of the body? Whence? For which reasons? The questions are closely related to the physician's practical work, to prognosis, and presuppose a considerable number of doctrinal elements. They are not meant to modify any of the central constituents of the medical doctrine but to extend its validity to particular cases.

Another text resembling a research programme (in the form of incomplete indirect questions and very short notes[256]) is formulated in *Epidemics IV* 14 in connection with an individual case. The female household member of Nikostratos discharged three different kinds of urine which are described in detail. Only one of them is mentioned elsewhere in the Hippocratic Collection.[257] The wording of the 'research programme' following after this individual report cannot be reconstructed with any confidence.[258] It seems to consist of personal notes aimed at considering

---

[255] An example of a segregation (*apóstasis*) descending through the midriff and crossing over to the other side of the body is found at *Epidemics II* 2.8: A woman was paralysed at the right arm and the left leg after a slight cough (i. e., the origin of the 'harmful substance' was above the midriff). — Further examples may be the cases of "Apemantos and the father of the carpenter ... and Nikostratos," who did *not* cough, although they probably had been expected to do so. Their very inexplicit story, *Epidemics II* 2.9, seems to say that they had pain "in their kidneys at the [respectively] opposite sides" (ἑτέρωθι), perhaps in relation to symptoms in their upper body half. (*Epid. II* 5.88.3—12 Li. = Per. 15—18 La.; cf. above p. 182, and Nikitas, Untersuchungen 161—188.)

[256] Langholf, Syntaktische Untersuchungen 47—51.

[257] In *Epid. VII* 5.438.15—17, the words ξυσματώδεα ... ὑφίστατο refer to the sediment of the urine and mean something similar to ὑπόστασις ... ξυσματώδης in *Epid. IV*. For ὑπόστασις λευκὴ ὀροβώδης of *Epid. IV* one might compare *Acut. (Sp.)* 2.462.10—464.1 Li. = 1.164.7—8 Kw. = 1.84.16—17 Joly, but the colour is different there: ὑποστάσιας ὑπερύθρους ... ὁποῖον ὀρόβων. An "egg-yolk coloured sediment" (λεκιθώδεα) occurs nowhere else, although greasy matters standing on the surface of urine are mentioned several times in the Collection (cf. above p. 18 f., and Jouanna, Archéologie 130 f.).

[258] *Epid. IV* 5.152.3—15 Li. = Per. 107—113 La. οἷον τὸ ἐναιώρημα διεστηκός. οἷον (post οἷον add. ἔξω VHIR: fortasse delendum) ἐξ οἵου (οἵου V: οἵου οὐ HIR) τὸ ὑφιστάμενον ἔπειτα οὐρεῖται. καὶ τὸ μέν τι (μέν τι VIR: μέντοι H) τοιοῦτο· τὸ δὲ ἱδρυμένον ἄλλο τοιοῦτον ὀλίγον ἐπὶ πλατὺ διεσκεδασμένον, ἄλλο τεταραγμένον. ἕτερον τοιοῦτο ἐναιώρημα νεφελίου ὑπομέλανος δοκέοντος πάχος ἔχειν, χαύνου δέ (post δέ add. ἄλλο λεπτόν VHIR: delevi). ἄλλο ἐναιώρημα λεπτὸν τοιοῦτον. ἄλλο οἷον ἵππου. ἄλλο οἷον τὰ ζοφώδεα. πόσα. Cf. the tentative German translation and the comments given in Langholf, Syntaktische Untersuchungen 141 f.

possible cases of urinary sediments and suspensions probably for prognostic purposes, although it does not intend to be a universally applicable or exhaustive system. The following tentative paraphrase may give a rough idea of the content of these rather enigmatic lines: "How the suspended matters are dispersed. Which sediment is urinated after which chronologically ... The sediment[259] is of a different quality[260] when it is spread out only a little horizontally, and of a different one when it is stirred up. The suspension of the latter kind[261] consists of a darkish cloud which, although seeming to be thick, yet is loose ... Another suspension of this kind is thin. Another one is as from [the urine of] a horse. Another one is like the 'dark urine.' How many." Again, the questions formulated concern a rather marginal point of the doctrine, whose applicability is extended to special cases. The basic importance of the suspensions and sediments in the urine is not called into question.

Some of the questions are not only asked within the *framework* of a professional discussion involving certain theoretical concepts, but contain such concepts more explicitly. *Epidemics IV* 25 comprises a short case report on "the vine-dresser of Menandros," who, in explicit contrast to an aforementioned patient, "did discharge loose stool in the beginning. Then it ceased, and so did the urine. He had a *krísis* on the 7th day, no rigor [but the other patient did have rigor]; was it because he [the vine-dresser] had had a bowel movement before [the critical 7th day]? On the 7th day he had no bowel movement. The kinsman of Potamon had no rigor for two days before the *krísis*. Therefore the urine was not retained."[262] The question, which was certainly of rather marginal importance, seems to have been asked in a doctrinal context sketched by the aphorism *Epidemics VI* 1.8, "Those who have rigor do not have any segregations," cf. what has been said above p. 83f. From the passages quoted there, it can be inferred that the answer should have been (a cautious?) "yes."

One of the ubiquitous basic doctrines of the *Epidemics* and of other treatises of the Collection has it that the morbid matter may be excreted out of the body in the form of certain urinary sediments which were believed to be possible kinds of *apóstasis*. Consequently, a thin and watery

---

259 τὸ δὲ ἱδρυμένον.

260 ἄλλο τοιοῦτον.

261 ἕτερον τοιοῦτο ἐναιώρημα.

262 *Epid. IV* 5.168.3–5 Li. = Per. 179–180 La. ὁ (δὲ add. HIR: om. V) Μενάνδρου ἀμπελουργὸς ὡσαύτως πλὴν γαστὴρ κατ' ἀρχὰς λεπτὰ ἐδίδου. ἔπειτα ἔστη, καὶ τὸ οὖρον. ἐκρίθη, οὐκ ἐρρίγωσεν, ἑβδόμῃ, ἦρα ὅτι (ἡ add. HIR: om. V) γαστὴρ προεταράχθη; {ὁ ποτάμωνος} τούτου (τούτου V: τούτω HIR) κοιλίη οὐ διῄει ἑβδομαίῳ. ὁ Ποτάμωνος (ὁ Π. V: om. HIR) πρὸ κρίσιος δύο ἡμέρας οὐκ ἐρρίγωσε· διὰ τοῦτο οὐδὲ τὸ οὖρον ἔσχετο.

urine without a sediment was regarded as ineffective for the expulsion of the *materia peccans.*[263] If, however, the harmful matter was excreted through another 'outlet'[264] either before or after the discharge of urine, it was reasonable to expect a urine which was thin and yet of good omen. Thus clinical observations which apparently formed exceptions to the doctrine could be explained by the doctrine itself — an extension of its applicability. On the basis of the presupposed internal *apóstasis* mechanism, the question is asked in *Epidemics I* 8 (end) Li. (= 17 Kw., Jones): "For many, it [the disease] ended in *dysenteríē* after everything else had got to its *krísis*, e. g. for Xenophanes and Kritias. I will mention those who, after the *krísis* and after there had been a good sediment and after everything had got to its *krísis* in a favourable way, discharged much watery, clear and thin urine: Bion ..., Kratis ..., Areton's boy, Mnesistratos' wife. They all suffered from *dysenteríē* after it. Was it because they had discharged watery urine? To be investigated."[265] The historian would like to know how this ancient author intended to find out about the aetiology — perhaps through a rudimentary kind of statistics, and after the scheme *post hoc, ergo propter hoc*? The answer expected by the physician seems, in any case, to have been "yes."

A similar question occurs in *Epidemics VII* 79, the case history of "the fuller on Syros," who suffered from *phrenîtis*: "His urine was clear and without sediment. Was that because of his bowel movement effected through *thapsíē* [a laxative]? On the 18th day, it [the fever] disappeared without perspiration."[266] The answer would be "yes." The exceptional urine could be explained within the framework of the doctrine.

Yet another question formulated in *Epidemics IV* 27 (in a case description) presupposes the *apóstasis* doctrine: "He was fatigued from working.

---

263 Cf. *Aph.* 4.528.1 Li. = 4.154 Jones; *Coac.* 5.714.10—11.

264 Cf. above p. 80.

265 *Epid. I* 2.648.9—650.4 Li. = 1.193.22—194.7 Kw. = 1.170 Jones πολλοῖσι δὲ τῶν ἄλλων κεκριμένων ἐς δυσεντερίας ἐτελεύτα, οἷον Ξενοφάνει καὶ Κριτίᾳ. οὖρα δὲ (δὲ Gal. comm.: om. AVIR) ὑδατώδεα πολλὰ καθαρὰ καὶ (καθαρὰ καὶ VIR: καὶ A: om. Gal. comm.) λεπτὰ μετὰ κρίσιν (μ. κρ. A: καὶ μ. κρ. VIR: μ. κρ. καὶ Gal. comm.) καὶ ὑποστάσιος καλῆς (κ. AVIR: πολλῆς Gal. comm.) γενομένης (γε- AV, Gal. comm.: γι- IR) καὶ τῶν ἄλλων καλῶς κεκριμένων ἀναμνήσομαι οἷσιν ἐγένετο· Βίωνι ... [sequuntur nomina propria] ... μετὰ δὲ δυσεντεριώδεες ἐγένοντο οὗτοι πάντες· ἦρά γε (ἦρά γε VIR: ἆρά γε Gal. in cit. *De comate*, CMG V 9.2, 191 sq.: 'Man muß zusehen, ob ...' Galeni interpret. Arabica: ἦρα A: οὖρα Gal. comm.) ὅτι οὔρησαν ὑδατώδεα; σκεπτέον (ἦρα ... σκεπτέον delev. Ermerins, Jones).

266 *Epid. VII* 5.434.20—436.3 οὖρον καθαρὸν ὑπόστασιν οὐκ ἔχον· ἦρα διὰ τὴν ἀπὸ τῆς θαψίης ὑποχώρησιν; ὀκτωκαιδεκαταῖος ἀνῆκε μολυνθεὶς ἄνευ ἱδρῶτος. The masculine gender of ἀνῆκε μολυνθείς (μολύνομαι cannot be said of the patient but only of the disease or its signs) excludes any other symptom but fever, which is usual in *phrenîtis* and therefore not mentioned explicitly in this case history.

On the 20th day, into the feet [an *apóstasis*], and *krísis*. Does it [the *apóstasis*], with fatigued persons, go into the limbs and not into the eye?"[267] The question, which arose out of a prognostic interest in new special applications of the doctrine, seems to be connected with an assumption cautiously expressed under special conditions in ch. 25, "Those to whom segregations (*apóstasis*) go into the eyes during *kaúsos* fevers, have red jaws and nose-bleeding, but also those who have ear trouble; but perhaps the segregations go rather into the limbs: I do not know exactly,"[268] and with a number of other passages all discussing the conditions under which an *apóstasis* turns off into the eyes[269] and into the limbs.[270] The answer to the question should have been again "yes."

Epidemics VI 3.7 asks, "The concretion [formed] after urinating occurs rather in children. Is it because they are warmer?"[271] The question (which again concerns only a marginal detail) presupposes the warm/cold scheme. Its answer must have been "yes," cf. *On the Nature of Man*, ch. 12, and *On Airs, Waters, Places*, ch. 9, where the mechanism of the development of the stone is described at length.[272]

The following text was, it seems, originally a notebook entry, perhaps to be used for medical instruction: *Epidemics VI* 2.20, "About the serous blood: that shy persons have that kind, or persons who have suffered from insomnia; and whether it is bad or good. Those whose spleen tends downward have their feet and knees and hands warm and their nose and ears always cold. Is it because the blood is thin? Do they have it also naturally?"[273] It is scarcely possible to determine even in its outlines the

---

267 *Epid. IV* 5.172.3–4 Li. = Per. 200 La. κοπιώδης ἐξ ἔργων. εἰκοσταῖος, ἐς πόδας, καὶ κρίσις. ἦρα τοῖσι κοπιώδεσιν ἐς ἄρθρα καὶ οὐκ ἐς ὀφθαλμόν;

268 *Epid. IV* 5.168.12–15 Li. = Per. 185–186 La. οἷσιν ἐς τοὺς ὀφθαλμοὺς ἀποστάσιες ἐν καύσοις, ἐξέρυθροι γνάθους καὶ αἱμορραγικοί, ἀτὰρ καὶ οἷσι παρὰ τὰ ὦτά ἐστιν· ἴσως δὲ καὶ ἀποστάσιες ἐς ἄρθρα μᾶλλον· οὐ μὴν σάφα οἶδα.

269 Segregations into the eyes seem to have been a specialty of the author of *Epid. IV*: cf., in addition, 5.166.12–168.12 Li. = Per. 177–184 La.; 170.2–7 Li. = Per. 191–192 La.; 172.19–174.9 Li. = Per. 208–214 La.; 178.7–16 Li. = Per. 228–231 La. Cf. also the general remark in *Epid. II* 5.78.3–4, where the eyes are listed as a potential seat of an *apóstasis* (see also above p. 80 f.).

270 Particularly in persons or fevers being κοπιώδης, *Aph.* 4.512.11–12 Li. = 4.142 Jones; *Hum.* 5.486.16–17 Li. = 4.76 Jones; cf. also *Epid. IV* 5.190.11–15 Li. = Per. 280–281 La.; *VI* 5.270.6–8; and below p. 192.

271 *Epid. VI* 5.296.3–4 τὸ μετ' οὔρησιν σύναγμα παιδίοισι μᾶλλον, ἦρ' (ἦρ' MV: ἆρα Gal. comm.: ἆρά γε Gal. in cit. *De comate*, CMG V 9.2, p. 192.4–5: om. Pall) ὅτι θερμότερα (θερμ- MV, Gal. comm., Pall.: ἔνθερμα Gal. in cit.);

272 *Nat. Hom.* 6.62.21–64.3 Li. = 4.36 Jones; *Aer.* 2.36.20–42.6 Li. = 1.46.14–48.15 Kw. = 1.94–98 Jones; cf. *Coac.* 5.700.7–12: calculi are not formed in old (i. e., colder) people.

273 *Epid. VI* 5.288.5–9 περὶ τοῦ αἵματος τοῦ ἰχωροειδέος, ὅτι ἐν τοῖσι πτοιώδεσι τὸ τοιοῦτον ἢ (ἢ MV, Pall.: καὶ ἐν Gal.) τοῖσιν ἠγρυπνηκόσι, καὶ εἴτε φλαῦρον εἴτε

discussion underlying this question. *Prognostics*, ch. 2, when dealing with the *facies Hippocratica*, mentions a relationship between cold ears and insomnia,[274] and a gynaecological text describing symptoms of the face similar to the ones of *Prognostics* explains that "white ears" are due to watery blood.[275] An individual case history (the case of Skopas, *Epidemics II* 3.11, cf. shortly below) exhibits a combination of insomnia, a "spleen which tended downward," and a discharge of watery blood,[276] but unfortunately says nothing about the temperature of the patient's extremities. It is useless to speculate about the details of any underlying theory. The problem touched upon in the questions may have been left inexplicit because it was regarded as of little importance.[277]

In *Epidemics II* 3.11, at the end of the description of the individual case of Skopas, a question (grammatically speaking, an elliptical indirect question[278]) is formulated: "Whether an excretion of this kind is critical, [an excretion] which was also present in the case of the member of the Antigenes household in Perinthos."[279] Part of the text tradition has the sentence not as a question but as an affirmative statement: "There came an excretion of the kind which was critical in the case of ..." etc. It is not possible to decide which version is the authentic one.[280] Either reading implies an opposition to doctrines propounded in one of the 'handbooks' of the Hippocratic Collection. The whole chapter on Skopas (who recovered from his disease) seems to refer to what the doctrine formulated in

---

χρηστόν. οἷσιν ὁ σπλὴν ἐστι κατάρροπος, πόδες καὶ γούνατα καὶ χεῖρες (γ. κ. χ. MV, Pall.: χ. κ. γ. Gal.) θερμά, ῥὶς καὶ (καὶ Gal., Pall. ed. Di.: om. MV, Pall. cod. U) ὦτα ἀεὶ ψυχρά. ἦρα διὰ τοῦτο ὅτι (ὅτι Gal.: om. MV, Pall.) λεπτὸν τὸ αἷμα; ἦρα καὶ φύσει τὸ (φύσει τὸ Gal.: φύσις MV: φύσιν Pall.) τοιοῦτον οὗτοι ἔχουσιν; There follows another question (?), the meaning of which is not quite certain, *Epid. VI* 2.21 (5.288.10–11), cf. above p. 31, notes 91 f.

274 *Prog.* 2.114.3, 8–9 Li. = 1.79.15, 21–22 Kw. = 2.8 Jones ὦτα ψυχρά ... ἠγρύπνηκεν.

275 *Superf.* 8.484.21–486.6 Li. = 78.31–80.7 Lienau τὰ ὦτα λευκά (for the construction cf. Langholf, Syntaktische Untersuchungen, p. 51), ... ταύτῃσι τὸ αἷμα ἐξυδατώθη. (In the last sentence, ἔνσιμος has to be read with the manuscripts, in contrast to the ῥὶς ὀξεῖα of *Prog.* 2.)

276 *Epid. II* 5.112.9–114.9 Li. = Per. 51–59 La. ἄγρυπνος ..., σπλὴν ... κατάρροπος ..., αἷμα ἐξ ἀριστεροῦ ὑδαρές.

277 As to the answer expected by the author, one can only guess. Flashar (transl.), [Aristoteles], Problemata, p. 299 contends that the two questions have to be taken in the sense of cautious positive answers rather than hints for further inquiry: they constitute "eine Antwort, die ... ganz im Stil der für die Probl. charakteristischen Doppelantwort gehalten ist."

278 Langholf, Syntaktische Untersuchungen 47–51.

279 *Epid. II* 5.114.8 τὸ τοιοῦτον εἰ (εἰ scripsi: ἤει, i. e. ἤει, VHIR: 'Man muß untersuchen, ob' Gal. in comm. ad loc.) κρίσιμον (-ον V: -ως HIR) ὅ τι καὶ τῷ (τῷ V: τὸ HIR) Ἀντιγένεος ἐν Περίνθῳ.

280 Cf. Langholf, Syntaktische Untersuchungen 127–129, where the complete text of the report is edited.

Prognostics says about urine (ch. 12), stool and flatulence (ch. 11).[281] Some of the formulations are quite similar. The "descent" of Skopas' flatulence is favourable according to the standards of *Prognostics*,[282] and so is his urine, but only as far as it is described *directly* within this case history. Skopas' discharges are said to have been identical with those of the "member of the Antigenes household," who is mentioned in other passages of the *Epidemics*. According to *VI* 4.2, this Antigenes kinsman had a "thick, white urine" which is said to have been favourable because it saved him from a worse *apóstasis* (into the joints, it seems, i. e. from arthritis or arthrosis).[283] This contradicts *Prognostics* 12, where the "thick" urine is regarded as a fatal sign.[284] Since the urine of Skopas must have been "thick" as with Antigenes' kin, Skopas' case, with a favourable outcome, contradicts *Prognostics* indirectly through the comparison. Another point of opposition towards *Prognostics* can be found in the description of Skopas' stool, which is said to have been "slightly viscous," "scanty, viscous ..." on the day of the *krísis*.[285] Skopas' recovery contrasts with the doctrine of *Prognostics* which has it that "it is bad if [the stool] is scanty and viscous."[286] It seems that *Prognostics* or its literary or oral sources had set a certain standard for evaluating prognostic signs. In Skopas' case, some observed facts contradicted the commonly accepted doctrine. Skopas exhibited symptoms which were supposed to be of bad omen, but he recovered. Hence the question, to be answered in the affirmative (or the explicit statement, if one follows the other textual tradition), and the reference to another 'exception,' whose case, although nowhere described

---

281 The following interpretation implies that the respective *doctrines* contained in *Prognostics*, not necessarily the treatise as such, are older than *Epidemics II* 3.11; for the chronological distinction between the treatise and its doctrines, see above p. 159, n. 146; cf. p. 222—231, 250 f.

282 Cf. Langholf, *loco cit.*

283 *Epid. VI* 5.306.7—10 οὖρον παχὺ λευκὸν οἷον τὸ (τὸ V, Pall.: τῷ M: τὸ supra scripto ῷ Gal. cod. U) τοῦ Ἀντιγένεος (ἀντιγένεος Pall. cod. U, Galeni interpr. Arab., Joh. [qui habet etiam ariugeneo]: ἀμφιγένεος MV, Pall. ed. Di.: ἀρχιγένεος Gal. cod. U) ἐπὶ τοῖσι κοπιώδεσι ... ῥύεται τῆς ἀποστάσιος. The context of the preceding and following paragraphs is on affections of the joints, cf. *Aph.* 4.528.7—530.3 Li. = 4.154 Jones and the passages collected p. 186 f., 192, on segregations into the limbs. The same "white, thick" urine is mentioned for the household member of Antigenes in *Epid. IV* 5.160.11—12 Li. = Per. 151 La. (but without an evaluation): οὖρον οἷον τῷ (τῷ praetulerim: τὸ VHIR) Ἀντιγένεος (ἀντ- V: ἀρτ- HIR)· λευκόν, παχύ.

284 *Prog.* 2.142.1—2 Li. = 1.90.14—15 Kw. = 2.26 Jones θανατωδέστερα δὲ τῶν οὔρων τά τε δυσώδεα καὶ ὑδατώδεα καὶ μέλανα καὶ παχέα. Here καὶ is synonymous with ἢ because "watery" excludes "black" as well as "thick." Also *Epid. III* 3.90.9—10 Li. = 1.229.9—10 = 1.250 Jones contradicts *Prog.* in this respect.

285 ὑπόγλισχρον..., ὡς ὀλίγων ἐόντων, γλίσχρα.

286 *Prog.* 2.136.12 Li. = 1.88.20 Kw. = 2.24 Jones πονηρὸν δὲ καὶ σμικρόν τε ἐὸν καὶ γλίσχρον.

in an individual report of its own, must have been a didactic paradigm.[287] The medical problem discussed (a point of minor relevance within the framework of the *apóstasis* doctrine) was solved by introducing, or 'detecting,' two new forms of *apóstasis*. Instead of falsifying the doctrine of *Prognostics*, the bad signs of this treatise were re-interpreted as 'critical.' This is an extension of the doctrine, for 'critical' may in fact be good or bad.[288]

In summation: a survey of all explicit theoretical questions formulated in the *Epidemics* yields the result that they have certain typical features. Without exception, all questions presuppose the medical theories expounded in the *Epidemics* and in other treatises of the Collection. None of the questions raises doubts about any of the principal constituents of the theories or aims at falsifying them.[289] On the contrary, several questions explicitly contain the main theoretical terms and concepts. Sometimes the outlines of a larger theoretical discussion can be reconstructed. Whenever the questions aim at modifying the medical theories, the modifications concern only marginal constituents of the theories. In a number of questions we observe that they were asked out of an interest in prognosis and in order to extend the applicability of the medical theories either generally or to special cases or even to apparent exceptions, and thereby to confirm the validity of the theories. Never does a question restrict the validity or applicability of any medical theory. The constructive attitude, in which the questions were asked, can be realized by the fact that the answers which they prompt are most often easy to predict, and that the answers are mostly in the affirmative. Never can 'no' be expected, never can scepticism be found in a question.

Doctrinal Statements with 'Perhaps' in the *Epidemics*

The explicit theoretical questions asked by the authors of the *Epidemics* indicate to the medical historian the directions in which these ancient physicians tried to extend their professional knowledge, and what the doctrinal guidelines and limitations were that defined their research. Similar information can be drawn from those doctrinal aphorisms of the *Epidemics* which contain the qualification "perhaps." In some texts, the authors do

---

[287] Nikitas, Untersuchungen 238, with more material on this patient.

[288] Even within the system of *Prognostics*, the prognostical value of individual disease signs is never absolute: *all* signs, it is said there, must be calculated in their mutual relationships (last chapter of the treatise). Therefore the contradiction to *Prognostics* implied in the *Epidemics* passage is of little consequence.

[289] On the falsification of medical theories, see also above p. 118 and below p. 208–215.

not just reproduce established tenets, but tentatively state something new, although in most of these passages the statements containing "perhaps" refer to tiny details of the doctrine: to the feasibility of provoking heartburn artificially, and to the possibility that heartburn stops diarrhoea;[290] to the likelihood of certain segregations turning off into the limbs;[291] to the quality ("perhaps hot") of a particular mucous discharge through the nose;[292] to the probability of suppurations under certain limited conditions;[293] to the possibility that a certain form of urine retention is due to the form of the accompanying fever and to preceding exercises;[294] to the chance that a particular type of patient (whitish complexion) catches a fever;[295] to another form of fever, *Epidemics VI* 8.21, "The fevers in which the lips get ulcerous, are perhaps intermittent and cool off on the third day."[296] Twice "perhaps" is used in discussions of the aetiology of individual disease cases.[297] Nowhere does the "perhaps" formulation question the validity of the doctrine; on the contrary, the doctrine is presupposed by the formulations, and nowhere can be made out any reservations vis-à-vis the doctrine. Some of the passages aim at *extending* the validity, or applicability, of theoretical concepts. Not one single passage can be found which restricts their validity. All this accords with what has been observed in the preceding section concerning the questions asked in the *Epidemics*.

The doctrine is tentatively extended in the following passages, which, in contrast to those mentioned, do not refer to insignificant details but are of a more general importance. None of them contradicts any other doctrine. *Epidemics VI* 3.23, "Those who have haemorrhoids are not seized with pleuresy or pneumonia or canker or furuncles or knobby growths, nor perhaps with *léprē*, nor perhaps with anything else (variant reading for 'anything else:' *alphós*)."[298] The aphorism belongs to a doctrinal

---

290 *Epid. II* 5.92.13–16 Li. = Per. 32–33 La. For the effect of changes, cf. *Epid. II* 5.84.5–7.

291 *Epid. IV* 5.168.12–15 Li. = Per. 185–186 La. (cf. above p. 186 f. and below p. 192).

292 *Epid. IV* 5.182.1–5 Li. = Per. 242–243 La.

293 *Epid. IV* 5.186.18–188.2 Li. = Per. 267 La.

294 *Epid. VI* 5.270.2–5.

295 *Epid. VI* 5.350.1–2.

296 *Epid. VI* 5.352.3–4 οἱ πυρετοὶ ἐν οἷσιν ἐφελκοῦται χείλεα, ἴσως διαλείποντες (διαλείποντες V: διαλιπόντες M, Pall.), καὶ τριταίοισι ψύξιες.

297 *Epid. IV* 5.170.5–7 Li. = Per. 192 La.; *VI* 5.308.7–10 Li. = Per. 322–323 La.

298 *Epid. VI* 5.304.2–4 οἱ αἱμορροΐδας ἔχοντες (-ες M, Gal., Pall.: -ας V) οὔτε πλευρίτιδι οὔτε περιπλευμονίῃ οὔτε φαγεδαίνῃ οὔτε δοθιῆσιν οὔτε τερμίνθοισι (οὔ. τερμ. Gal.: om. MV, Pall.), ἴσως δὲ οὐδὲ λέπρῃσιν, ἴσως δὲ οὐδὲ ἄλλοισιν (ἄλλοισιν MV: ἀλφοῖσιν Gal., Pall.). For the reconstruction of the wording cf. the parallel version in *Hum.* 5.500.8–11 Li. = 4.92 Jones; it reads οὔτε τερμίνθοις and ἄλλοισιν in its more conservative cod. A, οὔτε τερμίνθοισιν ἁλίσκονται and ἀλφοῖσιν in its cod. M. Palladios has ἁλίσκονται after πλευρίτιδι. The text is perfectly understandable without this verb,

context which assumed that haemorrhoids were something beneficial (cf. *Aphorisms VI* 11 and 21: they help against *melagkholíē, nephrîtis* and *maníē*[299]), and that treating them was dangerous because it provoked other diseases (cf., e. g., *Epidemics IV* 58,[300] *Aphorisms VI* 12[301]). The other passage which proposes a tentative extension of a rather general doctrine is *Epidemics II* 1.6, "All continuous or intermittent protracted [fevers] and wounds and painful expectorations and growths, and whatever else manifests itself later, perhaps even other things too, have this in common: what develops quicker lasts shorter, what develops slower lasts longer."[302] Other "perhaps" formulations on not very special topics of the doctrine have already been quoted in other contexts. A passage discussed earlier[303] states, "I believe that the sanguineous and bilious [body] is affected with heartburn. Perhaps it results in 'the black' with these [patients]" (*Epidemics II* 3.15). Either of the possible two interpretations of 'the black' fits well into the doctrine of *On Diseases II* and *Epidemics*. Another text mentioned above, *Epidemics VI* 1.9, cautiously states that degenerations of the legs are "perhaps" brought about by a segregation which, after excessive exercises, has turned off into the limbs.[304] This assumption agrees with a number of other passages in the *Epidemics* and elsewhere.[305]

---

whose absence or changing position respectively seems to indicate that it has intruded into the text as a gloss from the margin or from between the lines. — The words *léprē* and *alphós* denote diseases of the skin. As Professor Grmek has informed me in a letter, they do not correspond to leprosy in the modern sense but rather to a benign dermatosis such as psoriasis.

299 *Aph.* 4.566.7–8 Li. = 4.182 Jones; 568.7–8 Li. = 4.184 Jones. More material above p. 111.

300 *Epid. IV* 5.196.10–11 Li. = Per. 306 La.

301 *Aph.* 4.566.12 Li. = 4.182 Jones. More testimonies on this doctrine can be found in Littré's "Table alphabétique," vol. 10, p. 631 f., s. v. 'hémorrhoïdal, le flux,' and 'hémorrhoïdes.' The proverb mentioning a notorious quack, Ἀκεσίας τὸν πρωκτὸν ἰάσατο, seems to presuppose the same doctrine (Zenob. *I* 52; Corpus Paroemiographorum edd. Leutsch/Schneidewin I, where parallel passages are listed; Aristoph. frg. 903 Kock, Edmonds).

302 *Epid. II* 5.74.16–76.1 πάντων δὲ τῶν συνεχέων ἢ διαλειπόντων {τῶν} χρονίων καὶ τρωμάτων καὶ πτυέλων ὀδυνωδέων καὶ φυμάτων {φλεγμοναὶ} καὶ ὅσα ἄλλα ἐπιφαίνεται (-εται V: -ονται HIR) ὕστερον, ἴσως δὲ καὶ ἄλλων πρηγμάτων κοινόν (-όν Deichgräber e Gal. "ist gemeinsam": κοινῶν VHIR)· τὰ μὲν θᾶσσον βραχύτερα, τὰ δὲ βραδύτερα μακρότερα.

303 Cf. above p. 136.

304 *Epid. VI* 5.270.6–8 αἱ (αἱ M, Gal.: ἐκ V: ἀλλ' οἷς ἐκ Pall.) τῶν σκελέων ἐκθηλύνσιες (-ύνσιες M, Gal., Pall.: -ύσηες V), οἷον ἢ πρὸ νούσου ὁδοιπορήσαντι ἢ ἐκ νούσου αὐτίκα (αὐτίκα M, Gal., Pall.: om. V), διότι ἴσως τὸ ἐκ κόπων (τὸ ἐκ κόπων M, Gal., Pall.: τὸ ἐκκόπτον V: τῶν ἐκκόπτων Gal.) ἐς ἄρθρα ἀπέστη, διὸ αἱ (αἱ Gal.: καὶ MV, Pall.) τῶν σκελέων ἐκθηλύνσιες (-ύνσιες M, Gal., Pall.: -ύσηες V). Palladios has some additional variants.

305 See above p. 186 f., notes 267–270, where parallel passages are quoted.

Verbs Denoting Mental Processes in the *Epidemics*

Besides the authors' usage of "perhaps" and their questions, their use of words denoting mental activities can reveal something about their research methods. "In the classical period, there is no exact equivalent, in Greek, for our 'observation'."[306] The verb most frequently used in the *Epidemics* is *skopéomai* (with the collateral forms *sképtomai, skeptéon*), 'to look to,' 'to consider,' 'to examine:' its meaning is ambiguous.[307] In most of the text passages the action denoted consists in inspecting or considering concrete cases, or objects, according to, or in the light of, certain rules or theories or standards (and *never* in examining abstract rules or theories in the light of concrete cases). Some instructive examples: *Epidemics I*, ch. 5 Li. (= ch. 11 Kw., Jones), "You should consider all favourable coctions of the evacuations from all parts, or good and critical segregations."[308] Ch. 5 Li. (= ch. 11 Kw., Jones), "Raw and uncooked matters forming bad segregations signify an absence of *krísis* or pains or delays or fatal outcomes or relapses. Which of these possibilities is the most likely [in an individual case] has to be considered with the aid of other signs."[309] Ch. 11 Li. (= ch. 25 Kw., Jones), "After considering [the individual cases] in the light of these [aforementioned general rules on fever development] one has to prescribe the patient's diet."[310] Ch. 12 Li. (= ch. 26 Kw., Jones), "One must consider [in the concrete cases, and starting from the aforementioned rules] in which *períodoi*[311] the irregular fevers and the quartan, quintan, septan, and nonan fevers come to their crises."[312] *Epidemics III*, ch. 16, "Starting from these [theoretical details] it is easy to consider the order of the critical days [in the individual cases] and to prognosticate from them [i. e., either from the details, or the days, or

---

306 Lloyd, Magic 129 f.

307 Cf. above p. 179 f.

308 *Epid. I* 2.632.12–634.2 Li. = 1.189.18–20 Kw. = 1.162 Jones πεπασμοὺς τῶν ἀπιόντων πάντας πάντοθεν ἐπικαίρους ἢ καλὰς καὶ κρισίμους ἀποστάσιας σκοπεῖσθαι.

309 *Epid. I* 2.634.3–6 Li. = 1.189.21–24 Kw. = 1.164 Jones ὅ τι δὲ τούτων ἔσται μάλιστα, σκεπτέον ἐξ ἄλλων.

310 *Epid. I* 2.676.10–11 Li. = 1.201.9–10 Kw. = 1.182–184 Jones δεῖ δὲ καὶ τὰ διαιτήματα σκοπεύμενον ἐκ τούτων προσφέρειν. Jones's translation, "It is necessary also to consider the patient's mode of life and to take it into account when prescribing," is grammatically correct but unparalleled for its content. Prescriptions in acute diseases are scarcely made dependent on the patient's former mode of life. The idea expressed (diet made dependent on the crises) is the subject of *Acut.*

311 Cf. above p. 95–105.

312 *Epid. I* 2.680.9–682.2 Li. = 1.202.8–10 Kw. = 1.184 Jones πλάνητες δὲ πυρετοὶ καὶ τεταρταῖοι καὶ πεμπταῖοι καὶ ἑβδομαῖοι καὶ ἐναταῖοι, ἐν τίσι (τίσι scripsi: τῇσι A: ᾗσι VIR) περιόδοισι κρίνονται, σκεπτέον. Jones's translation suggests that the author considered these fevers exceptions to his rule, but the text gives no hint of such an interpretation.

both]."[313] *Epidemics II* 1.6, "At the beginnings of the diseases one must consider whether they culminate immediately."[314]

Besides the group of verbs related to *skopéomai*, there are several other verbs expressing mental activities.[315] Like the former verbs they most often denote activities concerning concrete cases or concerning objects with which the physician deals (or is advised to deal) according to, or in the light of, certain rules or theories or standards. Nowhere in the *Epidemics* do they denote activities which consist in examining abstract rules or theories in the light of concrete cases.

'Types' and 'Groups' in the *Epidemics*

A passage which contains verbs denoting mental processes and which is particularly characteristic of the research method is *Epidemics I*, ch. 10 Li. (= ch. 23 Kw., Jones). Syntactically the text is an enumeration of various viewpoints borne in mind by the author(s) during his, or their, medical activity (the passage is not a 'sentence' with a predicate[316]). "The circumstances of the diseases, from which we used to form our judgement and to differentiate,[317] learning from the common nature of all [persons and things] and from the individual nature of each [person and thing]; from the disease, from the patient, from the things administered, from the one who administers (because this, too, contributes to an easier or more difficult development);[318] from the *katástasis*[319] of the weather and of each country, both universally and with respect to the parts; from the custom, regimen, occupational activities, and age of each [patient]; through utterances, manners, silence, thoughts, sleep, insomnia, dreams — what kind?

[313] *Epid. III* 3.102.7–8 Li. = 1.232.16–17 Kw. = 1.256 Jones. For the Greek text, cf. below p. 207, note 371.

[314] *Epid. II* 5.74.12–16 πρὸς τὰς ἀρχὰς σκεπτέον τῶν νούσων, εἰ αὐτίκα ἀνθεῖ. Cf. the parallel passages *IV* 5.158.7–8 Li. = Per. 139 La.; *VI* 5.272.2–4; more examples are *Epid. II* 5.80.4–11, 82.12–14; *VI* 5.350.3–4 τὸ σῶμα ἔργον ἐς τὴν σκέψιν ἄγειν. (Cf. above p. 51.) *Hum.* 5.500.3–7 Li. = 4.92 Jones σκεπτέον δὲ ἐξ ὧν ἴσμεν ... περὶ χροιῶν, "One must judge by what we know about complexions."

[315] Examples: *Epid. I* 2.678.1 Li. = 1.201.13–14 Kw. = 1.184 Jones διαλογιζόμενον δοκιμάζειν καὶ σκοπεῖσθαι. *III* 3.102.2 Li. = 1.232.10 Kw. = 1.256 Jones καταμανθάνειν. *II* 5.76.11 θεωρεῖν. 78.17–18 ἐγίνωσκον. 88.13 γνοίη (V: διαγ- HIR). *VI* 5.342.11 καταμαθητέον. *Hum.* 5.482.13 Li. = 4.70 Jones ἐπιθεωρέειν (A: τὰ διαιτήματα M). 494.17–18 Li. = 4.86 Jones προσλογιστέον.

[316] Further examples in Langholf, Syntaktische Untersuchungen 51; cf. 47 ff.

[317] διεγινώσκομεν, imperfect, implies a habit (Galen's δια- is lectio facilior). The verb means 'to recognize by differentiating.'

[318] Cf. the truism in Seneca rhet., *Controv. IV* 5: Nihil magis aegris prodest quam ab eo curari a quo volunt.

[319] Cf. above p. 169 ff.

when? –; plucking, itching, tears; from the paroxysms, stools, urines, expectorations, vomits; the successions [or: transformations] of diseases and segregations – how many? what was first? what followed? – towards death or *krísis*; sweat, rigor, chill, cough, sneezing, hiccups, breaths, belchings, flatulence – with or without a noise? –, nose-bleedings, haemorrhoids. Starting from these things one has also to consider what happens under their effect."[320]

This enumeration is the sum of professional experience although not a programme of 'empiric' or 'positivist' research. "Each country" implies that the author(s) practised his, or their, craft in more than just one or two places. "We" is unclear. It either includes other people who accompanied the itinerant author, and who might have been co-authors; or it is a *pluralis modestiae* of one single author. 'Forming one's judgement by differentiating' is described as a complex activity. In a concrete disease case, each of the signs (symptoms) and facts (physiological, meteorological, and others) has to be evaluated in the context of the other signs and facts; moreover, for each of them the aetiological relationship to the other ones has to be assessed: "What does each of them effect?" This implies, of course, the inverse question: "Under which effect does each of them occur?" It appears that the method outlined in this chapter of *Epidemics I* is compatible with Plato's famous description of Hippocrates' method in the *Phaedrus* (269 c–272 b), which can be paraphrased: *(i)* First one should consider whether a thing consists of one or many forms, and then *(ii a)* if it consists of only one form, one should examine what its capacity for acting or being acted upon is, or *(ii b)* if it consists of many forms, [*a'*] enumerate its forms and then [*b'*] ask the same question of each of the forms.[321] The Greek word for 'form' could just as well be rendered by 'type' in this and other contexts.

---

[320] *Epid. I* 2.668.14–670.15 Li. = 1.199.9–200.2 Kw. = 1.180 Jones τὰ δὲ περὶ τὰ νοσήματα, ἐξ ὧν διεγινώσκομεν (διε- AVIR: δια- Gal.), μαθόντες ἐκ τῆς κοινῆς φύσιος ἁπάντων καὶ τῆς ἰδίης ἑκάστου, ἐκ τοῦ νοσήματος, ἐκ τοῦ νοσέοντος, ἐκ τῶν προσφερομένων, ἐκ τοῦ προσφέροντος – ἐπὶ τὸ ῥᾷον γὰρ (γὰρ AVIR: om. Gal.) καὶ χαλεπώτερον (-τερον VIR, Gal.: -τατον A) ἐκ τούτων (τούτων VIR: τούτου A, Gal.) –, ἐκ τῆς καταστάσιος ὅλης καὶ κατὰ (καὶ κατὰ VIR, Gal.: κατὰ, mut. in καὶ τὰ A) μέρεα τῶν οὐρανίων καὶ χώρης ἑκάστης, ἐκ (AVIR: καὶ Gal.) τοῦ ἔθεος, ἐκ τῆς διαίτης, ἐκ τῶν ἐπιτηδευμάτων, ἐκ τῆς ἡλικίης ἑκάστου, λόγοισι, τρόποισι, σιγῇ, διανοήμασιν, ὕπνοισιν, οὐχ ὕπνοισιν, ἐνυπνίοισι, οἵοισι (οἵοισι A: τοίοισι VR, τοιοῖσι I: τισὶν οἷσι Gal.) καὶ ὅτε, τιλμοῖσι, κνησμοῖσι, δάκρυσιν, ἐκ τῶν παροξυσμῶν, διαχωρήμασιν, οὔροισιν, πτυάλοισιν (πτυάλοισιν AVIR: πτύσμασιν Gal.), ἐμέτοισι, καὶ ὅσαι ἐξ οἵων ἐς οἷα διαδοχαὶ νοσημάτων καὶ ἀποστάσιες ἐπὶ τὸ ὀλέθριον καὶ κρίσιμον, ἱδρώς, ῥῖγος, ψύξις, βήξ, πταρμοί, λυγμοί, πνεύματα, ἐρεύξιες, φῦσαι σιγῶσαι, ψοφώδεες (φ. σ. ψ. A: φ. σιγώδεες ψ. VIR: φύσεσι ψοφώδεσι χολώδεες Gal.), αἱμορραγίαι, αἱμορροΐδες. ἐκ τούτων (δὲ add. Gal.: om. AVIR) καὶ ὅσα διὰ τούτων σκεπτέον.

[321] The paraphrase is borrowed from Lloyd, Hippocratic question, with some changes,

Plato's description refers to a method of *classification*.[322] The question whether a thing consists of one or many 'forms' primarily means, "Which 'types' (*eídē*, singular *eídos*) does the thing consist of?", and it is asked in the context and in the terms of Platonic philosophy, with *eídos* referring not directly to the concrete phenomena observable in a given case but to the idea (abstract type) of the thing or item under consideration. To quote Jouanna (in translation):[323] "What do the *eídē* of the body mean? ... According to the parallelism established by Plato between the body and the soul, the *eídē* of the body do not mean the different elements of the body but the different species ('espèces') which constitute the class ('genre') body, i. e. the different types of constitution, for instance the dry and wet, or bilious and phlegmatic constitutions. After the enumeration of the *eídē*, says Plato, one has to determine the *dýnamis* of each *eídos*, in other words the passive and active natural properties." "Following the parallelism between the method of the orator and of the physician, one must conclude that Plato's Hippocrates has to make a classification of the different types of foodstuffs or remedies parallel to the different types of constitution, and to establish a causal relationship between the two series."[324]

---

particularly in the translation of πολυειδές ('of many forms'), which was proposed by Jaap Mansfeld, Plato and the method of Hippocrates, Greek, Rom., and Byz. Stud. 21 (1980), 341–362 (350).

322 Antje Hellweg, Untersuchungen zur Theorie der Rhetorik bei Platon und Aristoteles (Hypomnemata, 38), Göttingen, 1973, 181–232, with bibliography. Hans Herter, The problematic mention of Hippocrates in Plato's *Phaedrus*, Illinois Class. Stud. 1 (1976), 22–42, with comprehensive bibliography.

323 Jacques Jouanna, La *Collection hippocratique* et Platon (*Phèdre*, 269c–272a), Rev. Ét. Grecques 90 (1977), 15–28 (in partic. 24f.; my translation).

324 Jouanna contends that φύσις throughout this Platonic passage refers strictly to "le tout de l'objet considéré" (p. 22), and that "l'interprétation cosmologique est irrecevable." According to him, the method of Plato's Hippocrates "n'exige pas une connaissance préalable de l'Univers" (p. 26). I think that this restriction of the meaning of φύσις, particularly of ἄνευ τῆς τοῦ ὅλου φύσεως (270c), creates unnecessary difficulties. As early as 270a, Pericles had been mentioned (somewhat ironically) as having been "filled up" with μετεωρολογία (270a), a word certainly meaning something like "discours élevés," albeit with an allusion to cosmological studies (for the oscillation in meaning, cf. *Cratyl.* 396c, 404c); this collateral sense of 'natural philosophy' is emphasized by the addition of φύσεως πέρι, which is not redundant, although Jouanna, p. 19, thinks so. It emphasizes one of the two possible meanings of μετεωρολογία ('celestial phenomena') without suppressing the other one ('lofty discussion'); cf. Herter 26, note 14. That the word 'nature' (φύσις) has the broadest possible sense here (and perhaps in the whole context 269c–272b) becomes evident from φύσιν Νοῦ τε καὶ διανοίας ..., ὧν δὴ πέρι τὸν πολὺν λόγον ἐποιεῖτο Ἀναξαγόρας. This philosopher was concerned not only with a classification of what constitutes the *Nous* but primarily with the aspect of its being a constitutive (even the most essential) part of Nature as a whole. The possible meanings of Plato's τῆς τοῦ ὅλου φύσεως (270c) have been summarized by Lloyd, Hippocratic question: "At least four interpretations are possible, namely that it means (1) the whole

The passage in *Epidemics I*, ch. 10 Li. (= ch. 23 Kw., Jones) quoted above can very well be interpreted in the light of the *Phaedrus* testimony on Hippocrates' method: "The circumstances of the diseases" were recognized on the basis of a *classification* of the individual cases according to the following 'headings:' First, "the common nature of all persons and things" (i. e. universals of the highest hierarchic level) and "the individual nature of each person and thing" (i. e. less universal characteristics found, as for example, only in a group of patients or under specific weather conditions). Second, according to 'headings' referring to subject matter: "From the disease" (i. e. types of diseases, or nosological units), "from the patient" (i. e. types of body constitution etc.), "from the things administered" (i. e. types of food, drugs, applications of all sorts), "from the one who administers," "from the *katástasis* of the weather and of each country, both universally and with respect to the parts," "from the custom, regimen, occupational activities, and age of each patient." All this can be meant to refer to certain 'types' (the number of which may have been left undetermined), to a classification in the sense of Plato's description. (There follow in the *Epidemics* passage some viewpoints for analysing the concrete complexes of phenomena in order to establish the various 'types': "Through utterances [of the patient], manners, silence, thoughts, sleep, insomnia ..., stools, urines ..." etc.)

Of course one should not read Plato's terms and philosophy into texts of the Hippocratic Corpus. To some extent (but to what extent?), Plato did what has ever since been done with 'Hippocrates:' He interpreted the available information about Hippocrates' method on the basis of his own

---

of nature or the universe, (2) the whole of the body, (3) the whole of the body-soul complex, or (4) the whole of whatever subject happens to be under discussion." Probably the broadest meaning should be accorded to this phrase. περὶ ὁτουοῦν φύσεως (270 d) means either "about any nature" ("about the nature of anything," Jouanna, p. 20) or rather "about anything in the field of nature" (Kühner/Gerth, vol. 1. 278 f., 338–340). Plato's expression τὸ ὅλον probably refers to cosmology, as Joly has contended; see Joly, Question hippocratique; Robert Joly, Platon, Phèdre et Hippocrate: Vingt ans après, in: Formes de pensée 407–422; Fernand Robert, Rev. Ét. Grecques 95 (1982), p. XVIII–XXII. Joly's additional inference that Plato overinterpreted Hippocrates, because obviously nowhere in any one treatise of the Corpus the method of classification is used together with cosmological speculation, is unjustified: Plato does not say that both features (cosmology plus classification) are found *together* anywhere in one and the same treatise; in fact he does not even speak of *treatises* in that context. Note, however, that *Flat.*, which seems to have been regarded genuine by three influential authors of the fourth and third centuries B. C. (Aristotle, Antiphanes, and Callimachus; cf. Langholf, Kallimachos), and which in its doctrines appears to be compatible with *Epid. I* and *III*, *has* cosmology (religious or quasi-religious function of the air, cf. below p. 244). A remarkable oscillation in the meaning of τὸ ὅλον (body/universe) is found in *Hebd.* 8.672–673 Li. = 79 Roscher = 4.218–221 Jones: The patient, when dying, ἀποπνέει ἀθρόον τὸ πνεῦμα τοῦ θερμοῦ, ὅθεν περ ξυνέστη τὸ ὅλον, εἰς τὸ ὅλον πάλιν. Cf. above p. 165, note 169.

system of thought.[325] Nevertheless it is a significant fact that some aspects of the method recoverable from the *Epidemics* and from other treatises of the Collection can be described in Platonic terms without essentially being distorted.[326] Were none of these medical treatises extant, Plato's short characterization would be misleading if one tried to reconstruct them according to it. But since, as will be demonstrated shortly below, the *Phaedrus* passage is so very compatible with several surviving medical texts, it is plausible that Plato had them in mind (and/or related texts now lost, which may have been more explicit about the method). It is even imaginable that Hippocrates himself had talked about methods and demonstrated them during a sojourn in Athens:[327] His method must have been widely known there at Plato's time, as can be inferred from the fact that Plato not only represented Phaedrus as being well informed about the method, but was even able to use it as an example for rhetoric without having to describe it to his reading public. Since, however, Plato does not say that Hippocrates was the first or the only one to use the method, its application in treatises of the Hippocratic Collection, for instance in the *Epidemics*, is no evidence for authenticity.[328]

When observing concrete disease cases, the authors of the *Epidemics* either started from *a priori* types of patients, diseases, weather, etc., and tried to subsume the cases to them, or they tried to determine new types on the basis of an analysis of the concrete phenomena after a given set of 'headings' or categories. As will be demonstrated below, the two procedures of classification could be, and usually were, combined: Besides the traditional types which are taken over from contemporary or earlier medicine, there are new ones obviously formed by the authors themselves.[329] The 'groups' of patients thus formed were intellectual constructs: since there were no hospitals, it is unlikely that any patients were physically gathered together according to their diseases. The authors do not even use a word for 'group.'

Patients are 'grouped' according to traditional types whenever they are labelled with term-like expressions taken from the current systems of

---

325 This was also Galen's procedure, cf. Smith, Hippocratic tradition *passim*. Iain M. Lonie, Hippocrates the iatromechanist, Med. History 25 (1981), 113–150 describes the phenomenon for the 17th and 18th centuries; Lonie's results have been modified by Ingo W. Müller, Klassische Fassade oder ernsthafter Hippokratismus?, Medizinhist. Journ. 22 (1987), 62–79.

326 Diller, Ausdrucksformen 149 f. (= Kleine Schriften Medizin 122 f.).

327 This possibility is suggested by Plato's λέγει Ἱπποκράτης (270 c; but λέγει can, of course, also mean 'write,' cf. Langholf, Kallimachos, note 69).

328 The basis of argumentation in Lichtenthaeler, Eid 313–324 is, therefore, contestable.

329 Vincenzo Di Benedetto, Tendenza e probabilità nell' antica medicina greca, Critica storica 5 (1966), 315–368. Dittmer, Konstitutionstypen.

nosology or humoral pathology (e. g. *dysenteriṓdēs*, 'suffering from *dysenteríē*,[330] or 'phlegmatic,' 'bilious,' etc.). This happens so frequently in the *Epidemics* that no examples need to be given here. Also sex and age are traditional criteria, *Epidemics I*, ch. 8 Li. (= ch. 16 Kw., Jones): "Many women fell ill, but they were fewer than the males, and their mortality was less ... To most of them menstruation occurred during the fever, and many virgins menstruated then for the first time."[331] The age-group of children is subdivided, *Epidemics I*, ch. 4 Li. (= ch. 10 Kw., Jones): "Children just weaned, and older ones of eight or ten years, and children approaching puberty."[332]

The 'group' described in the following text is formed on the basis of the three criteria 'sex,' 'age,' and 'sports activities,' and of further criteria furnished by the patients' symptoms: *Epidemics I*, ch. 1 Li. (= ch. 1 Kw., Jones), "This happened to male persons in and shortly after puberty, in their youth, and in their best years; and of them particularly to many who frequented wrestling places and gymnasia. Few women were affected."[333] Although all of the former three criteria and many of the symptoms were traditional, their combination in one 'group' of patients may have been the finding of the author(s). The members of the 'group' were characterized by the fact that each of them was simultaneously a member of certain larger 'groups;' the 'group' described was the field of intersection of other larger ones. Or in Plato's terms: The type of patients described "consisted of many forms" because it consisted of several sub-types ('sex,' 'age,' 'sports activities,' symptoms). Each of the features considered had its own capacity for acting or being acted upon (cf. above p. 195).

Sometimes a word for 'type' is used, *eídos* (plural *eídē* or *eídea*),[334] which, however, has some other connotations than its modern translation. It is

---

[330] Cf. above p. 150–164.

[331] *Epid. I* 2.646.10–648.1 Li. = 1.193.6–12 Kw. = 1.170 Jones γυναῖκες δὲ ἐνόσησαν μὲν πολλαί, ἐλάσσους δὲ ἢ ἄνδρες, καὶ ἔθνῃσκον ἧσσον... τῇσι μὲν οὖν πλείστῃσιν ἐν τοῖσι πυρετοῖσι γυναικεῖα ἐπεφαίνετο καὶ παρθένοισι πολλῇσι τότε πρῶτον ἐγένετο.

[332] *Epid. I* 2.630.4–5 Li. = 1.188.24–189.1 Kw. = 1.162 Jones παιδία ὅσα ἀπὸ γάλακτος ἤδη, καὶ πρεσβύτερα, ὀκταετέα καὶ δεκαετέα, καὶ ὅσα πρὸ ἥβης. Cf. *Epid. III* 3.84.11–12 Li. = 1.228.10 Kw. = 1.246 Jones.

[333] *Epid. I* 2.602.2–5 Li. = 1.181.4–6 Kw. = 1.148 Jones ἐγίνετο δὲ ταῦτα μειρακίοισι, νέοισιν, ἀκμάζουσι, καὶ τούτων τοῖσι περὶ παλαίστρην καὶ γυμνάσια πλείστοισι· γυναιξὶ δὲ ὀλίγῃσιν ἐγίνετο.

[334] The same word occurs in Plato *Phaedr.* 270 d, 271 d (bis), 272 a; cf. πολυειδής 270 d, 271 a; the word γένος seems to be used synonymously with εἶδος 271 b. In the fifth and fourth centuries B. C., *eídos* belonged to colloquial language (Hans Diller, Zum Gebrauch von εἶδος und ἰδέα in vorplatonischer Zeit, in: Medizingeschichte in unserer Zeit, Festgabe for E. Heischkel und W. Artelt, Stuttgart, 1971, 23–30), so it is legitimate to assume that some 'Platonic' connotations can be traced already in the pre-Platonic medical treatises of the Collection, particularly since Plato must have found in this literature a

etymologically related to a Greek word for 'to see,'[335] a semantical connection still strongly felt in the fifth and fourth centuries. In the *Epidemics*, *eídos* has a meaning oscillating somewhat between 'appearance,' 'look,' and 'type.' In fact, the 'types' of the *Epidemics* were defined on the basis of criteria recognizable through the senses.[336] *Epidemics III*, ch. 14, "The 'type' [*eídos*] of those suffering from consumption was: smoothness,[337] whitish, freckled, reddish complexion, blue-grey colour of the eyes,[338] disposition to white phlegm,[339] projection of the shoulder-blades like wings. Women the same way. People with [a disposition to ?] a prevalence of black bile and of blood were attacked with *kaúsos, phrenîtis*, and *dysenteríē*.[340] Young individuals with [a disposition to ?] a prevalence of phlegm suffered from *teinesmós*. Long *diárrhoia*[341] and acrid, greasy stools affected persons with [a disposition to ?] a prevalence[342] of acrid bile."[343] The

---

procedure comparable to, and perhaps even foreshadowing, his own one. Cf. also C. M. Gillespie, The use of Εἶδος and Ἰδέα in Hippocrates, Class. Quart. 6 (1912), 179–203. Fernand Robert, Hippocrate, Platon, Aristote et les notions de genre et d'espèce, Hist. and Philos. of the Life Sciences 4 (1982), 173–201. For the meaning of Hippocratic εἶδος/ἰδέη as compared to τρόπος cf. Laín Entralgo, Historia clínica 38 f.; Laín Entralgo, Medicina hipocrática 231–234.

335 εἶδον.

336 Diller, *op. cit.* This holds true even with regard to the humoral 'types' of patients such as the "people with [a disposition to?] a prevalence of black bile" (cf. below); these 'types' were recognized by certain manifest characteristics (e. g. of the stool or urine etc.).

337 The neuters τὸ λεῖον etc. have an abstract meaning, perhaps best rendered as 'smooth*ness*' etc.

338 On τὸ χαροπόν cf. Jones's note *ad loc.*

339 On λευκοφλεγματίαι cf. above p. 154.

340 On these diseases, cf. above p. 153 ff.

341 Cf. above p. 153.

342 The words λευκοφλεγματίαι, τὸ μελαγχολικόν, τὸ ὕφαιμον, φλεγματώδεσιν, and πικροχόλοισιν are difficult to translate because one does not know exactly the humoral doctrine implied. I have tentatively interpreted them in analogy to the doctrine of *Nat. Hom./Salubr.*, with which there seems to be some relationship, although no identity. (φλέγμα λευκόν, a disease name current in the nosological treatises, might as well be a specific humour; it is absent from *Nat. Hom./Salubr.*; so is πικρόχολος, and χολή is never called πικρή there; ὕφαιμον is unclear.) According to *Nat. Hom./Salubr.*, diseases occur whenever one of the four humours, which are always present in the body, prevails at the expense of the other ones. Although this doctrine (which expressed ideas popular in fifth and fourth century Greek medicine) is compatible with *Epid. I* and *III* in the sense that it can largely be read into these treatises (and *vice versa*), there might be differences unknown to us because of the inexplicitness of the *Epid.* texts. The obvious parallelism between *Epid. I/III* and *Nat. Hom./Salubr.* justifies the insertion of "[a disposition to?] a prevalence of" in the translation. The prevalence may have been latent or manifest. Cf. above p. 136 f.

343 *Epid. III* 3.96.4–98.5 Li. = 1.231.12–18 Kw. = 1.254 Jones εἶδος δὲ τῶν φθινωδέων ἦν τὸ λεῖον, τὸ ὑπόλευκον, τὸ φακῶδες, τὸ ὑπέρυθρον, τὸ χαροπόν, λευκοφλεγματίαι, πτερυγώδεες· καὶ γυναῖκες οὕτω. τὸ μελαγχολικὸν καὶ ὕφαιμον – οἱ καῦσοι καὶ τὰ

'types' of patients described here are determined by a complex medical theory involving physiognomical characteristics[344] and body humours. The passage exemplifies again that the modern historian can sometimes hardly answer the question whether a certain 'type' was taken over from an older tradition or whether it was the original finding or construction of the authors of the *Epidemics*. Indeed, the procedure observable in these treatises consists in determining 'groups' of patients on the basis of an individual's being part of *various* other types or 'groups.' For instance, the individuals who suffered from consumption during one particular year belonged to seven other 'groups' (either to all, or to some, or to one of them; the text is not clear in this respect). Although some of the other 'groups' occur also in other treatises of the Collection and must, therefore, have been traditional, the description of one 'group' as the field of intersection of other 'groups' may have been the discovery of the author(s) of the text passage.[345]

One would certainly go too far if he said that the method of classification exhibited by the authors of the *Epidemics* relied primarily on 'types' of patients, or 'body-types,' and only secondarily on 'types' of diseases, symptoms, etc. A clear logical distinction between the patient and the

---

φρενιτικὰ καὶ τὰ δυσεντεριώδεα τούτων ἥπτετο. τεινεσμοὶ νέοισι φλεγματώδεσιν. αἱ μακραὶ διάρροιαι καὶ τὰ δριμέα διαχωρήματα καὶ λιπαρὰ πικροχόλοισιν.

[344] For physiognomical and other individual features, cf. also *Epid. II* 5.80.1–14; 128.2–13; 132.14–21 (in 132.17 παχύγλωσσοι should probably be read instead of the manuscripts' [VHIR] ταχ- and of Galen's "mit schneller Zunge" [transmitted only in Arabic]; likewise in *Epid. IV* 5.186.3 Li. = Per. 259 La. [ταχ- VHIR], where προπετέως means 'protruding,' cf. *Epid. II* 5.96.7–8); 136.2–5; *Epid. VI* 5.266.7–11; 334.8–11; 352.16–354.2. Elizabeth C. Evans, Physiognomics in the ancient world, Philadelphia, 1969 (Transact. of the Amer. Philos. Society, N. S. 59.5), 17–28. See also below p. 249 with notes (divination from signs of the body). Physiological and pathological features are, of course, not distinguished in the sense of modern medicine. A theory underlying medical physiognomical doctrine is set forth in *VM* 1.626.6–634.11 Li. = 1.26.18–30.2 Kw.

[345] A passage in *Epid. VI* 7.6 explicitly attributes a passive (?) or active (?) rôle to the *eídos* in cases of consumption. The ambiguous text, which is extremely concise (in fact a sort of notebook entry), can be paraphrased as follows: "[Consider] if somebody naturally, without being angry, has a voice like angry persons; or [consider] those who naturally have excited eyes, resembling the eyes of normal angry people [ὅταν ὀργίζωνται οἱ μὴ τοιοῦτοι]; and the other things analogously. And as to diseases: for instance, consumption produces the *eídos* [one might also translate: 'for instance, the *eídos* produces consumption' or: 'what form of consumption is produced by the *eídos*']. If he [the patient] is of this or that nature, this or that disease will befall him. And so on analogously." 5.340.8–12 φωνὴ οἵη γίνεται ὀργιζομένοισιν, ἣν τοιαύτη ᾖ μὴ ὀργιζομένῳ φύσει, ἢ καὶ ὄμματα οἷς (οἷς V: οἵ' M: οἷα Pall.) ἂν ᾖ φύσει ταραχώδεα, οἷα ὅταν ὀργίζωνται οἱ μὴ τοιοῦτοι, καὶ τἄλλα κατὰ λόγον, καὶ νούσων (νούσων M, Gal., Pall.: νοῦς V), οἷον τὸ φθινῶδες ποιέει τὸ εἶδος· ἢν τοιοῦτος φύσει ὑπάρχῃ, ἐς τοιοῦτον νόσημα παρέσται, καὶ τἄλλα οὕτως. Galen's text, extant only in an Arabic version, seems to differ in the second half of the paragraph.

disease was not made because it was unnecessary for practical purposes.[346] When, however, studying the 'types' present in the *Epidemics*, one can observe that those of the body are the most numerous ones. The authors probably did not follow a strict logical method. Their procedure was not the result of a deductive process or even of primarily theoretical considerations, but had arisen from practical observations made on the basis of the accepted medical doctrines such as *krísis, pépsis*, and *apóstasis*, particularly during epidemics with their conspicuous syndromes. Still the method exhibits a remarkable uniformity, namely a preference for grouping patients and not diseases or symptoms. Traditional nosology is presupposed in the *Epidemics* but tends to be considered only on a subordinate level.[347]

The following description of 'groups' is instructive for the wide range of bodily features involved, *Epidemics I*, ch. 9 Li. (= ch. 19 Kw., Jones): "There was a large number of diseases. Out of the patients, particularly the following died: male persons in and shortly after puberty, in their youth, and in their best years; smooth ones, with whitish complexion, straight-haired, black-haired, black-eyed, the ones who had lived planlessly and carelessly, thin-voiced, rough-voiced, lispers, irascible ones. Also the women who died belonged mostly to this *eídos*."[348] Again it cannot be said whether an individual of any of the age-groups belonged to all or only some (perhaps only one?) of the other 'groups.' In a pharmacological passage, *Epidemics II* 3.2, an enumeration of various viewpoints to be kept in mind by the physician, the 'type' of the patient is mentioned together with some other features: "... How many [remedies] are indicated for each [patient], and in which diseases, and when during the disease; considering the age, the 'types' (*eídea*), the regimen; which season of the year, what is it like, what is its tendency? And so on."[349] The passage makes it evident that the underlying method is not so systematic as a reader of Plato's account in the *Phaedrus* might be inclined to infer. *eídos* seems to be

---

[346] The medical language often did not make this distinction, cf. the syntactical examples collected in Langholf, Syntaktische Untersuchungen 103 f. (cf. 59 f., 68 f.).

[347] This can probably not be explained in moral terms as an increased human interest in the patient.

[348] *Epid. I* 2.656.1–7 Li. = 1.195.15–20 Kw. = 1.174 Jones πλῆθος μὲν οὖν τῶν νοσημάτων ἐγένετο. ἐκ δὲ τῶν καμνόντων ἀπέθνῃσκον μάλιστα (μάλιστα VIR, Gal.: om. A) μειράκια, νέοι, ἀκμάζοντες, λεῖοι, ὑπολευκόχρωτες (ὑπ- AV, Gal.: λευκ- IR), ἰθύτριχες, μελανότριχες, μελανόφθαλμοι, οἱ εἰκῇ (οἱ εἰκῇ AVIR: ἡσυχῇ Gal.) καὶ ἐπὶ τὸ ῥᾴθυμον βεβιωκότες (post βεβ. add. ὑψώφωνοι IR: om. AV, Gal.), ἰσχνόφωνοι, τρηχύφωνοι, τραυλοί, ὀργίλοι. καὶ γυναῖκες (κ. γ. AV, Gal.: γ. δὲ IR) πλεῖσται ἐκ τούτου τοῦ εἴδεος ἀπέθνῃσκον.

[349] *Epid. II* 5.104.10–12 ὁκόσα ἑκάστῳ καὶ ἐφ' οἷσι νοσήμασι, καὶ ὁπότε τοῦ νοσήματος, ἡλικίην, εἴδεα (εἴδεα V: (ε)ἰδέαν HIR), δίαιταν, ὁκοίη ὥρη ἔτεος, καὶ ἥτις καὶ ὁκοίως ἀγομένη, καὶ τὰ τοιαῦτα. For the beginning of this passage, cf. above p. 138, note 15.

mentioned on the same logical level[350] as the patient's age, although in other contexts the age seems to be one characteristic of the *eídos*. The historian should, therefore, avoid trying to reconstruct a definition of *eídos* in the *Epidemics*. The word was not a technical term but had largely kept its colloquial meaning.

Besides 'types' of patients, the word *eídos* can also denote 'types' of diseases, fevers, etc., *Epidemics III*, ch. 12: "Many other 'types' (*eídea*) of fevers arrived,[351] tertian, quartan, nocturnal, continuous, protracted, irregular, causing nausea, fevers without any tendency."[352] Even relapses have their 'types:' *Epidemics I*, ch. 9 Li. (= ch. 20 Kw., Jones), "All [patients] whom I know, to whom the relapses happened according to this [aforementioned] 'type' (*eídos*), recovered."[353] The context of this passage has already been dealt with above (p. 115–117). Evidently, the author(s) discovered these 'types' of relapses by forming 'groups' out of patients who exhibited the same chronological features in their diseases. 'Types' of patients and 'types' of diseases coincided in the individual cases. For some passages one can hardly determine whether *eídos* refers to the body or to the disease.[354] In the majority of contexts describing types or groups, the word *eídos* does not even occur at all.[355]

The authors display some virtuosity in forming 'groups.'[356] In *Epidemics III*, ch. 9, we find: "All [patients] under all aforementioned conditions were without appetite to a degree which I had never encountered before;

---

350 'Logical level' is an anachronistic expression.

351 *epidēméō*, lit. 'to arrive at a population' (*dḗmos*).

352 *Epid. III* 3.92.5–7 Li. = 1.229.19–21 Kw. = 1.250 Jones πολλὰ δὲ καὶ ἄλλα πυρετῶν ἐπεδήμησεν εἴδεα, τριταίων, τεταρταίων, νυκτερινῶν, συνεχέων, μακρῶν, πεπλανημένων, ἀσωδέων, ἀκαταστάτων.

353 *Epid. I* 2.664.7–9 Li. = 1.197.20–21 Kw. = 1.178 Jones διεσῴζοντο πάντες, οὓς κἀγὼ οἶδα, οἷσιν αἱ ὑποστροφαὶ διὰ τοῦ εἴδεος τούτου γενοίατο.

354 This is the case in *Epid. III* 3.70.11–12 Li. = 1.225.7–9 Kw. = 1.240 Jones ἑκάστου δὲ τῶν ὑπογεγραμμένων εἰδέων ἦσαν οἱ κάμνοντες, καὶ ἔθνῃσκον πολλοί, where πολλοί possibly refers not only to ἔθνῃσκον but also to ἦσαν οἱ κάμνοντες. *Hum.* 5.494.6–8 Li. = 4.86 Jones ὅταν οὖν καὶ ἔαρ οὕτως ἀγάγῃ (i. e., like summer), καὶ ἦρος γίνονται ἴκτεροι (as in summer)· ἐγγυτάτη γὰρ αὕτη ἡ κίνησις (i. e., the internal movement of bile) τῇ ὥρῃ κατὰ τοῦτο τὸ εἶδός ἐστιν, "as to this 'type'," namely either this type of humour (bile) and its pathological effects, or this type of season (a spring which is like summer).

355 On the other hand, *eídos* could be used in quite different contexts: In *Epid. II* 5.102.15 it refers to the 'manner' of covering the patient with blankets. 74.4 ἐν τῷ ἄνω εἴδει is unclear (the 'type' of weather?).

356 The 'groups' foreshadow how Aristotle uses the correlations of features, particularly in his biological treatises, e. g. *Hist. an. II* 502 b 28–503 a 8, 504 a 31–b 9, 506 a 12–20, 507 b 34, *III* 511 a 3–8, 517 a 30–33, 519 b 34–520 a 5, 521 b 29–32, 523 a 15–17, *IV* 532 a 20–22, *Part. anim. III* 664 b 20–26, 674 a 21–30, 676 a 11–14, *IV* 688 a 32–b 1, 692 b 22–693 a 10, b 5–8 (cf. *Progr. anim.* 711 a 2–5), *Gener. anim. I* 728 a 34–b 2, *II* 745 b 30–34, *IV* 774 b 5–10.

but particularly so were the latter ones [namely the ones with digestive troubles], and again of them and of the others those who were to die."[357] *VI* 7.1 "The combinations [literally: 'the allotments of the combinations'] of the affections were as has just been described [cf. the preceding lines of the account]: the first-described affections occurred also without the latter ones, but the latter ones not without the ones described first."[358] The description of the 'groups,' however, is occasionally unclear, probably because the text lacks a final revision: *Epidemics I*, ch. 4 Li. (= ch. 10 Kw., Jones), "Of all [groups of patients] some died, but most of the cases of death occurred among the aforementioned [patients; i. e. those who had *(i)* digestive troubles and *(ii)* unfavourable segregations, cf. the preceding lines], and of them in particular children died who were just weaned, and older ones of eight or ten years, and children approaching puberty. This [*(ii)*?] occurred to them [all patients? or children?] not without what has been described before [*(i)*], but to many the aforementioned features [*(i)*] occurred without the latter ones [*(ii)*]."[359]

A specialty of *Epidemics I*, when forming 'groups,' is the counter-proof whether there were any exceptions from the "allotment of combinations" in the 'groups,' for instance ch. 4 Li. (= ch. 10 Kw., Jones), "These all survived, and I do not know anyone of them who died."[360] Ch. 8 Li. (= ch. 14 Kw., Jones), "I know of none who died during this *katástasis* if he had had a good nose-bleeding."[361]

---

[357] *Epid. III* 3.90.1–4 Li. = 1.228.26–229.2 Kw. = 1.248–250 Jones ἀπόσιτοι δὲ πάντες μὲν ἐγένοντο (δὲ π. μ. ἐ. I: π. μ. ἐ. R, Gal.: δ' ἐ. π. μ. V) καὶ ἐπὶ πᾶσι τοῖσι προγεγραμμένοισιν, ὡς ἐγὼ οὐδὲ πώποτε ἐνέτυχον, πολὺ (πολὺ VI: πολλοὶ R, Gal.) δὲ μάλιστα οὗτοι (οὗτοι R, Gal.: αὐτοὶ VI) καὶ οἱ ἐκ τούτων καὶ (οἱ post καὶ add. V: om. IR, Gal.) ἐκ τῶν ἄλλων δὲ οἳ καὶ ὀλεθρίως ἔχοιεν (οἳ ... ἔχοιεν VI: οἱ ὀλ. ἔχοντες R, Gal.). Blass's athetesis of οἱ before ἐκ τούτων makes the text smoother but is unnecessary.

[358] *Epid. VI* 5.336.3–5 ὡς γὰρ γέγραπται, οὕτως αἱ ξυγκληρίαι τῶν παθημάτων ἦσαν· τὰ μὲν πρῶτον (-τον Pall.: -α MV) γεγραμμένα καὶ ἄνευ τῶν ὕστερον γεγραμμένων ἐγίνετο· τὰ δ' ὕστερον οὐκ ἄνευ τῶν πρότερον. The word ξυγκληρίη is derived from κλῆρος, 'allotment,' and refers to persons metaphorically. It signifies either the participation of one person in several lots, or of several persons in one lot, or both.

[359] *Epid. I* 2.630.3–7 Li. = 1.188.22–189.3 Kw. = 1.162 Jones ἔθνῃσκον δὲ (ἐκ post δ' add. VIR: om. A, Gal.) πάντων μέν, πλεῖστοι δὲ (ἐκ post δ' add. VIR: om. A, Gal.) τούτων, καὶ τούτων (κ. τ. VIR, Gal. interpr. Arab.: om. Gal. codices Graeci) παιδία ὅσα ἀπὸ γάλακτος ἤδη, καὶ πρεσβύτερα, ὀκταετέα καὶ δεκαετέα, καὶ ὅσα πρὸ ἥβης (ἦσαν post ἥβ. add. Gal.: om. VIR). ἐγίνετο δὲ τούτοισι ταῦτα οὐκ ἄνευ τῶν πρώτων γεγραμμένων, τὰ δὲ πρῶτα πολλοῖσιν ἄνευ τούτων.

[360] *Epid. I* 2.632.10–11 Li. = 1.189.16–17 Kw. = 1.162 Jones περιεγένοντο δὲ πάντες οὗτοι, καὶ οὐδένα τούτων οἶδα ἀποθανόντα.

[361] *Epid. I* 2.642.6–8 Li. = 1.191.21–22 Kw. = 1.166 Jones οὐδένα οἶδα, εἰ καλῶς αἱμορραγῆσαι, ἐν τῇ καταστάσει ταύτῃ ἀποθανόντα. Other passages with this typical "I do not know of anyone" expression are *Epid. I* 2.606.1–3 Li. = 1.181.18–20 Kw. = 1.148 Jones; 620.5–6 Li. = 185.22–186.2 Kw. = 156 Jones; 648.4–6 Li. = 193.16–

In a methodological passage, the "way" by which the 'groups' were formed is described: *Epidemics VI* 3.12, "The essential [follows, results] from the genesis and from the point of departure [of the diseases] and from very much information obtained little by little, by gathering and learning in what respect they [the disease cases] are similar to each other; secondly, in what respect the features dissimilar to them are similar to one another, so that one [new] similarity comes out of the dissimilarities. This is obviously the way. This is the [positive] proof for things correct, and the refutation of things wrong."[362] The text is, again, extremely concise,[363] but the principal points are clear enough. The main criterion for forming 'groups' is similarity, and the author tries to find similarities even among cases not conforming to a given 'group;' he determines new 'groups,' either independent ones or sub-'groups' (he is not explicit here about hierarchic levels). It seems certain that the observation of some cases featuring a *krísis* on the 17th day (*Epidemics I*, ch. 9 Li. = ch. 20 Kw., Jones; see the discussion above p. 115–117) is based on this method, whether or not the method had then been formulated in such abstract terms as in *Epidemics VI* 3.12. These cases form one 'group' consisting of several sub-'groups.'[364]

A text outside the *Epidemics* explains that in detecting the similarities and dissimilarities, the senses are important. It forms the initial lines of *In the Surgeon's Office*. Although it is highly condensed in its diction, it is nevertheless at the same time redundant. One gets the impression that the text passage with its awkward repetitions represents a conglomerate of various stages of the author's attempt to formulate a medical aphorism as clearly as possible – as though he repeatedly cancelled lines which he

---

18 Kw. = 170 Jones; 658.9–10 Li. = 196.10–11 Kw. = 174 Jones; 664.5–10 Li. = 197.18–23 Kw. = 178 Jones; cf. *Epid. II* 5.96.17–98.1, 18–19.

[362] *Epid. VI* 5.298.4–9 Κεφάλαιον (scil. γίνεται) ἐκ τῆς γενέσιος καὶ ἀφορμῆς καὶ πλείστων λόγων καὶ κατὰ σμικρὰ γινωσκομένων συνάγοντα καὶ καταμανθάνοντα ᾗ (ᾗ scripsi: ἥ Gal.: ἡ M: ἣ V: εἰ edd.) ὅμοιά ἐστιν ἀλλήλοισιν, αὖθις τὰς ἀνομοιότητας τούτοισιν (αὖθις ... τούτοισιν Gal.: om. MV) ᾗ (ᾗ scripsi: ἥ Gal.: ἣ V: καὶ ἡ M: εἰ edd.) ὅμοιαι ἀλλήλῃσίν εἰσιν, ὡς (ὡς MV: om. Gal.) ἐκ τῶν ἀνομοιοτήτων ὁμοιότης γένηται μία· οὕτως ἂν ἡ (ἡ MV: εἴη Gal.) ὁδός· οὕτω καὶ τῶν ὀρθῶς ἐχόντων δοκιμασίη καὶ τῶν μή (post μὴ add. ἐχόντων Gal.: om. MV), ἔλεγχος.

[363] Deichgräber, Die Epidemien 39. Diller, Ausdrucksformen 147–149 (= Kleine Schriften Medizin 120 f.). Manetti/Roselli *ad loc.* – The transmitted η (= ᾗ, 'how') makes the sense more nuanced than εἰ ('whether,' which implies an alternative question that could be answered only by 'yes' or 'no').

[364] Cf. also the literature quoted in the preceding note. It is possible that Aristotle's description of *definition* in *Anal. post. II* 13 (97 b 7–27) has been influenced by the *Epid.* passage or by similar discussions on method in medicine. He even gives a medical example.

found too imprecise, and replaced them with better formulations.[365] "Either similar or dissimilar." Then the sensual means of recognizing (dis)similarities are listed.[366] Another methodological passage in *Epidemics VI* (a teacher's concept?) gives some concrete examples of what constituted the 'groups,' 8.26: "For good physicians, similarities mean puzzles and embarrassment, but also the contrary. [It has to be considered] what the reason is; that there is a difficulty of evaluation, [even] if one knows the method; e. g., if he [the patient] is peaked in the head, flat-nosed, sharp-nosed, bilious, vomits with difficulty, has black bile, is young, has lived without a plan. Evaluate all this together, taking into account also the quantitative degrees."[367] Despite some uncertainties about the authentic wording[368] and about details of the interpretation, the overall sense of the

---

[365] Gal. *In Hp. Off. comm.* 18 B. 863 K. = vol. 2, p. 194 f. Reinhold (Ἱπποκράτης, κομιδῇ Caroli H. Th. Reinhold, Athens, 1866); Arabic text and English translation in CMG, Suppl. orient. 1 (ed. M. Lyons), Berlin, 1963: "It often happens in a book like this [namely Hp. *Off.*], where the author is explaining many ideas and facts succinctly, that he jots down for his own purposes the same ideas and facts in different words, in order to decide for himself which is the best method of expression. Afterwards the copyist finds some of these phrases written in the margin, and he transcribes them all in the text itself ..." Cf. also Gal. *In Hp. Epid. I comm.* p. 43.23–29 Wenkebach; Emonds, Zweite Auflage 20 f.

[366] Cf. above p. 51 f. The autograph draft may have looked like this (the square brackets used in print ⌊ ⌋ indicate possible cancellations by the author himself which might have been scrupulously copied by the ancient editor of these notes; for the sake of clarity, Kühlewein's text is reproduced here without the variant readings):
Ἢ ὅμοια ἢ ἀνόμοια ἐξ ἀρχῆς
⌊ἀπὸ τῶν μεγίστων, ἀπὸ τῶν ῥηΐστων⌋
ἀπὸ τῶν πάντη πάντως γινωσκομένων,
⌊ἃ καὶ ἰδεῖν καὶ θιγεῖν καὶ ἀκοῦσαι ἔστιν⌋
⌊ἃ καὶ τῇ ὄψει καὶ τῇ ἀφῇ καὶ τῇ ἀκοῇ καὶ τῇ ῥινὶ
καὶ τῇ γλώσσῃ καὶ τῇ γνώμῃ ἔστιν αἰσθέσθαι⌋
ἃ οἷς γινώσκομεν ἅπασιν ἔστιν γνῶναι.
Translation of the lines not bracketed: "Either similar or dissimilar from the beginning, according to what can be recognized in every case and with certainty; what can be recognized through all means of cognition we possess." (*Off.* 3.272.2–6 Li. = 2.30.2–7 Kw. = 3.58 Withington.) "From the beginning" corresponds to ἐκ τῆς γενέσιος καὶ ἀφορμῆς in the preceding text (*Epid. VI* 3.12) and to πρόφασις in the following one, 8.26.

[367] *Epid. VI* 5.352.16–354.2 ἀγαθοῖσι δὲ ἰητροῖσιν αἱ ὁμοιότητες πλάνας καὶ ἀπορίας, ἀλλὰ ⟨καὶ⟩ τἀναντία (ἀ. κ. τ. Deichgräber, Die Epidemien, p. 39: "in dem Anderen und dem Gegenteil" Gal. pars memoriae, i. e. τἄλλα καὶ τἀναντία: ἀλλὰ τἀναντία MV, Pall.)· ἡ πρόφασις οἵη (οἵη MV, Gal. pars mem.: οἶδα Pall., Gal. pars mem.)· ὅτι χαλεπόν ἐστιν ἐκλογίσασθαι εἰδότα τὰς ὁδούς, οἷον εἰ φοξός, εἰ σιμός, ὑπόξυρος, χολώδης, δυσήμετος, χολώδης μέλας, νέος, εἰκῇ βεβιωκώς· ἅμα ταῦτα πρὸς ἄλληλα ξυνομολογήσασθαι καὶ ἐπὶ τὸ μᾶλλον καὶ ἧσσον (καὶ ... ἧσσον Gal. pars mem., Pall.: om. MV). Cf. Deichgräber, Die Epidemien 39 f.; Diller, Ausdrucksformen 145–147 (= Kleine Schriften Medizin 118–120); Manetti/Roselli *ad loc.*

[368] Galen has additional variant readings.

passage is clear. The physician has, according to the "method," to correlate various features of the patient, in order to find similarities with other cases.[369]

The aims in 'grouping' the patients are formulated in *Epidemics III*, ch. 16 = *On Critical Days*, ch. 1: "I think it is an important part of medical science and activity [*tékhnē*] to be able to consider correctly also what has been written. I think he who knows and uses written information will not make great mistakes in medical science and activity [*tékhnē*]. One must inform oneself accurately about each *katástasis*[370] of the seasons and about the disease: Which common element in the *katástasis* or in the disease is good? Which common element in the *katástasis* or in the disease is bad? Which disease is protracted and fatal, which is protracted and benign? Which acute one is fatal, which acute one is benign? Starting from these [details] it is easy to consider the order of the critical days and to prognosticate from them [i. e., either from the details, or the days, or both]. The one who has knowledge about this can know whom, and when, and how he should treat through regimen."[371] The context suggests that the written information alluded to must have comprised notes or literature *(i)* about the weather and its effects ("*katástasis* of the seasons"), *(ii)* about diseases (nosology), and about prognostic signs in *(iii)* chronic

---

[369] The Greek text, as it is reproduced above, contains two ambiguities: What does "but also the contrary" mean? Contrary to "similarities" or to "puzzles and embarrassment?" And what is the signification of "reason:" "reason for the situation just described" or "reason of the disease," "aetiology?" On πρόφασις, see generally Fernand Robert, Rev. des ét. gr. 89 (1976), 317—342. Anastasios A. Nikitas, Zur Bedeutung von ΠΡΟΦΑΣΙΣ in der altgriechischen Literatur, Akademie der Wissenschaften und der Literatur, Abh. d. geistes- und sozialwiss. Klasse, no. 4, Mainz/Wiesbaden, 1976. Jean Irigoin, Préalables linguistiques, in: Formes de pensée 173—180.

[370] Cf. above p. 169—179.

[371] *Epid. III* 3.100.7—102.10 Li. = 1.232.7—19 Kw. = 1.256 Jones (≈ parallel version in *Dieb. judic.* 9.298.2—10, cod. M) μέγα δὲ (δὲ VIR: om. *Dieb. judic.*: deest Gal.) μέρος ἡγεῦμαι τῆς τέχνης εἶναι τὸ δύνασθαι σκοπεῖν καὶ (σκ. κ. VIR: κατασκοπέεσθαι *Dieb. judic.*) περὶ τῶν γεγραμμένων ὀρθῶς· ὁ γὰρ γνοὺς καὶ χρεόμενος τούτοις οὐκ ἄν μοι δοκέει (δοκέει Foesius: δοκέῃ VIR: δοκέοι *Dieb. judic.*) μέγα (μέγα VIR: μεγάλα *Dieb. judic.*) σφάλλεσθαι ἐν τῇ τέχνῃ (ἐν τ. τ. VIR: κατὰ τὴν τέχνην *Dieb. judic.*). δεῖ δὲ (δὲ VIR: δὴ *Dieb. judic.*) καταμανθάνειν τὴν κατάστασιν τῶν ὡρέων ἀκριβῶς (τὴν … ἀκρ. V, *Dieb. judic.*: ἀκρ. τὴν κ. τ. ὡ. IR) ἑκάστην καὶ τὸ νόσημα (ἑ. κ. τὸ ν. VIR: κ. τῶν νούσων ἑκάστη [sic] *Dieb. judic.*), ἀγαθὸν ὅ τι κοινὸν ἐν τῇ καταστάσει ἢ ἐν τῇ νούσῳ, κακὸν ὅ τι κοινὸν ἐν τῇ καταστάσει ἢ ἐν τῇ νούσῳ (ἀγαθὸν … νούσῳ VIR [sed καὶ pro κακὸν I; κακὸν ὅ τι καίριον V; κακὸν … νούσῳ om. R]: ὅ τι τὸ νόσημα ἀγαθόν, ὅ τι καὶ κινδυνῶδες ἢ ἐν τῇ καταστάσει ἢ ἐν τῇ νούσῳ *Dieb. judic.*)· μακρὸν ὅ τι νόσημα καὶ θανάσιμον· μακρὸν ὅ τι καὶ (καὶ VIR: om. *Dieb. judic.*) περιεστικόν· ὀξὺ ὅ τι θανάσιμον· ὀξὺ ὅ τι (καὶ post ὅ τι add. VIR: om. *Dieb. judic.*) περιεστικόν. τάξιν τῶν κρισίμων ἐκ τούτων σκοπέεσθαι καὶ (τὸ post καὶ add. *Dieb. judic.*: om. VIR) προλέγειν ἐκ τούτων εὐπορέεται. εἰδότι περὶ τούτων ἔστιν εἰδέναι (εἰδότι … εἰδέναι VIR: ἔτι δὲ ἀπὸ τουτέων ἔστιν *Dieb. judic.*) οὓς καὶ (καὶ VIR: om. *Dieb. judic.*) ὅτε καὶ ὡς δεῖ διαιτῆν.

and *(iv)* acute diseases. The Hippocratic Collection gives an idea of what might be meant, because it comprises entire books about nosology (no. *ii*; some of the nosological and gynaecological texts must be older than the *Epidemics*) and about the prognosis of acute diseases (no. *iv*; in particular *Prognostics*, whose chronological relationship to parts of the *Epidemics* is unknown,[372] and prognostic aphorisms such as contained in *Prorrhetics I, Koan Prognoses*, and *Aphorisms*, which at least in parts may be older than the Epidemics[373]). No particular work on the prognosis of chronic diseases (no. *iii*) is extant or known to have existed, but many treatises contain scattered information on the subject. The weather and its effects (no. *i*) are dealt with in *On Airs, Waters, Places* and in various writings of the Collection including the *Epidemics*.[374] All of the categories or 'types' of patients, diseases, weather etc. found in these various branches of medical literature could, theoretically, be adopted for forming 'groups' of patients, and many of the categories can, in fact, be retrieved in the extant collective and individual case reports of the *Epidemics*. Not all 'groups' of patients described in the *Epidemics* can, however, be found in the other medical works, because part of the method of the *Epidemics* consisted in finding new 'groups.' The practical aim of the grouping procedure was, according to the passage quoted (*Epidemics III*, ch. 16 = *On Critical Days*, ch. 1), "to know whom, and when, and how he should treat," a programmatical phrase which must have been regarded as important because it recurs in *Epidemics I*, ch. 11 Li. (= ch. 25 Kw., Jones),[375] *Epidemics VI* 2.16,[376] and Plato's *Phaedrus*.[377]

Criticism and Scepticism in the *Epidemics*

The authors of the *Epidemics* were not positivists, who induced new knowledge by generalizing about *raw* data. One short glimpse at the case material as recorded by them makes it immediately evident that they saw their disease cases (individual and collective) always through a filter of preconceived ideas such as *krísis*, *pépsis*, *apóstasis*, and of traditional nos-

---

[372] Cf. above p. 159.

[373] Cf. below p. 222–231. For the relative chronology of *Prog.* and *Coac.*, see Langholf, Symptombeschreibungen; Jones (ed.), Hippocrates, vol. 2, p. XX–XXIX.

[374] Cf. above p. 164–179.

[375] *Epid. I* 2.678.3–4 Li. = 1.201.16–17 Kw. = 1.184 Jones.

[376] *Epid. VI* 5.286.3–4.

[377] 268 b ἐρέσθαι εἰ προσεπίσταται καὶ οὕστινας δεῖ καὶ ὁπότε ἕκαστα τούτων ποιεῖν, καὶ μέχρι ὁπόσου. Similarly Aristot. *NE* 1137 a 13–17.

ological concepts.[378] There is scarcely a case description which does not contain these dogmas. The doctrines were very persistent, as can be inferred, for example, from the numerous instances where the *krísis* of a disease case is said to have occurred "around" the *n*th day (this day being 'critical' according to the doctrine). When the dogma was not supported by the facts, the physicians felt entitled to adapt the facts to the doctrine. Here are a few examples implying day-numbers (many more instances could be quoted from the *Epidemics*):[379] *I*, ch. 3 Li. (= ch. 3 Kw., Jones), "At its quickest, the *krísis* came around the 20th, in most cases around the 40th day, in many around the 80 days."[380] *III*, 2nd series, case 9, "Around the 14th day ..., around the 60th day ..., around the 80th day ..., around the 100th day."[381] *IV* 3, "Around the 40th day."[382]

Sometimes one gets the impression that the "around" has been simply omitted by the author(s). This seems to be the case whenever decisive disease signs are said to have occurred on a day with a high number (i. e. in a numerical range where the critical days are only sparse according to the doctrine). Examples are *Epidemics I*, case 5, "She vomited some bilious matter on the 40th day; the final *krísis* with the end of the fever was on the 80th day."[383] Case 6, "Around the 30th day ..., around the 40th day ..., on the 60th day ..., on the 70th day."[384] *III*, 2nd series, case 1, "On the 40th day ..., she died within 120 days (variant reading: on the 120th

---

378 Grensemann, Krankheit der Tochter *passim*; Lloyd, Magic 128 f., 154 f.; Grmek, Les maladies 409–425. Diller's statement that, when starting to treat a patient, the physician of the *Epidemics* "steht zunächst vor einer tabula rasa," is mistaken (Ausdrucksformen 136 [= Kleine Schriften Medizin 109]).

379 Occasionally, however, περί indicates only that the author(s) did not know the exact point of time, e. g. *Epid. IV* 5.192.6–7 Li. = Per. 285–286 La. περὶ ἑβδόμην ἢ ὀγδόην ...· περὶ ὀγδόην, οὐκ οἶδα σαφέως.

380 *Epid. I* 2.612.3–6 Li. = 1.183.10–12 Kw. = 1.152 Jones ἔκρινε τούτων, οἷσι τὰ βραχύτατα γίνοιτο, περὶ εἰκοστήν, τοῖσι δὲ πλείστοισι περὶ τεσσαρακοστήν, πολλοῖσι δὲ περὶ τὰς ὀγδοήκοντα. For the cardinal number, cf. above p. 61–65 and 133 f.

381 *Epid. III* 3.128.8–20 Li. = 1.239.13–240.4 Kw. = 1.272 Jones περὶ δὲ τεσσαρεσκαιδεκάτην ..., περὶ δὲ ἑξηκοστὴν ..., περὶ ὀγδοηκοστὴν ..., περὶ δὲ ἑκατοστήν. The 100th day, however, is not regarded critical in the theory.

382 *Epid. IV* 5.146.3 Li. = Per. 75 La. περὶ τεσσαρακοστήν. – In *Epid. VII* 5.452.2–3, the awkward syntactic structure of the transmitted text appears to be due to a mixture of two constructions and should not be altered by editors: ἢ πρότερον ἢ ὕστερον τεσσαράκοντα ἡμέρῃσιν (sic codd. MV; the author had in mind τεσσαράκοντα ἡμέρῃσιν "within 40 days" *plus* ἢ πρότερον ἢ ὕστερον τεσσαράκοντα ἡμερέων [Littré's wording] "either before or after 40 days"). The inconsistency could be reproduced as: "within either before or after 40 days."

383 *Epid. I* 2.698.4–5 Li. = 1.208.2–4 Kw. = 1.196 Jones τεσσαρακοστῇ ἤμεσεν ὀλίγα χολώδεα· ἐκρίθη τελέως, ἄπυρος, ὀγδοηκοστῇ.

384 *Epid. I* 2.698.14–700.8 Li. = 1.208.13–209.1 Kw. = 1.198 Jones περὶ δὲ τριακοστὴν ..., περὶ δὲ τεσσαρακοστὴν ..., ἑξηκοστῇ ..., ἑβδομηκοστῇ ..., ὀγδοηκοστῇ.

day)."[385] Similar expressions occur in cases 2 and 9.[386] Other examples of a tendency to present reality in conformity with theory are the frequent breaches and recommencements in counting days in the individual case-descriptions (above p. 108–112).

Whenever the case descriptions contain words like *krísis*, 'critical,' 'segregation' (*apóstasis*), 'cooked(ness),' 'ripe(ness)' etc. (which happens very frequently), an interpretation by the authors is implicitly given. Sometimes, however, the Hippocratic physicians even explicitly interpret the pathological occurrences in terms of the internal humoral mechanism postulated by them, as in *Epidemics IV* 25, where it is described how a woman had a segregation into the eye around the 8th day and got her *krísis* around the 20th day, whereas her husband, who otherwise had the same symptoms, got to the *krísis* on the 7th day, but "his eye troubles occurred only on the 80th day and lasted longer, perhaps because they began *after* the *krísis*, even a long time after it."[387] Another instance is *IV* 26, "While there was the upward movement [i. e. the vomiting], she felt better ...; this was because she vomited bad substances," viz. the *materia peccans*.[388] In *IV* 47 somebody develops a skin affection "instead of the ensuing cough: for he did not cough [afterwards], although he had done so before." The segregation, which in other individuals appeared in the form of the second (or ensuing) cough, came as a skin affection in his case.[389] *IV* 53, "I think he did not have the ear affection [by which the others were seized] because he had vomited thick matters" [in other words, because the *materia peccans* was contained in the vomit and could, therefore, not harm the ear].[390]

---

385 *Epid. III* 3.106.3–12 Li. = 1.233.13–23 Kw. = 1.258 Jones τεσσαρακοστῇ ..., ἐν εἴκοσι καὶ ἑκατὸν ἔθανε (εἴκ. κ. ἑ. ἔθ. V: δὲ τῆι ρκ′ ἡμέρη ἀπέθανε IR: ἑκατοστῇ ... καὶ εἰκοστῇ ἀπέθανεν Gal. in explic.).

386 Furthermore, let it be kept in mind that with numeral adjectives of the -αῖος type, which so frequently occur in the *Epidemics* to denote day numbers, it was linguistically impossible (or at least awkward) to express "around;" e. g. *Epid. I* 2.668.6–7 Li. = 1.198.23–199.1 Kw. = 1.180 Jones εἰ δέ τινες ἐπερρίγουν περὶ τὴν εἰκοστήν, τούτοισιν ἔκρινε τεσσαρακοσταίοις (τεσσ. A: μ′ VIR: deest Gal.). *VI* 5.330.16–17 τεσσαρακοσταίους. 308.9 ἑξηκοσταῖον. *IV* 5.170.6 Li. = Per. 192 La. ὀγδοηκοσταίῳ.

387 *Epid. IV* 5.170.2–7 Li. = Per. 191–192 La. γυναικὶ καρηβαρικῇ ἰσχυρῶς, ταύτῃ ἐκρίθη περὶ εἰκοστήν. εἰκοστῇ καυσώδης ὑποχόνδρια... ἐς ὀφθαλμὸν δεξιὸν περὶ ὀγδόην. ἀνδρὶ ταὐτά, πλὴν ἑβδόμης ἐκρίθη... ὀγδοηκοσταίῳ καὶ χρονιώτερα τούτῳ τὰ τοῦ ὀφθαλμοῦ, ἴσως ὅτι ὕστερον τῆς κρίσιος, καὶ ὅτι πολλῷ (-ῷ V: -ά HIR).

388 *Epid. IV* 5.170.12–14 Li. = Per. 196 La. καὶ ἐπεὶ ἐχώρει ἀνωτέρω, τούτου γενομένου βελτίων ἐγένετο ..., ὅτι ἄνω ἤμει ἔμετον κακόν.

389 *Epid. IV* 5.188.19–190.2 Li. = Per. 275 La. τοῦτ' ἀντὶ τῆς βηχὸς τῆς ὕστερον· οὐ γὰρ ἔβηξε, τὸ δὲ πρότερον.

390 *Epid. IV* 5.194.3–4 Li. = Per. 292 La. οἶμαι (οἶμαι scripsi: "ich glaube" Gal.: οἱ καὶ VHIR) παρ' οὓς οὐ γενέσθαι, ὅτι πέπονα ἔπτυσεν.

The ancient physicians' endeavour to understand the concrete disease cases by interpreting them (implicitly or explicitly) in terms of the theories available to them can legitimately be called 'research work,'[391] in spite of the fact that this medical approach was not essentially critical or sceptical.

Another tendency of 'research' that can be seen in the *Epidemics* consists in the modification of traditional theories and methods. Examples of new doctrinal details have been quoted above: the doctrine on odd/even critical days (p. 103–118); the theoretical questions asked, and the cautiously formulated assertions ('perhaps,' p. 179–192). Examples of new methods of inquiry are the combinations of symptoms after a 'check-list' (p. 157–164); the investigation into the influence of the seasons on the diseases (p. 164–179); 'types' and 'groups' found on the basis of (dis)similarities (p. 194–208).[392] In fact, 'research' would be a fairly correct modern label for these activities traceable in the *Epidemics*, although, surprisingly enough for modern physicians and scientists, it never occurs in these books that existing theories are submitted to criticism[393] or modified in a negative way by restricting their range of applicability or even abolishing them either in part or as a whole. Whenever there are modifications, they imply an extension of the range of applicability. This holds good of doctrines as well as of methods.[394] Never does any text in the *Epidemics* declare that this or that sign or body discharge traditionally regarded as 'critical' or as a segregation (*apóstasis*) does *not* generally have the property attributed to it; instead, several new critical signs and new forms of *apóstasis* are detected (see, in particular, above p. 179–192), and there is a marked tendency to ask only constructive theoretical questions which extend the validity of the existing doctrine, and which prompt an affirmative answer. The same applies to the theoretical statements qualified by 'perhaps.' The number of potentially critical days is systematically increased by including also the even days in addition to the traditional odd ones. With regard to methods of inquiry, a similar extension is manifest: Older methods are not abolished but integrated into new ones and thus given a wider range of applicability. The above-mentioned 'check-list' is a highly flexible method and, unlike the nosological description of whole diseases, applicable to virtually *any* disease case; but traditional nosology is neither abolished nor even criticized: instead it remains part of the new method (p. 150–164). The meteorological approach of *Epi-*

---

391 Although this expression does not occur in the Collection, cf. above p. 179 f., 193.

392 On *Epid. IV* 5.196.1–4 Li. = Per. 301–302 La. see Langholf, Syntaktische Untersuchungen *ad loc.*: this obscure passage seems to modify a doctrine set forth in *Prog.* ch. 14 ≈ *Coac.* § 384.

393 On criticism generally, see Deichgräber, Geschichte der wissenschaftlichen Kritik; Ducatillon, Polémiques.

394 Only occasionally, *therapeutic* methods are criticized: Herodikos "killed" the feverish patients with exercises and fomentations, *Epid. VI* 5.302.1–4; cf. Manetti/Roselli *ad loc.*

demics I and *III* is considerably more flexible than the one of *On Airs, Waters, Places* (and of *On the Sacred Disease*); but the traditional method is not criticized: instead, the new method of *Epidemics I* and *III* is formulated in a way that no contradictions to the older one can occur (p. 172–179). New 'types' and 'groups' are found by using also traditional ones (p. 198 ff.).

In the *Epidemics*, there is a strong tendency to explain *everything* with the underlying doctrines and methods, which are formulated and applied flexibly enough to cover all of the phenomena observed by the medical authors (sometimes via small adjustments, either of the doctrine or, as indicated shortly above, of the phenomena). The image of building a house suggests itself. One stone is added[395] to the other, and whenever any part of the construction proves not to be entirely sufficient for the purpose, the construction is extended. Nothing is ever dismantled in the *Epidemics*, the steadfastness of the foundation walls is never doubted.[396] An instructive example of the procedure is the way clinical observations are dealt with which ought to have led to re-examining the validity of the doctrine. Such possible counter-evidence is neither allowed to invalidate the theory, nor is it, on the other hand, simply neglected. Instead, the doctrine is formulated so as to cover also the apparent exceptions: it is extended by introducing, for instance, quantifying premises. *Epidemics II* 1.7 lists rash and other affections of the skin as possible forms of segregation. The author says that they are useful only on the condition that their extension on the body surface corresponds to the heaviness of the disease. The niece of Timenes died, he explains, because her finger, where the segregation (an abscess?) occurred, was too small an organ to receive the peccant matter, which thereupon flowed back into the body and caused the exit.[397] In similar words, *Epidemics I*, ch. 4 Li. (= ch. 9 Kw., Jones) mentions a rash which developed in some patients; its lack of efficacy as a segregation is interpreted as the consequence of its small extension.[398] Yet another form of segregation is mentioned in *Epidemics II* 1.7 (*in fine*). The text is particularly interesting because it appears to imply that this

395 This concurs with general observations made by Edelstein, Idea of progress 33 f., about the way progress was conceived of in the classical period of Greece: "Progress was ... understood in merely additive terms. The various periods were thought of as knowing more or less, and the inventor was assumed to have added to the fund of knowledge at his disposal ... The change is treated not as qualitative but as quantitative, and the various inventions and additions taken together are like stones in a mosaic ..." Cf. Dodds, Concept of progress 1–25; also below p. 225 f.

396 This is done in other treatises, whose relationship to the *Epidemics* is only very imprecisely known, for instance in *On Ancient Medicine*.

397 *Epid. II* 5.78.4–10. For the wording, see above p. 80 f.

398 *Epid. I* 2.628.11–14 Li. = 1.188.17–20 Kw. = 1.160–162 Jones.

segregation was not acknowledged by all physicians; this *apóstasis* may have been a medical discovery of the author, who did not fail to quantify: "Abundant nosebleeds lead mostly to recovery, as in the case of Heragoras. The physicians did not recognize this."[399] Accordingly in *Epidemics I*, ch. 8 Li. (= ch. 13 Kw., Jones) the fact that Philiskos, Epameinon, and Silenos died despite a nosebleed is explained by stating that it was not abundant.[400] In ch. 9 Li. (= ch. 19 Kw., Jones) of the same book, the daughter of Philon ought to have survived because she had not only an ordinary nosebleed, but even an *abundant* one; still she died. This is explained by an untimely dinner she had on the seventh day.[401] If a segregation was followed by the patient's recovery, this very fact could be taken as confirming that the segregation had been successful, and that the doctrine was correct; if, however, he died, either the segregation itself or the organ receiving it were too small, or some other cause such as wrong diet was responsible. The physician could not be held accountable.

Deichgräber speaks of the "consciously empirical character" in the research of *Epidemics* (in particular books *II, IV, VI*),[402] the essential feature of which is, according to him, the use of the senses ("Autopsie"). He believed that there is a "sceptical attitude," a "profound scepticism." For Deichgräber, the general doctrinal aphorisms were arrived at by sceptical induction from observation. This view cannot be substantiated, as will be demonstrated below.[403] Although there is some plausibility in the assumption that some of the doctrines were in fact 'induced' or 'generalized,' one does not know when and by whom and how it was done. With regard to 'scepticism,' Deichgräber found in *Epidemics II, IV, VI* a small number of general statements containing a 'perhaps' (*II* 1.6; *VI* 3.23; *IV* 25 = Per. 185–186 La.[404]); moreover, he found many uses of 'perhaps' in the descriptions of concrete historical observations.[405] From

---

399 *Epid II* 5.78.17–18 αἱμορραγίαι λαῦροι ἐκ ῥινῶν ῥύονται πολλά, οἷον τὸ (τὸ VI, 'wie bei der Krankheit des' Gal.: τῷ HR) Ἡραγόρεω· οὐκ ἐγίνωσκον οἱ ἰητροί. The sense cannot be that the doctors did not *notice* the nosebleeding.

400 *Epid. I* 2.642.4–10 Li. = 1.191.19–24 Kw. = 1.166 Jones.

401 *Epid. I* 2.658.9–12 Li. = 1.196.10–13 Kw. = 1.174 Jones.

402 Die Epidemien p. 35; cf. 35–40.

403 p. 219–221.

404 Quoted above p. 190–192, where further instances are cited.

405 Deichgräber, Die Epidemien p. 36 f., has collected passages where cautiousness is expressed towards one's own observations or towards reports taken over from others, or where ignorance is admitted. Here is a list supplementing his quotations by passages not previously referred to: "I think" (this verb does, of course, not always necessarily express cautiousness): *Epid. IV* 5.162.1–2 Li. = Per. 154 La.; 194, 3–4 Li. = Per. 292 La.; 196.1–4 Li. = Per. 301–302 La.; *VI* 5.284.12; 294.3–4; *VII* 5.398.14–15; 408.22; 436.10–11; 448.12–13 ᾤετο, "he thought." – "It seems:" *Epid. II* 5.90.7–9 Li. = Per. 21 La.; 124.13, 17. – "I do not know:" *Epid. II* 5.124.1–2; *IV* 5.170.9 Li. = Per.

this evidence he concluded that the *Epidemics* made sceptical generalizations on the basis of sceptical observation.

The conclusion, however, ought to have been quite different considering the scarcity of 'perhaps' in general statements and of the relative insignificance of these general statements (cf. above on theoretical questions and 'perhaps,' p. 179–192). Since none of the basic doctrines in the *Epidemics* is ever questioned or restricted in its validity by a 'perhaps' or by similar qualifications, and since general formulations are only very rarely so (a dwindling number as compared to the hundreds of apodictic aphorisms claiming to be generally true in the *Epidemics*), one cannot but infer that the authors of the *Epidemics* were audacious in drawing (or taking over from others) the basic outlines of the doctrine, as well as both careful and scrupulous in dealing with the details. It is possible that the basic outlines were the work of an individual or of a *group* of physicians who took over tenets hallowed by tradition and by universal acceptance (such as nosology), and who amalgamated them with a new doctrine, whose main features were *krísis*, *pépsis*, and *apóstasis*. If it was a group, it may have been a rather close-knit community, probably with a leading personality in its midst, and perhaps with some sort of medical school attached. A small *pólis*, where the expectations of the population were more likely to converge on new doctrinal elements (*krísis, pépsis, apóstasis*) than in a large city, may have been the ideal environment for the public acceptance of innovation in medical doctrine, and the itinerant life of fifth and fourth century physicians must have been an ideal way of propagating newly established and publicly accepted doctrines to other towns. The detailed work on the practical application of the doctrine must have been predominantly the task of individuals (members or non-members of the group), not the task of the group as a whole. The individual members were anxious to do good work with careful examination and anamnesis, and they were particularly intent on not contradicting the *basic* doctrinal consensus of their group. To employ the house-building metaphor[406] again: the outlines of the building were determined by pre-existing structures (which were not to be dismantled but to be incorporated, perhaps to serve new functions) and by a closely coordinated team of architects. The details were executed possibly by the same persons (but individually, not as a group), or possibly by other individuals. While there was total concurrence on the 'master plan' within the group, considerable uncertainty arose as soon as an individual was faced with the details. Hence the relatively high

193 La. – "He [the patient] said:" *Epid. VII* 5.462.23. – "It escaped my notice:" *Epid. V* 5.226.10–12. Some of these passages have been quoted by Deichgräber in other sections of his book.

[406] Lonie, A structural pattern 241 f.

frequency of 'perhaps' in texts describing particular details of anamnesis or dealing with insignificant doctrinal details. Scepticism existed, but it was confined to such details. The main approach was not sceptical and was determined by factors inherent not primarily in the subject matter but in the pre-existing structures, in the organization of the group, and in the expectations of the public. There is no attempt at falsifying one's own doctrines or theories,[407] there is no "productive scepticism"[408] in the *Epidemics* but simply the intent of the good craftsman to do good work without error and in harmony with the colleagues of his group. To work with all one's senses, together with a willingness to recognize errors of detail and, if possible, to correct them, is a prerequisite of any craft. This attitude is acquired during apprenticeship. The apparent 'scepticism' of the *Epidemics* is, therefore, a rather trivial feature. It should not be called scepticism.

Applicability as a Proof of the Doctrines in the *Epidemics*

No attempt is made in the *Epidemics* to offer evidence in support of any of the fundamental general assumptions. Proofs for the validity of a four humours doctrine (phlegm, bile, black bile, and blood) are put forward in another treatise (whose doctrines are kindred but probably not quite identical with the ones of the *Epidemics*), namely in *On the Nature of Man*, ch. 5–6.[409] There, however, as in the case of other 'proofs' in the Hippocratic Collection, "the tests were interpreted solely in terms of the author's own assumptions."[410] According to modern standards, "what was needed was for those assumptions to be *tested against others*. The function of these tests was to *corroborate* the theories in question, not to provide data to *decide between* competing theories."[411] "Their investigations were

---

[407] Grmek, Les maladies 423; cf. above p. 118, 190.

[408] Deichgräber, Die Epidemien p. 37. In a more general context, Lloyd, Magic 234 has characterized the situation: "... although much Greek work is critical in the sense that the writers reject both popular assumptions and their colleagues' opinions, it is often anything but self-critical: on the contrary there is frequently a distinct incaution and dogmatism in the statement of the writer's own position, a failure not just to examine, but even to recognize, its weak points."

[409] *Nat. Hom.* 6.40.15–46.8 Li. = 4.12–18 Jones. The chronological relationship of *Nat. Hom.* to *Epid. I* and *III* is unknown. That Polybos was the author of the whole treatise does not necessarily imply that it is more recent. Jouanna's assumption that *Nat. Hom.* was an important medium for the introduction of the concept of black bile into the "school of Kos" is not supported by any evidence. (Jouanna [ed.], Hippocrate, La nature de l'homme, p. 60).

[410] This and the following two quotations are from Lloyd, Magic 151.

[411] Two cases of alternative *questions* in the *Epidemics* have been quoted above p. 182 f., with notes 248, 254. They, however, do not constitute competing *theories*.

not open-ended, but designed specifically to provide support for theories that appear to have been adopted on the basis of general, often philosophical, considerations and arguments."

Concerning the basic assumptions in *Epidemics I* and *III*, Lichtenthaeler rightly remarked that many of the specific words and expressions used in the context of those doctrines occur so frequently from one case description to the next that they betray long-standing habitual use.[412] This holds true also of the other books of the *Epidemics*. Evidently no need was felt for proving, within these treatises, the basic assumptions. In all probability, these authors were able to produce evidence in favour of their theories. If they were medical teachers, they may have done so when giving their lectures. Perhaps one or the other argument had been written down by them without later being incorporated into these books. But the very fact that *no proof at all* occurs in the *Epidemics* shows sufficiently how firmly the fundamental theories were established within the group of physicians from whom the texts originated.

For the modern reader, a strange contrast exists between, on the one hand, the absence of proofs, and on the other hand, the large number of passages which serve as implicit corroborations of the medical doctrines. In the *Epidemics* the validity of the underlying theories is confirmed in two ways: *(i)* By the explicit application of medical doctrines to concrete historical cases of disease; *(ii)* by the explicit application of historical cases of disease to theoretical contexts. These two kinds of short digressions cannot, of course, have been meant to be *proofs* (in any strict sense) of the underlying doctrine, yet it seems that they served a similar purpose.

An example of a general insertion on doctrinal matter into a case description[413] occurs in *Epidemics III*, ch. 10, in the midst of a description of an epidemic: "With many, it is a favourable sign if there are good evacuations through the bladder." (In the epidemic described, however, the urine was never good, and many, therefore, died).[414] In *Epidemics IV* 16, the definite articles refer to a doctrine put forward in other books of the Epidemics (*II* 1.3 and *VI* 1.11), a doctrine with which this case matched: "In autumn, the [household member] of Eumenes vomited black bile, and odours were prominent, and *the* fevers with rigor and *the* heartburn ... and *the* intestinal worm. [She had] a loose stool all the

[412] Le troisième Épidémique 49.

[413] For further examples, cf. Nikitas, Untersuchungen 48–50, 120–122. Grensemann, Krankheit der Tochter 78.

[414] *Epid. III* 3.90.10–11 Li. = 1.229.10–11 Kw. = 1.250 Jones ἐπὶ πολλοῖσι γὰρ αἱ κατὰ κύστιν καθάρσιες χρησταὶ γενόμεναι ἀγαθόν (ἐπὶ ... ἀγαθόν VIR, Gal.: del. Ermerins, Kw., Jones).

time."[415] At 30, "Her shanks were full of hard, white, scabby swellings, and so were her feet, but less. The same was found in the lower sections of her thighs (for most patients this means an unfortunate outcome), and also in the loins." In fact, the woman died.[416] At 33–34, "On the 8th day, when being purged with laxative drugs, she had symptoms like patients who endure it [the purging] easily when they are not unexpectedly weakened, [stool] of the type which is neither foamy nor bloody, but like eggs, like the one of Herakleides. She excreted much through the purging and endured it easily."[417] At 35, after an enumeration of some symptoms in an individual case, "... such patients get a reddish complexion. She was rather reddish ..."[418] At 45, "Similarly the other one: In the beginning he had slightly viscous excrements, out of which the thick one is critical. After that, while suffering from insomnia, he had slightly viscous, slightly bilious excrements, thick, not of the loose type. (Whenever the stool begins to get solid, the crises are near.) ... He had the *krísis* around the 9th day."[419] Nikitas,[420] who has collected the relevant material, correctly explains these insertions, which are found almost exclusively in book *IV*, by saying that the special disease case motivated the author (or redactor) of *Epidemics IV* to intercalate theoretical passages into the chapter, and that these passages on doctrinal matter are not abstractions made from the special case under consideration, but due to the author's trying to apply what he had learned, and to draw connections between his observations and his theoretical knowledge.

---

[415] *Epid. IV* 5.154.6–9 Li. = Per. 118 La. τοῦ φθινοπώρου ἤμεσε χολὴν μέλαιναν ἡ Εὐμένεος, καὶ (αἱ add. HIR: om. V) ὀδμαὶ δὲ πρόδηλοι καὶ οἱ φρικώδεες πυρετοὶ καὶ αἱ καρδιαλγίαι ... καὶ τὸ ἑλμίνθιον. διαχωρήματα λεπτὰ πάντα τὸν χρόνον. Cf. Langholf, Syntaktische Untersuchungen *ad loc.*; Nikitas, Untersuchungen 189–192.

[416] *Epid. IV* 5.172.19–174.9 Li. = Per. 208–214 La. ἡ γραίη ἡ κατὰ Σωσίλεω λευκοφλέγματος, κνῆμαι σκληροῖσιν οἰδήμασι λευκοῖσι φολλικώδεσι, καὶ πόδες, ἧσσον δέ. ἦν δὲ καὶ ἐν τοῖσι κάτω τῶν μηρῶν (τοῖσι δὲ πολλοῖσι δυσέξοδον τοῦτο), ἀτὰρ καὶ ὀσφύϊ. Note that the words in parenthesis admit just as well of the translation: "for most patients this *meant* an unfortunate outcome." On the ambivalent meaning of certain syntactical constructions (general *versus* historical meaning) see Langholf, Generalisationen.

[417] *Epid. IV* 5.176.13–178.6 Li. = Per. 225–227 La. ὀγδόῃ, ἐν τῇσι τῶν φαρμάκων καθάρσεσι κάτω, σημεῖα οἷα εὐφόρως φέρουσι, κἂν μὴ παρὰ λόγον γυιῶνται, καὶ μήτε ἔπαφρα μήτε ὕφαιμα, ἀλλ' οἷα ᾠά ἐστιν, οἷα Ἡρακλείδεω. ἐκαθάρθη πολλὰ καὶ ῥηϊδίως ἔφερε. (For μήτε, which implies a type, cf. below on *Epid. IV* 45, this page, note 419.)

[418] *Epid. IV* 5.178.7–16 Li. = Per. 228–231 La. οὗτοι καὶ ἐξέρυθροι γίνονται. μᾶλλόν τι ἐξέρυθρος ἐοῦσα ...

[419] *Epid. IV* 5.186.10–15 Li. = Per. 262–264 La. ὁμοίως ὁ ἕτερος· ἐν ἀρχῇσιν ὑπόγλισχρα ὑποχωρήματα, ἐξ οἵων τὸ παχὺ κρίσιμον. ἀγρύπνῳ μετὰ ταῦτα ὑπόγλισχρα ὑπόχολα πέπονα {χολώδεα} μὴ λεπτά. (ἐπὴν δὴ ἄρξηται συνίστασθαι, ταχεῖαι αἱ κρίσιες.) ... ἐκρίθη περὶ ἐνάτην. (The negation μὴ indicates that the stool has a *typical* consistency; cf. Langholf, Syntaktische Untersuchungen *ad loc.* and above, this page, note 417, on *Epid. IV* 33–34.)

[420] Untersuchungen 120 f., cf. 50, 97, 101.

The other kind of short digression consists of remarks that can be reduced to the formula: "... as, for instance, happened to the patient so-and-so." Again, Nikitas[421] has collected the numerous passages from the *Epidemics* books and classified them under three categories of types, of which the more important are the second and third type.[422] Most of the short references to the individual cases serve to illustrate *historical observations* in a group of patients ("such and such symptoms occurred, as, for instance, ..."), or to illustrate *general remarks* on what can always be expected ("such and such symptoms occur, as, for instance, ..."). It should suffice here to quote just one representative passage for each of the two categories. *Epidemics I*, ch. 9 Li. (= ch. 20 Kw., Jones), "The feverish and painful swellings at the ear neither ceased nor suppurated with some patients, although their fever stopped. With them, a diarrhoea of bilious matters or a dysentery or a sediment in thick urine dissolved [the swellings], as, for instance, happened with Hermippos of Klazomenai."[423] *IV* 41, "A sign, whether the segregations (*apóstasis*) in the diseases bring a *krísis*: If the patients, after being feverish, are not fevered any more, and after feeling unwell feel well; as, for instance, happened to Kharon with his affection at the anus."[424]

Nikitas is again certainly right in concluding that these inexplicit examples, which illustrate general doctrinal remarks or historical descriptions of collective disease cases, presuppose that the original individual case descriptions, out of which the names were taken, were accessible to the reader; for a reader who did not know the cases alluded to, the names of the patients meant only that the symptoms mentioned had in fact been observed in these patients.[425] A detailed description of the case of Hermippos the Klazomenian is included among the individual reports of *Epidemics I* (case 10),[426] but for most of the cases used as examples the full details are not extant.

---

421 Untersuchungen 55–58.

422 The passages of Nikitas' first type can be comprised within the two other types and are not relevant here.

423 *Epid. I* 2.660.1–5 Li. = 1.196.19–23 Kw. = 1.176 Jones τὰ (τὰ AVIR: om. Gal.) παρὰ τὰ ὦτα ἐν πυρετοῖσιν ἐπαιρόμενα μετ᾽ ὀδύνης ἔστιν οἷσιν ἐκλείποντος τοῦ πυρετοῦ κρισίμως (ἔστιν post κρ. add. Gal.: om. AVIR) οὔτε καθίστατο οὔτε ἐξεπύει· τούτοισι διάρροιαι (-αι AVIR: -α Gal.) χολωδέων ἢ δυσεντερίη ἢ παχέων οὔρων ὑπόστασις γενομένη ἔλυσεν (ἔλ. A, Gal.: λύει VI: λείη R), οἷον Ἑρμίππῳ τῷ Κλαζομενίῳ.

424 *Epid. IV* 5.182.6–8 Li. = Per. 244–245 La. αἱ ἐπὶ τῇσι νούσοισιν ἀποστάσιες εἰ κρίνουσι, σημεῖον, εἰ (εἰ V: ἢν HIR) πυρώδεα ἐόντα μὴ πυρεταίνωσι καὶ δύσφορα ἐόντα εὐφόρως φέρωσιν· οἷον τὰ ἐν τῇ ἕδρῃ Χάρωνι.

425 Untersuchungen 58. The reader might have known the cases also personally or through oral descriptions.

426 *Epid. I* 2.704.15–708.5 Li. = 1.210.15–211.14 Kw. = 1.202–204 Jones.

Another inference, however, which Nikitas has made, is problematic, albeit essentially correct. It implies more questions than it answers. He asserts that the general statements on doctrinal matter found in the *Epidemics* are generalizations based on a large number of individual cases, of which the inexplicit examples are relics.[427] In this opinion, he follows Deichgräber, who had contended that the author of *Epidemics II, IV*, and *VI*[428] tried to induce generally valid scientific rules from his observational material in order to establish a system.[429] Certainly, there must have been some amount of generalization or 'induction,'[430] particularly for those doctrinal statements which independent medical research today would call 'correct.' The extant material, however, does not permit any proof that 'induction' was carried out on a large scale by the authors of the *Epidemics*. As can be shown, they tried to form 'groups' of cases similar or dissimilar to each other,[431] and there is some *plausibility* in the assumption that they made doctrinal generalizations on the basis of such groups during epidemics, when the similarity of many cases is obvious to every observer, as well as independently from epidemic diseases. But there is not one single instance of the cognitive process postulated by Deichgräber and Nikitas for the *Epidemics* treatises, namely that the observation of cases resulted in a general doctrinal statement. Although sometimes observed disease cases lead the physicians to ask general questions[432] which look like the first step toward a generalization, the extant evidence about these cases is always so scant that the modern medical historian cannot know on what observational basis the questions were formulated. Often they appear merely as an appendix to *one* case description.[433]

---

[427] Nikitas, Untersuchungen 58; cf. 50, 82 f.

[428] According to Deichgräber, one author has written the three books. This is possible, but cannot be substantiated considering the disparities of style and content even within single books.

[429] Die Epidemien p. 36: "... wenn der Verfasser nun, ähnlich wie in Epidd. I und III, den Versuch macht, aus dem Beobachtungsmaterial wissenschaftliche Erkenntnisse von einer gewissen Allgemeingültigkeit abzuleiten ..." This physician had the desire "zum System vorzudringen." Cf. p. 51: "Die Beobachtung am Krankenbett ist der Ausgangspunkt. Die wiederkehrenden Erscheinungen ordnen sich zu Regeln und finden ihre literarische Formulierung in Aphorismen."

[430] For the concept of 'induction,' cf. above p. 113, 164.

[431] Cf. above p. 194–208.

[432] Cf. above p. 179–190.

[433] In an earlier paper, I have said that "in den Epidemien können wir bis ins Detail verfolgen, wie Ärzte Krankheitsdaten gesammelt, deren Korrelationen beobachtet und aus solchem Korrelieren des Datenmaterials Theoreme induziert ... haben; die Bücher von Deichgräber und von Nikitas geben genügend Beispiele für dieses Verfahren der Epidemien-Verfasser." (Die parallelen Texte 264 f.) I now think that this proves erroneous. In fact, we can see that the physicians collected case material, and that they tried to form 'groups' out of the cases. We also find a considerable number of doctrinal passages

The medical historian's most important and central questions, as far as the 'research methods' of the authors of the *Epidemics* are concerned, can, therefore, not be answered: How were the general statements ('aphorisms') arrived at? Was it by the authors of the *Epidemics*, or by other, earlier physicians? Was the 'induction' made on the basis of many or just a few cases, or even only one single case as in the anatomical description of *Epidemics II* 4.1–2? How systematic was the process of 'induction'?[434] Was it carried out by comparing, one by one, single cases (from one epidemic, or from various places)? Or were the generalizations found intuitively during a long professional activity, perhaps even during more than one generation, and then passed on from master to apprentice (who perhaps modified them)? The historian can ask these questions from passage to passage but should give up any hope of answering them. He can only speculate. The inexplicitness of the *Epidemics*[435] is an obstacle which he cannot surmount. Some methodological passages of the *Epidemics* quoted above[436] suggest that at least some of the generalizations were arrived at systematically, but the bulk of universally valid statements of the *Epidemics* was probably not laid down as the result of just one standard procedure.

It is tempting to speculate why the *Epidemics* do not contain any proof of their doctrines. The principal dogmas held by the group of physicians were, it seems, not questioned within this group; at least no traces of any such doubt occur in the *Epidemics*. Questions were asked, and investigations were made, strictly according to, or in the light of, the accepted doctrines.[437] Even 'reality' was seen strictly through the filter of the *krísis*, *pépsis*, and *apóstasis* dogma and of the other approved medical tenets.[438] As one consequence, the concept of contagion or infection from one person to the other, which was familiar in contemporary thought,[439] is

---

claiming to be universally true. It is *plausible* that at least some of these latter 'aphorisms' were formulated by the authors of the *Epidemics* on the basis of such 'groups,' but it cannot be proved because there is no such instance which shows the whole mental process with regard to the same case material.

434 Cf. above p. 145–149. For evidence of unsystematic and rash generalization, see Langholf, Generalisationen.

435 Cf. above p. 136 ff.

436 In connection with the procedure of these authors to form 'groups' of patients, p. 194 ff.

437 Cf. above p. 179–194.

438 See above p. 108–112, 208–215, where the example of the adaptation of historical critical days to the doctrine is given. How often *krísis*, *pépsis*, and *apóstasis* as well as other concepts are mentioned in the case descriptions will be seen immediately by inspecting any of the *Epidemics* books.

439 Apart from ritual pollution, for which see Parker, Miasma (*passim*), contagion in a medical sense is mentioned, e. g., in Thuc. *II* 50 f.; Plat. *Phaedr.* 255 d; Isocr. *Aegin.* (19) 29; [Aristot.] *Probl. I* 7, *VII* 8. Cf. below p. 244.

nowhere explicitly mentioned in the Collection: It was unnecessary for the prevailing doctrines and not easily compatible with them. Deichgräber was mistaken in writing that the starting-point of the method (in *Epidemics II, IV, VI* particularly) was pure observation, and that together with this pure observation some speculative concepts and ideas are present.[440] Observation was rather subordinated to the doctrines and supposed to support them; some of the exemplary cases of patients alluded to so frequently in the *Epidemics* may have served the same purpose.

As Regenbogen[441] has pointed out, pre-Aristotelian Greek science in the fifth and fourth centuries widely used analogies as proofs for hypotheses. The method consisted in comparing an hypothesis or an imperceptible object or process, *a* (the *explanandum*), to a perceptible object or process, *b* (the *explanans*), which was considered analogous; sometimes a second and third perceptible object or process b_1, b_2 were added.[442] The purpose

---

[440] Die Epidemien p. 40. The formulation is rather vague: "Mag die Methode auch, so wie sie theoretisch formuliert ist [namely in some methodological passages of the *Epidemics*], ins Gebiet der Logik übergehen, ihr Ausgangspunkt ist und bleibt die reine Beobachtung... Um so mehr überrascht den modernen Leser, wie jetzt auch in diesen Büchern neben die Ergebnisse der Beobachtung und der methodischen Ordnung und Erklärung ein Begriffsmaterial tritt, dessen erkenntnistheoretische Grundlage z. T. in der naiv rationalen Spekulation zu suchen ist." This seems to be something like a *communis opinio*. Other scholars before and after Deichgräber have expressed similar views. According to Roscher, Hebdomadenlehren 69, *Epid. I* and *III* are unique among the Hippocratic treatises because their author admits only practical experience and discards all speculative theories. It is true that in the fifth century B. C. "medical men clamoured for facts, and yet more facts" (Jones [ed.], Hippocrates, vol. 2, p. XXVI f.). But their task of a "collection and classification of phenomena" was not their "first interest." It was subordinated to the requirements of their practical work and of the doctrines according to which they worked. They did in fact have "embracing theories and constructive ideas." But unlike theories of natural philosophy of their epoch, these theories were not, and did not need to be, made explicit in every text, because the professional physician knew them anyhow, or was supposed to know them. Cf. Lloyd, Magic 146–169 on "The development of empirical research."

[441] Regenbogen, Forschungsmethode (Kleine Schriften p. 153). His material is drawn primarily from the Hippocratic treatise *Genit./Nat. Puer./Morb. IV*. For more material see Lonie, Hippocratic treatises *passim*. Moreover, his chapter "The author's scientific method" (*ibid.* 72–86) is instructive. See also Wenskus, Vergleich und Beweis. Lloyd, Polarity and analogy 341–360. An explicit example not mentioned hitherto is *Epidemics II* 6.4 (5.134.4–5), τῆς φωνῆς λυομένης πάντα λύεται· ἡ γὰρ φύσις (φύσις VHIR: λύσις Li.) τῇ φθέγξει ὁμοίη. Nature and "all" are only imperfectly perceptible, but speech is perceptible.

[442] This method is comparable to a particular technique of divination which aimed at revealing a future event (the *explanandum*) by utilizing 'symbolic' omens that were considered analogous to the future event (a portent or a dream could serve as such an *explanans*). The technique occurs in *Genesis* 40–41 (dreams of Pharaoh, his butler, and his baker) and in Greek and Roman sources from Homer onward, e. g. *Iliad II* 305–329; *Odyssey XV* 160–178, 525–534; for parallels in medical prognosis (dreams in *Vict.*

was to prove, in this way, the correctness of the assumption concerning *a*. The same form of thinking underlies, it seems, some of the passages mentioned above, in which the authors of the *Epidemics* quote individual cases as examples exhibiting analogies either to the cases under discussion (individual or collective) or to general doctrines already formulated. The validity of the medical interpretations of 'reality' was in some of these passages to be confirmed by the analogies.[443]

Moreover, each analogous case of disease (or rather each case which admitted of being interpreted analogously by the ancient physician) corroborated the general applicability of the medical doctrines. Similarly the intercalations of general reflexions into case material, a typical feature of *Epidemics IV*, can be accounted for. Each application of the doctrine and each case applicable to it confirmed the correctness of the doctrine and enhanced its value.[444] Observation of disease cases confirmed the theory, and the theory guided the physician's observation — a circular method resulting in a one-sided feedback which could not but corroborate the doctrine.

Prognostic Doctrines Applied in the *Epidemics*

The feedback just mentioned is particularly obvious in the structural characteristics and practical application of the prognostic aphorisms. The aphorisms were *(i)* supplemented during practical use by annexing extensions to their structural 'nucleus,' and were *(ii)* applied by the medical practitioner(s) who wrote individual case histories in the *Epidemics*.

As far as prognostic aphorisms are concerned, the following remarks will be confined to the treatise *Prorrhetics I* because, despite its composite character, it is still considerably more homogeneous than the other collec-

---

IV) see below p. 237 f., 245—247; generally, Jean Bayet, Présages figuratifs déterminants dans l'antiquité gréco-latine, in: Mélanges Franz Cumont, Annuaire de l'institut de philologie et d'histoire orientales et slaves, vol. 4 (1936), Bruxelles, 1936, 27—51; Lloyd, Polarity and analogy 181 f.; see also, for additional material, Cic. *De div. I* 39—59; 72; *II* 63 and Pease *ad loc.* — The function of certain proverbs may be similarly viewed, when a given situation of life (the *explanandum*) is interpreted or elucidated by a proverb (the *explanans*) which presents analogies to the situation.

443 This does not preclude other modern interpretations of these passages as proposed by Nikitas, *loc. laud.*

444 Smith, Galen on Coans 585 has drawn a parallel between the method of Hippocratic physicians and the method of modern Hippocratic scholarship. Another parallel could be drawn to psychoanalysis; about his own method, Sigmund Freud stated: "Die Psychoanalyse macht eine Grundvoraussetzung, deren Diskussion philosophischem Denken vorbehalten bleibt, deren Rechtfertigung in ihren Resultaten liegt." (Abriss der Psychoanalyse, Frankfurt am Main, 1953, first sentence.)

tions of aphoristic texts, *Aphorisms* and *Koan Prognoses*.[445] Perhaps, *Prorrhetics I* was compiled from fewer sources and/or during a shorter period, thus allowing conclusions as to the state of the development of Greek medicine reached by one author, or group of authors, at one point of time around 400 B.C.

Before dealing with the above-mentioned topics *(i)* and *(ii)*, some general remarks about the medical doctrines of *Prorrhetics I* are necessary. This treatise exhibits doctrinal similarities with the *Epidemics*, but also characteristic differences. A medical concept or approach presupposed by *Prorrhetics I* and shared with *Epidemics* is nosology in the sense of the nosological treatises. The following disease-names are used: *dysenteríē*, § 143 (cf. *On Affections*, ch. 23); *eileós*, § 158 (for descriptions in the nosological treatises, cf. the tableau in Jouanna, Archéologie, p. 519 f.); *íkteros*, §§ 32, 146, 154, 164 (cf. Jouanna, *loco cit.*); *kaûsos*, §§ 18, 81, 90 (cf. Jouanna, *loco cit.*); *kholérē*, § 37 (cf. *On Affections*, ch. 27); *leienteríē*, § 138 (cf. *On Affections*, ch. 24); *melagkholíē*, §§ 14, 18, 123 (cf. *On Diseases I*, ch. 3); *opisthótonos*, § 88 (cf. Jouanna, *loco cit.*); *phrenîtis*, §§ 1, 3, 4, 5, 6, 9, 11, 12, 13, 15, 27, 28, 31, 34 (cf. Jouanna, *loco cit.*).

Other concepts are less prominent in *Prorrhetics I*. Body humours in the sense of those doctrines of the Collection which postulate two (bile and phlegm) or four humours (namely, in addition to bile and phlegm, the humours blood and black bile, or blood and water) occur rarely. Blood is mentioned mainly in the context of nosebleeding, bile several times in adjectives derived from *kholḗ* (§§ 21, 53, 79, 92, 97, 98, 139, 166). Black bile is not referred to except rudimentarily in the disease name *melagkholíē* (cf. above), which was however traditional and does not necessarily presuppose an autonomous humour.[446] Phlegm is not mentioned at all; it either played only an insignificant rôle in the outlook of the author(s) and redactor(s) of *Prorrhetics I*, or was not recognized as an important agent, or was unknown. The absence of phlegm can be taken as an indication that *Prorrhetics I* is either relatively ancient or otherwise doctrinally dissociated from the *Epidemics*. As Jouanna has demonstrated cogently, phlegm is a more recent humour than bile.[447]

---

445 For an assessment of the homogeneity of *Prorrh. I*, *Coac.*, and *Aph.*, compare the information given on *similia* by Littré in his edition of the three treatises (*passim*). On *Prorrh. I* see also Perazzi, Ippocrate (in particular p. 131–222). — The most important treatises dealing with prognosis in aphoristic form are *Prorrhetics I* (Littré vol. 5), *Aphorisms* (Littré vol. 4, Jones vol. 4), and *Koan Prognoses* (Littré vol. 5). Treatises dealing mainly with prognosis in other literary forms are *On Airs, Waters, Places* (Littré vol. 2, Jones vol. 1), *Prognostics* (Littré vol. 2, Jones vol. 2), and *Prorrhetics II* (Littré vol. 9). For other treatises touching the subject, see Edelstein, Περὶ ἀέρων, ch. II.

446 Cf. above p. 46–50 and Wittern (ed.), Hippocrates, *De morbis I*, p. 192 f.

447 Archéologie 141 f.

The *krísis*, *pépsis*, and *apóstasis* concept is present, but references to it are few. The word *krísis* occurs in §§ 36, 105, 107, 117; 'critical' in §§ 61, 134, 149, 'uncritical' in § 102; *pépsis* is represented by 'ripe,' § 102, and 'ripen,' §§ 133, 149, 153, *apóstasis* by its synonym *apóstēma*, § 122.[448] The scarcity of passages in *Prorrhetics I* which imply body humours or the *krísis*, *pépsis*, and *apóstasis* doctrine must be taken as an indication that the bulk of that work, or the majority of its aphorisms, dates from an epoch when these concepts were still nonexistent or not recognized.[449] It goes without saying that, if this conclusion is correct, the aphorisms of *Prorrhetics I*, or the majority of them, cannot have been 'induced' from case descriptions such as those contained in the *Epidemics*, which presuppose and constantly use the *krísis*, *pépsis*, and *apóstasis* doctrine.

(i) Structure of Prognostic Aphorisms

Many, but not the majority, of the aphorisms exhibit a simple structure: "Signs A, B (, ... K) indicate [or: provoke][450] L, M (, ... X)." It is plausible that this simplest form reflects an ancient type of prediction, a type perhaps rooted in popular lore.[451] Other types most often represented are more complex. A bipartite structure occurs frequently: "Signs A, B (, ... K) indicate [or: provoke] L, M (, ... P); if associated with sign(s) Q, R (, ... U), they indicate [or: provoke] V, W (, ... Z)."[452] Sometimes the second part

---

[448] Cf. also λύω, 'to dissolve' (a disease or symptom), §§ 57, 90, 118, 152, and ἄκρητος, 'unmixed,' 'untempered' (of excretions), § 111. In § 91, ἀκρασίης should be read instead of ἀκρισίης: the other symptoms clearly suggest it.

[449] The work must, however, have got its final form (arrangement of the aphorisms in four sections according to subject matter, cf. below p. 225, note 456) after the *krísis*, *pépsis*, and *apóstasis* doctrine had gained influence, because traces of this doctrine are found in all four sections of the work and in all structural elements that make up single aphorisms (nuclei, additions). — For the relatively early date of prognostic aphorisms cf. Langholf, Symptombeschreibungen 115–119; Jones (ed.), Hippocrates, vol. 2, p. XX–XXIX.

[450] 'To indicate' and 'to provoke' are almost synonymous in the prognostic treatises of the Collection. The same holds true of pre-astrological Greek star-lore (Pfeiffer, Studien zum Sternglauben 1–16) and of divination generally (Pease [ed.], Cic., *De div.*, Book I, p. 297 f. [= repr., p. 139 f.]; Book II, p. 316 f., 410 [= repr., p. 498 f., 592]). Cf. also above p. 60; 168; 169, note 189.

[451] This applies to the form, not necessarily to the content, which may be more recent despite an archaic form. Generally on the development of prognostic aphorisms in the Hippocratic Collection see Ermerins, De Hippocratis doctrina 5–12 *et passim*. Although Ermerins' speculations about the cult of Asklepios are obsolete, his philological observations on the structure and content of the aphorisms remain very valuable. In *Prorrh. I*, the simple structure occurs in §§ 3, 5, 9, 10, 20, 23, 24, 26, 28, 33, 35, 40, 44, 45, 47, 49, 50, 51, 52, 55, 56, 57, 62, 65, 68, 74, 76, 77, 84, 86, 96, 97, 106, 108, 126, 134, 137, 142, 150, 151, 157, 161, 162, 166, 167, 168, 169, 170.

[452] Examples taken from *Prorrhetics I*: §§ 4, 11, 12, 15/16, 19, 21/22, 32, 36, 39, 43, 46, 53, 58/59, 61, 64, 66, 67, 70, 71, 79, 83, 89, 90, 92, 94, 98, 99, 100, 105, 106/107, 109, 113,

contains a gradation: "Signs A, B (, ... K) indicate [or: provoke] L, M (, ... P), particularly if associated with sign(s) Q, R (, ... Z)."[453] Another frequent bipartite structure has a question: "Signs A, B (, ... K) indicate [or: provoke] L, M (, ... T); do they also indicate [or: provoke] U (, ... Z)?"[454] Or the second part may consist of an addition in the form: "... as, for instance, happened to the patient so-and-so."[455]

It would appear that most of the more complex aphorisms are expansions of the simple type. The formal nucleus is an affirmation. Various *additions* were made, but it cannot be determined whether they originated with the author of the nucleus or with later physicians. Obviously the method was additive.[456] In many cases a short and simple traditional

---

114, 117, 120, 123, 125, 127, 128, 129, 131, 140, 141, 142, 153, 156, 159/160. 'If' is rarely expressed by a Greek conditional clause.

[453] Examples from *Prorrhetics I*: §§ 2, 7, 21, 37, 48, 73, 79, 81, 104, 111, 112, 135, 136, 143, 155, 159. Only in 9 of these aphorisms 'if' is expressed by a Greek conditional clause.

[454] Examples: *Prorrhetics I*, §§ 13, 25, 29, 42, 53, 72, 92, 98, 114, 116 (question, plus: "if so, I would not be surprised"), 117, 118, 120/121, 122, 123, 127, 133, 136, 138, 140, 146, 154, 155, 156, 162/163 (if forming a unit). There may be more than one question in one aphorism. — Kindred are formulations without a question, but with "perhaps:" § 103, 143, 154; with "I believe:" § 122, 130, 146, 149, 156; with a restriction, "as a rule," § 139; "sometimes," § 72.

[455] Examples are *Prorrhetics I*, §§ 8, 13, 17, 27, 32, 34, 72, 78, 82, 99, 104, 119, 123.

[456] Cf. above p. 212. How the simple type of prognostic aphorisms was complemented through text additions is described in its outlines and with striking examples by Ermerins, De Hippocratis doctrina. — An additive method characterizes also the disposition of some of the prognostic treatises, which are just accumulations of more or less developed aphorisms arranged in sections (chapters) according to subject matter. For the disposition of *Coac.*, see the headings in Littré's translation; in *Prorrh. I*, the disposition of the aphorisms in sections (chapters) is less easily distinguishable than in *Coac.*, because the disease signs common to the single aphorisms of a section are not necessarily mentioned at the *beginning* of each aphorism (as they usually are in *Coac.*), but may occur anywhere in the aphorism. Therefore, Daremberg (in his translation, p. 77) complained: "Trouver dans cet opuscule un enchaînement d'idées, un plan, un système, y tracer des divisions bien nettes, en faire une analyse méthodique, me semble une chose tout à fait impossible: je l'ai essayé plusieurs fois sans pouvoir y parvenir; j'y renonce." But in fact *Prorrh. I* consists of four sections of similar length (this length of text units occurs also in other treatises of the Hippocratic Collection, cf. Langholf, Struktur): *§§ 1—38, amentia, delirium* (on *phrenītis* cf. *Morb. I*, §§ 30 and 34), 480 words after Polack's edition; *§§ 39—96, unfavourable signs*, 745 words; *§§ 97—124, spasms*, 597 words; *§§ 125—170, nosebleeding* (§§ 125—152) *and parotitis* (§§ 153—170), 752 words. The modern paragraph numbers printed in Littré's edition (and consequently in that of Polack) are sometimes arbitrary. Quite often text units which clearly belong together are divided. On the condition that §§ 23/24 belong(s) to 25; 33 to 32; 45 to 43/44 (cf. *Coac.* 50/51); 85 to 83/84; 97/98 to 99; 108 to 106/107 (cf. Galen's commentary), only 5 paragraphs do not fit into the aforesaid disposition: §§ 7, 29, 30, 75, 92. — Two facts prove that the questions asked in *Prorrh. I* are older than this arrangement: first, that the symptom common to the paragraphs of one section is sometimes found only in the question attached; second, that the symptom common to a section may be contained in a question forming a whole

aphorism may have occasioned reflexions, perhaps observations, on the part of a practitioner, who then appended additions. Some of the aphorisms contain several such extensions belonging to one or more of the above-mentioned types.[457] The medical terms referring to doctrinal concepts such as *krísis*, *pépsis*, and *apóstasis* occur in the nuclei as well as in the extensions. The types of questions and case-examples attached are very similar to those found in the *Epidemics*.[458] No appendix ever contradicts the nucleus or questions its validity. Whenever questions are asked in these extensions, they extend the thought in such a way that no incompatibility between the nucleus and the question's answer can arise. All this agrees with what has been said above on the research methods of the *Epidemics*. The feedback was exclusively positive, the doctrine contained in the aphorisms could not but become more and more acceptable, applicable, and 'true.'

(ii) Application of Prognostic Aphorisms

We have hitherto considered a positive feedback (aphorism > application of aphorism > extension of aphorism) only as far as it is inferable from the structures of the prognostic aphorisms. There are, however, also traces of the application of prognostic texts in anamnesis, i. e. in individual case-descriptions. Grensemann has demonstrated how the treatise *Prognostics* has been used in *Epidemics VII*.[459] Similarly it appears that some of the material contained in *Prorrhetics I* has influenced the case descriptions

---

paragraph by itself (§§ 1, 30, 63, 85, 121 [if not forming a unit with 120], 163 [if not forming a unit with 162], or in a question opening a paragraph, but not in the ensuing text. — The significance of the limited range of variations in the forms of the aphorisms can be evaluated against the background of the many other possibilities. The following list of unrealized or very rarely realized forms is far from being complete. For the sake of brevity, single letters are used here:

- A indicates [or provokes] B, unless C.
- Unless C, A indicates B.
- A, unless C, indicates B.
- A indicates B, but only if C.
- A indicates either B or C.
- It can be recognized by D whether A indicates B or C.
- It can be recognized by C whether A indicates B or not.
- A does not indicate B.
- A indicates neither B nor C.
- Neither A nor B indicates C.
- A, but not B, indicates C.
- Not A but B indicates C.
- If A, then B. (This type with a Greek conditional clause occurs only in extensions, never in a nucleus. For a Stoic discussion about this type, "Si cui venae sic moventur, is habet febrim," see Cic. *De fato* 12–16 = Stoic. vet. fragm. II 954.)

457 Therefore, there is some overlapping in the references given in the preceding notes.

458 Cf. above p. 179–190, 215–222.

459 Krankheit der Tochter.

of the *Epidemics*,[460] whose author(s) may have watched for certain combinations of symptoms on the basis of generally valid prognostic texts (written or oral[461]).

Let us now examine some examples by comparing passages of *Prorrhetics I* and of the *Epidemics*. *Prorrhetics I*, § 79: "Vomiting bilious matter in small quantities is bad, particularly if followed by insomnia. If in these cases blood drips from the nostril, it is fatal."[462] All of these symptoms appear in the individual case description *Epidemics III*, 1st series, case 12: "... On the 8th day ... she vomited bilious, light-greenish matter in small quantities; at night in a bad condition, did not sleep ... On the 9th day ... towards the evening ... she vomited bilious matter in small quantities. On the 10th day ... she did not sleep at all ... On the 14th day nosebleeding. She died."[463] Cf. *Epidemics I*, case 12, where however nosebleeding does not occur[464] in congruence with the version of the aphorism in *Koan Prognoses*, § 547 (it ends with the remark on sleeplessness).[465]

Another example is *Prorrhetics I*, § 32: "Deafness and very red urine and suspensions [in the urine] which do not settle indicate delirium. If such [patients] get affected with *íkteros*, it is bad. It is also bad if the *íkteros* is followed by amentia. It happens that these [patients] lose their voice without losing their comprehension. Some have a discharge of much loose stool, e. g. Hermippos, and he died."[466] All this is contained in *Epidemics*

460 The relationship between the prognostic aphorisms on the one hand (*Prorrh. I, Coac.*, and part of *Aph.*) and the cases of the *Epidemics* on the other hand would be a rewarding theme for a monograph, but collecting the material is a tedious task.

461 Oral tradition is likely to have left traces in *Prorrh. I*: many of the prognostic aphorisms are unclear to us. What, for example, does "and" in contexts like "symptoms A and B and C" mean? Does it signify the invariable combination of all these symptoms, or rather the facultative presence of one of them? An oral tradition of professional instruction was indispensable for a correct understanding. For a similar ambiguity in the descriptions of 'groups' of patients in the *Epidemics* see above p. 201 f. Other ambiguities that might be due to oral tradition concern therapeutic prescriptions, see above p. 69 f., and references to medicaments, p. 29 f.

462 *Prorrh. I* 5.530.5–7 Li. = 84.8–10 Polack τὰ μικρὰ ἐμέσματα χολώδεα κακόν, ἄλλως τε καὶ ἐὰν ἐπαγρυπνῶσι (-ῶσι I: -ήσουσι(ν) R, Gal.)· μυκτὴρ ἐν τούτοισιν ἀποστάζων ὀλέθριον. Cf. *Coac.* 5.708.16–17.

463 *Epid. III* 3.64.14–66.10 Li. = 1.223.18–224.3 Kw. = 1.236–238 Jones ἤμεσε χολώδεα σμικρά, ὑπόξανθα (ὑ. VIR: ξανθά Gal.). νύκτα δυσφόρως, οὐκ ἐκοιμήθη... ἐνάτῃ ... πρὸς δείλην ... ἤμεσε σμικρὰ χολώδεα. δεκάτῃ ... οὐχ ὕπνωσεν οὐδέν ... τεσσαρεσκαιδεκάτῃ αἷμα διὰ ῥινῶν· ἀπέθανε.

464 *Epid. I* 2.712.10–13 Li. = 1.213.4–7 Kw. = 1.208 Jones ἤμεσε μέλανα ὀλίγα (ὀλίγα A: ὀλίγω Gal.: om. VIR), χολώδεα ..., οὐχ ὕπνωσεν ... ἀπέθανεν.

465 *Coac.* 5.708.16–17 τὰ μικρὰ ἐμέσματα χολώδεα ⟨κακόν⟩ (κ. rec., edd.: om. A), ἄλλως τε κῆν ἀγρυπνέωσιν. That κακόν is missing here by a mere blunder is obvious not only from the parallel in *Prorrh. I* but also from the structure of the aphorism.

466 *Prorrh. I* 5.518.3–8 Li. = 78.9–13 Polack κώφωσις καὶ οὖρα ἐξέρυθρα, ἀκατάστατα (ἐξ. ἀκ. IR: ἀκ. ἐξ. Gal.) ἐναιωρήματα (-ήματα IR: -ούμενα Gal.) παρακρουστικόν·

III, 1st series, case 2: "Hermokrates ..., deafness right in the beginning ..., the urine was thick and red and, when left standing, did not settle ... Delirium. On the 6th day he got affected with *ikteros*. Amentia. [After the 17th day] he understood everything but could not talk ... He discharged much loose, thin stool ... He died."[467]

In other instances, the case descriptions of the *Epidemics* have most, but not all of the symptoms of the prognostic aphorisms, which, therefore, at least in these instances, cannot have been generalized from the *Epidemics*. *Prorrhetics I*, § 10: "During headache, vomit like verdigris with loss of hearing and with insomnia causes delirium quickly."[468] *Epidemics III*, 1st series, case 4, "... He had headache for a long time ..., the pain grew worse ...; he vomited ... matter like verdigris ...; the second day, loss of hearing ...; he fell into delirium around noon." Insomnia is not mentioned.[469] Similarly the preceding case, where insomnia occurs but deafness is missing: "... He felt a heaviness in his head and pain on the right side of his forehead for a long time ... On the 4th day he vomited ... matter like verdigris ..., at night he did not sleep, he was a little delirious. On the 5th day ... he did not sleep at night and was delirious ... On the 7th day, ... he did not sleep and was delirious ..."[470]

Individual case descriptions may feature the combination of symptoms contained in the sentence forming the nucleus of a prognostic aphorism while omitting those figuring in extensions of it. *Prorrhetics I*, § 1/2 (which clearly forms a unit) starts with a question which is the nucleus of the

---

τοῖσι τ⟨οι⟩ούτ{ε}οισιν ἰκτεροῦσθαι κακόν. κακὴ δὲ καὶ ἡ ἐπὶ ἰκτέρῳ μώρωσις (κακὴ ... μώρωσις Gal.: κακὸν δὲ καὶ ἡ ... κώφωσις IR). τούτους ἀφώνους (μὲν add. Gal.: om. IR), αἰσθανομένους δὲ (δὲ Gal.: δὴ IR) συμβαίνει γίνεσθαι· τοῖσι (τοῖσι IR: οἶμαι Gal.) δὲ καὶ κοιλίαι καταρρήγνυνται (τουτέοισιν add. Gal.: om. IR), οἷον (ἐγένετο add. Gal.: om. IR) Ἑρμίππῳ, καὶ ἀπέθανε. Cf. *Coac.* 5.626.6–10.

467 *Epid. III* 3.32.2–38.3 Li. = 1.215.17–216.18 Kw. = 1.218–220 Jones Ἑρμοκράτην ...· κώφωσις αὐτίκα ..., οὖρει παχέα ἐρυθρά, κείμενα οὐ καθίστατο ..., παρέκρουσεν. ἕκτῃ ἰκτεριώδης ..., οὐ κατενόει, ... κατενόει, διαλέγεσθαι οὐκ ἠδύνατο..., κοιλίη ὑγρὴ πολλοῖσι λεπτοῖσι..., ἀπέθανε. The similarity of the two names seems due to coincidence, unless one supposes that the last sentence in the extension of the prognostic aphorism (τοῖσι δὲ καὶ κοιλίαι ... ἀπέθανε) was added under the influence of the case (the καὶ after Ἑρμίππῳ is strange: was the original wording οἷον Ἑρμοκράτει· ἀπέθανε ?).

468 *Prorrh. I* 5.512.6–8 Li. = 76.2–4 Polack τὰ ἐν κεφαλαλγίῃσιν ἰώδεα ἐμέσματα μετὰ κωφώσιος ἀγρύπνῳ (ἀγρύπνῳ IR: ἀγρυπνώδεα Gal.) ταχὺ ἐκμαίνει. Cf. *Coac.* 5.620.3–4.

469 *Epid. III* 3.44.11–46.6 Li. = 1.218.23–219.6 Kw. = 1.226 Jones ... κεφαλὴν ἐπόνει χρόνον πολύν ..., ὁ πόνος παρωξύνθη ..., ἤμεσε ... ἰώδεα ...· δευτέρῃ κώφωσις, ... ἐξεμάνη περὶ μέσον ἡμέρης.

470 *Epid. III* 3.38.8–40.16 Li. = 1.216.22–217.19 Kw. = 1.222 Jones ... κεφαλῆς βάρος καὶ κρόταφον δεξιὸν ἐπωδύνως εἶχε χρόνον πολύν ... τετάρτῃ ἤμεσε ... ἰώδεα ..., νυκτὸς οὐκ (οὐκ VR, Gal.: om. I) ἐκοιμήθη, παρέκρουσε σμικρά. πέμπτῃ ... νύκτα (-τα VI: -τὸς R, Gal.) οὐχ ὕπνωσε, παρέκρουσεν ... ἑβδόμῃ ... οὐκ ἐκοιμήθη, παρέκρουσεν.

aphorism: "Are they affected with *phrenītis*, those who have *kōma* in the beginning together with pain in the head, the loin, the abdomen, and the neck, and with insomnia?" The aphorism continues with two statements: "If there is a little nosebleeding, it is fatal, particularly if early on the 4th day. An intensely red liquid around the stool is bad in any case, especially in the aforesaid ones."[471] The question — not the appendices — seems referred to, and answered in the affirmative, in *Epidemics III*, 1st series, case 11: "... She had *kōma* in the beginning, then insomnia, pain in the loin and heaviness of the head ..." Other symptoms from the prognostic passage are not mentioned, but at the end the diagnosis is given: "*Phrenītis*." Pain in the abdomen and the neck is missing.[472] Similarly, the symptoms named in the nucleus of *Prorrhetics I*, § 37 can all be found in *Epidemics III*, 1st series, case 3 (fever, pain in the thigh, suspension in the urine, delirium), but not the ones of the extension sentences.[473]

The content of prognostic aphorisms may appear in case descriptions with modifications other than omissions. In the following instance it seems as though the concept of black bile absent from the aphorism is referred to in the individual case description; this would imply that the case text is more developed than the prognostic one: *Prorrhetics I*, § 31, "During *phrenītis*, if there is flow of saliva with coldness, there will be vomit of black matter."[474] Cf. *Epidemics I*, case 12 (which has the symptoms of a *phrenītis*):[475] "... After waking up, he felt cold. Flow of saliva. In the evening he was very delirious, and shortly after it he vomited black, bilious matter, little."[476]

---

471 *Prorrh. I* 5.510.2—6 Li. = 75.2—7 Polack οἱ κωματώδεες ἐν ἀρχῇσι γενόμενοι (γε- IR: γι- Gal.) μετὰ κεφαλῆς, ὀσφύος, ὑποχονδρίου, τραχήλου ὀδύνης ἀγρυπνέοντες ἦρά γε φρενιτικοί εἰσιν; μυκτὴρ ἐν τουτέοισιν ἀποστάζων ὀλέθριον, ἄλλως τε καὶ ἢν τεταρταίοισιν ἀρχομένοισιν. κοιλίης περίπλυσις ἐξέρυθρος κακὸν μὲν ἐν πᾶσιν, οὐχ ἥκιστα δὲ ἐπὶ τοῖσι προειρημένοισιν. Cf. *Coac.* 5.620.20—622.4.

472 *Epid. III* 3.62.1—10 Li. = 1.222.15—223.2 Kw. = 1.234—236 Jones ἀρχομένη (δὲ add. IR, Gal.: om. V) κωματώδης ἦν, καὶ πάλιν ἄγρυπνος, ὀσφύος ὀδύνη, κεφαλῆς βάρος ...· φρενιτιαία (φρενιτιαία VR, φρενιτι... I [non bene exhibet finem verbi photographica taeniola]: φρενῖτις Gal.: φρενειτις Pap. Soc. Ital. no. 116: om. edd.).

473 *Prorrh. I* 5.518.14—520.2 Li. = 79.6—8 Polack τὰ κατὰ μηρὸν ἐν πυρετῷ ἀλγήματα ἔχει τι παρακρουστικόν, ἄλλως τε καὶ ἢν οὖρον ἐναιωρηθῇ λεῖον (τὰ ... λεῖον IR: Gal. codices alia; cf. *Coac.* 5.592.8—12). *Epid. III* 3.40.1—14 Li. = 1.217.1—16 Kw. = 1.222 Jones πῦρ ἔλαβε ..., οὖρα λεπτὰ ποικίλα, ἐναιωρήματα (-ματα R, Gal.: -μα VI) ἔχοντα κατὰ σμικρὰ οἷον κρίμνα, γονοειδέα ..., μηροῦ ὀδύνη ..., παρέκρουσε σμικρά ..., παρέκρουσεν.

474 *Prorrh. I* 5.518.2—3 Li. = 78.7—8 Polack τὰ ἐν (τοῖς add. Gal.: om. IR) φρενιτικοῖσι μετὰ καταψύξιος πτυελίζοντα μέλανα ἐμεῖται. The parallel version in *Coac.* § 101 (5.604.8—9) has φρενιτικοῖσι in IR, but πυρετοῖσι in the more conservative mscr. A.

475 Cf. above p. 156 f.

476 *Epid. I* 2.712.9—10 Li. = 1.213.3—5 Kw. = 1.208 Jones ἐξ ὕπνου ψύξις· πτυαλισμός. δείλης πολλὰ παρέκρουσε, μετ' ὀλίγον δὲ ἤμεσε μέλανα, ὀλίγα (ὀλίγα A: ὀλίγω Gal.: om. VIR), χολώδεα.

A question is asked after the nucleus of *Prorrhetics I*, § 118: "Paralysis like a hemiplegia, which goes upward from the loin to the neck and to the head, and which is accompanied by spasms, indicates delirium. Are such affections dissolved by spasms? After such affections, they [the patients] suffer variously and have relapses of the same [symptoms]."[477] All of the symptoms described appear also in *Epidemics I*, case 13, but the ones touched upon in the aphoristic *question* are only said to have *occurred*. The answer is given in the affirmative, but only to part of the question. No "dissolution" mechanism is suggested in the case description. Perhaps its author was too prudent to answer the complete question asked in the aphorism. "... Right in the beginning she felt pain in her loin. On the 3rd day, pain in the neck and in the head near the right-hand key bone. Soon after, her tongue became mute, her right arm was paralyzed as in hemiplegia, with spasm, she was delirious all the time... On the 4th day her tongue was unclear [when articulating], [this affection] was dissolved, spasms." The wording is not "*by* spasms." Subsequently, some relapses of pain in the corresponding regions of the other body half are reported. She recovered.[478]

Another question, equally asked after the nucleus of an aphorism, refers not to an internal mechanism but to observable features, *Prorrhetics I*, § 29: "Urine which is discharged only after others have reminded [the patient] is fatal. Is the urine of these [patients] as if one stirs up a urine sediment?"[479] This question seems referred to in an individual case description. The author is very explicit in his answer, which is, again, in the affirmative, *Epidemics I*, case 4: "... She discharged ... much urine at a time, but rarely, only after others had reminded her. It was thick and white, as it gets when a urine sediment is stirred up. Even when it [this

---

477 *Prorrh. I* 5.550.4–7 Li. = 92.1–4 Polack τὰ ἐξ ὀσφύος ἐς τράχηλον καὶ κεφαλὴν ἀναδιδόντα παραλύσαντα παραπληκτικὸν τρόπον σπασμώδεα παρακρουστικά· ἆρα (γε add. Gal.: om. IR) καὶ λύεται τὰ τοιαῦτα σπασμῷ; ἐκ τῶν τοιούτων ποικίλως διανοσέουσι διὰ τῶν αὐτῶν ἰόντες. Instead of ἐκ ... ποικίλως, the parallel version in *Coac.* 5.650.19–652.2 (only mscr. A is relevant there) has ἢ τῶν τοιούτων κοιλίαι. This, too, fits the case history in *Epid. I.*

478 *Epid. I* 2.712.15–716.3 Li. = 1.213.8–214.5 Kw. = 1.208 Jones αὐτίκα δὲ ἤρξατο πονεῖν ὀσφῦν. τρίτῃ πόνος τραχήλου καὶ κεφαλῆς κατὰ κληῖδα χεῖρα δεξιήν· διὰ ταχέων δὲ γλῶσσα ἠφώνει, δεξιὴ χεὶρ (-ὴ χεὶρ A, Gal.: -ὴν χεῖρα VIR) παρελύθη (-ελύθη AVIR: -έθη Gal.) μετὰ σπασμοῦ παραπληγικὸν τρόπον, παρελήρει πάντα ... τετάρτῃ γλῶσσα ἀσαφὴς ἦν (ἀ. ἦν AV: φωνῆς ἦν IR: σαφηνείας Gal.), ἐλύθη, σπασμοί (-οί AVIR: -ός Gal.).

479 *Prorrh. I* 5.516.12–518.1 Li. = 78.5–6 Polack τὰ οὐρούμενα {μὴ} ὑπομνησάντων ὀλέθρια· ἦρα (γε add. Gal.: om. IR) τουτέοισιν οὐρεῖται οἷον εἰ τὴν ὑπόστασιν (εἰ τὴν ὑ. Gal.: ἐπὴν ὑποστᾶσι H^1 IR) ἀναταράξειας (ἀνατ- Gal.: ταρ- H^1 IR); The negation is wrong here. The parallel version in *Coac.* § 584 (5.720.5–6 Li.) does not have it in its very conservative mscr. A (which is the only relevant one). Furthermore, A reads εἰ τὴν ὑπόστασιν.

urine] was left standing for a long time, it formed no sediment. Its colour and consistency was like cattle urine. This is what she urinated. I saw it myself."[480]

The application of the prognostic aphorisms in the case-histories of *Epidemics I* and *III* exemplifies, then, what could already be inferred from the very structure of the aphorisms: that these 'prognostic sayings,' either oral or written, were proved in practical use. There is no evidence that any prognostic aphorisms were ever formally disproved. Probably the useful ones among them were applied more often, whereas others were simply neglected, ignored, or even forgotten and not transmitted. With regard to aphorisms which we do *not* possess we can, of course, only speculate. Equally speculative is the answer to the question how the aphorisms were first formulated. It is reasonable to believe that there was not just one standard procedure such as 'induction,'[481] and it can in particular be ruled out that the aphorisms of *Prorrhetics I* have been 'induced' from *Epidemics I* and *III*. This possibility is precluded by the above-mentioned facts, especially that the doctrine of humours and of *krísis*, *pépsis*, and *apóstasis* is much less frequently mentioned in *Prorrhetics I* than in *Epidemics*. On the contrary, the inverse chronology is strongly suggested by the 'dialogue' held: with the aphorisms posing the questions, and the case-histories answering them. The inferable chronological relationship applies, however, strictly only to the *material* contained in *Prorrhetics I*, not necessarily to the treatise in its extant form (despite its relative homogeneity). Although its material, oral or written, should in all probability be older than *Epidemics I* and *III* (i. e. than ca. 410 B. C.[482]), the treatise itself, particularly the arrangement of its aphorisms,[483] might just as well be contemporary or more recent. 400 B. C. plus or minus several decades is probably the most precise guess one can make.[484]

---

480 *Epid. I* 2.692.10–15 Li. = 1.206.7–12 Kw. = 1.194 Jones ... οὖρει δὲ ... ἀθρόον πολὺ ὀλιγάκις ἀναμιμνῃσκόντων παχὺ λευκόν, οἷον γίνεται ἐκ (ἐκ AVIR: om. Gal.) τῶν καθισταμένων, ὅταν ἀναταραχθῇ· κείμενον πολὺν χρόνον οὐ καθίστατο (-το AVIR: -ται Gal.)· χρῶμα καὶ πάχος ἴκελον οἷον γίνεται ὑποζυγίου (-ίου AVIR: -ίων Gal.). τοιαῦτα οὖρει, οἷα (οἷα VIR, Gal.: ὅσα A) κἀγὼ (κ. AVIR: ἐγὼ Gal.) εἶδον. For ἀναμιμνῃσκόντων cf. σμικρὰ ὑπομιμνῃσκόντων ἔπινεν in *Epid. III* 3.142.10–11 Li. = 1.244.5 Kw. = 1.282 Jones. The parallel to *Prorrh. I* § 29 has already been noticed, but differently explained, by Ermerins, De Hippocratis doctrina 7.

481 Langholf, Generalisationen.

482 This is the date of *Epid. I* and *III*, cf. Deichgräber, Die Epidemien, p. 16, and above p. 77.

483 Cf. above p. 225, note 456.

484 For other estimates, see Perazzi, Ippocrate 140, 157–159, 162. – Grmek, Les maladies 424, quotes yet another aphorism from *Prorrh. I* parallel to case observations, but interprets the relationship *vice versa* (observation > aphorism).

IV. Prognosis and Divination

Prognosis was one of the most important activities of the Hippocratic authors. Some characteristics have already been dealt with above, particularly in connection with 'critical days' (p. 79–118) and with meteorology (p. 164–179). "The best thing a doctor can do is to exercise prognosis," begins *Prognostics*. "Knowing beforehand and telling beforehand, in the presence of the patients, what is, what has been, and what will be, and mentioning details which the patients do not mention, he will more easily be believed to know about the patients' condition, so that people dare to entrust themselves to the physician."[1] *Prognostics* continues that if the physician knows beforehand about the subsequent development of a patient's disease and announces it, he would not be held accountable in case of a fatal outcome.[2] He was then free to withhold treatment and to restrict himself to observing the patient and relieving his suffering.[3] This passage of *Prognostics* illustrates the social significance of prognosis in the relationship between "the disease, the patient, and the physician."[4]

It has plausibly been stated that ancient divination served the social function and purpose of achieving conformity of opinion.[5] Prognosis as a field of activity related to divination may be similarly viewed.[6] The relationship between the two fields was always felt: the expression "what is, what has been, and what will be" is a quotation from Homer. In the *Iliad*, Kalkhas, "the best of the diviners," is said to have known "what is,

---

[1] *Prog.* 2.110.2–7 Li. = 1.78.2–8 Kw. = 2.6 Jones Τὸν ἰητρὸν δοκεῖ μοι ἄριστον εἶναι πρόνοιαν ἐπιτηδεύειν. προγινώσκων γὰρ καὶ προλέγων παρὰ τοῖσι νοσέουσι τά τε παρεόντα καὶ τὰ προγεγονότα καὶ τὰ μέλλοντα ἔσεσθαι ὁκόσα τε παραλείπουσιν οἱ ἀσθενέοντες ἐκδιηγούμενος πιστεύοιτο ἂν μᾶλλον γινώσκειν τὰ τῶν νοσεόντων πρήγματα, ὥστε τολμᾶν ἐπιτρέπειν τοὺς ἀνθρώπους σφέας ἑαυτοὺς τῷ ἰητρῷ. Note the contrast to the *Knídiai gnỗmai* as they are represented in *Acut.*: In their description of details they reach only the level of a non-physician "if he skilfully asked the patients what they are suffering." (See above p. 14.)

[2] *Prog.* 2.110.7–112.11 Li. = 1.78.9–79.8 Kw. = 2.6–8 Jones ἀναίτιος.

[3] Detailed discussion of this issue by Edelstein, Περὶ ἀέρων, p. 100–102; Renate Wittern, Die Unterlassung ärztlicher Hilfeleistung in der griechischen Medizin der klassischen Zeit, Münch. med. Wochenschrift 121 (1979), no. 21, 731–734; Renate Wittern, Grenzen der Heilkunst, Stuttgart, 1982 (Robert Bosch Stiftung).

[4] See above p. 1.

[5] Burkert, Griechische Religion 184, 188; Dodds, The Greeks 75.

[6] Edelstein, Περὶ ἀέρων, ch. II; 100–102.

what will be, and what has been."[7] The verses are referred to also in *Epidemics I*, ch. 5 Li. = ch. 11 Kw., Jones: The physician should "say what has been, realize what is, and foretell what will be."[8] As the present chapter will demonstrate, other parallels between prognosis and divination concern the methods and forms of predictions; there were overlappings in terminology, too: in *Articulations*, ch. 9 it is, for instance, recommended that a physician should "prophesy" about the luxation of the shoulder by examining whether there is an inflammation or not.[9] In other passages to be quoted below, medical prognosis is even explicitly contrasted with divination. It must, however, be stated clearly here that such references to, or vestiges of, divination are by no means an outstanding feature of the Hippocratic Collection. The references are scarce, and the vestiges are not easily noted without careful scrutiny.

Even though for the medical craftsman of the Hippocratic Collection there appears to have existed a relatively clear-cut distinction between medical prognosis and divination (the latter craft being practised by other craftsmen), large parts of the population seem to have been rather indifferent to such a distinction. This situation is well illustrated by the occasional reference to the *iātrómantis*, 'physician and seer'[10] in sources outside of the Hippocratic Collection. He represents a more archaic stage when both activities, healing and divining, could be practised by one and the same person.[11] The word is never used of the Hippocratic medical practitioner, who is not a 'physician and seer' but a physician who prognosticates.

The scarcity of references made to divination concurs with the Collection's general lack of explicitness as to cults and religious beliefs, a lack of emphasis that is surprising, since religion and cult must have been socially quite important to these authors.[12] Kos, one of the centres of

---

[7] *Iliad I* 69–70 Κάλχας Θεστορίδης, οἰωνοπόλων ὄχ' ἄριστος, | ὃς ᾔδη τά τ' ἐόντα τά τ' ἐσσόμενα πρό τ' ἐόντα. The verse must have been a well-known formulaic description of the augur's activity because it occurs also in Hesiod *Theog.* 38. Later the idea became commonplace, cf. the collection of testimonia from throughout antiquity by Pease (ed.), Cic., *De div.*, Book I, p. 366 f. (= repr., p. 204 f.); Book II, p. 414 (= repr., p. 596).

[8] *Epid. I* 2.634.6–7 Li. = 1.189.24–190.2 Kw. = 1.164 Jones λέγειν τὰ προγενόμενα, γινώσκειν τὰ παρεόντα, προλέγειν τὰ ἐσόμενα. Realizing what has happened and what is going on within the body would not be called prognosis in modern terms, but rather (patho)physiology or aetiology. The doctor's ability to infer that certain symptoms are occurring or have occurred in an individual is today part of diagnosis.

[9] *Art.* 4.100.1–5 Li. = 124.7–13 Kw. = 3.218 Withington καταμαντεύσασθαι.

[10] As Liddell/Scott/Jones translate.

[11] Dodds, The Greeks 140 f., with note; Kudlien, Beginn 20 f., 58 f.; Kudlien, Primitive medicine 305–310; Parker, Miasma, *passim*, in partic. ch. 7 and 8; Burkert, Epoche 43 ff.; cf. φαρμακόμαντις in middle Attic comedy, Anaxandr. frg. 49 Kock, Edmonds.

[12] Lloyd, Magic 32–58.

Greek medicine around 400 B. C., may serve as an example. The physicians of the island were organized in the "Association of the Asklepiads of Kos and Knidos," if they belonged to the aristocratic clan.[13] Membership was defined by birth, not by profession. One of the activities of the organization must have been the worship of the common ancestor, Asklepios; another activity was to consult the oracle in Delphi, with which the Asklepiads maintained privileged relations. Some of the Koan physicians including Hippocrates himself and physicians in his family (who were Asklepiads) must have belonged to it.

The medical practitioners of Kos formed, moreover, a professional group. In an inscription[14] dated to the middle of the fourth century B. C., which preserves an official calender list of the religious events of the city of Kos, it is prescribed that at the religious festival for Zeus Polieus the physicians (*iātroí*) are to receive one portion of the meat left over from the offering, the flute-player also one portion, similarly the coppersmiths and the potters as groups.[15] The medical practitioners are referred to simply as "the physicians," without any further qualification. This indicates that they were organized as an officially acknowledged body, just like other craftsmen such as the coppersmiths and the potters.[16]

From another inscription[17] it can be inferred that the physicians of Kos had to comply with civic duties, some of which were religious. The text contains a decree passed by the public assembly of all citizens of Kos mandating that certain religious laws, which had long been used, be re-copied and published as inscriptions. One copy has been excavated. Since it dates from the first half of the third century B. C., its text should be used only with caution for the time around 400 B. C. Some conclusions may, however, be legitimately drawn on the grounds of an *a fortiori* argument. If the rather archaic dispositions formulated in the law were valid in the third century, they likewise should have been so 150 years earlier. The laws are about ritual pureness and purifications. For example, one law regulates the purity of the priestess of the goddess Damater Olympia. This priestess must never have anything to do with anything impure; she must not visit a tomb; she must not visit a house where a delivery has taken place until three days after the delivery; she must not visit a house in which somebody has died until three days have passed since the body has been carried out of the house; she must neither eat nor

---

[13] Cf. above p. 26.

[14] Franciszek Sokolowski, Lois sacrées des cités grecques, Paris, 1969, no. 151 A.

[15] χαλκέων καὶ κερα[μέ]|[ω]ν ἑκατέροις.

[16] Kudlien, Arzt Hellenismus 100; Poland, Vereinswesen 124 emphasizes that these organizations on Kos were not 'guilds' in the later sense.

[17] Sokolowski, *op. cit.*, no. 154; for the interpretation of details, see Parker, Miasma, *passim* (index, p. 402).

touch the meat of animals which have not been butchered. If she fails to observe any of these regulations, she has to be purified by being besprinkled with cereal grains out of a golden vessel. Under certain circumstances, similar purifications apply to persons not holding a priesthood.

These laws were, according to the decree of the public assembly, to be published by making two copies on steles, one of them to be erected in the temple of Damater, the other one in the temple of Asklepios. Beyond that, six copies were to be made on white wooden boards[18] and to be exhibited at various places, one of which was to be determined by the physicians.[19]

It would be rash to draw from this law any conclusions as to the religious attitude or 'Weltanschauung' of the physicians[20] of Kos, who possibly exercised political influence and were, therefore, especially apt to cooperate in the promulgation of the law. Its text perhaps does not even reflect the religious feeling of the average citizen of Kos in the first half of the third century or at the unknown time when the original legislation was passed: religious laws and ritual acts are never directly indicative of religious attitudes of individuals.[21] Still, the text, like other sacred regulations of Kos, is typical of the social environment the physicians were living in. Religion and cult were in the third as well as in the fifth and fourth centuries B. C. a very important and even basic factor in the social relations of the people, and between groups of people.[22] One can hardly overestimate the influence of religion and cult. Making offerings to the gods, consulting soothsayers, holding sacred processions, all was constantly being done, not only by state officials and on state occasions, but also in the framework of the many private associations, clubs, cooperatives, and clan organizations that existed, not to speak of strictly individual purposes. A cult of a deity or of a hero was the basis of almost every social

---

18 λευκώματα.

19 Literally: "[at the place] where the physicians determine among [or: for] themselves [to exhibit it]," εἶ τοὶ ἰατροὶ τάσσονται, with the verb in the middle voice. Rudolf Herzog translates, "in dem Lokal der Ärzte" (Vorläufiger Bericht über die koische Expedition im Jahre 1903, Archäolog. Anzeiger 1903, 196; cf. Archiv für Religionswiss. 10 [1907], 400–415; Heilige Gesetze 20–25), but this cannot be the meaning of the present tense form. Kudlien, Arzt Hellenismus 100f., suggests the possibility that ΙΑΤΡΟΙ is a misreading or misspelling instead of 'priest' (ΙΑΡΕΙΣ or ΙΕΡΕΙΣ, the dialect inscription using indiscriminately Α or Ε as second letter). I would prefer not to alter the transmitted text, since it in no way contradicts what we know about the public functions of physicians during that epoch.

20 For literature on this problem, see Nörenberg, Das Göttliche; Kudlien, Das Göttliche.

21 E. R. Dodds, The religion of the ordinary man in classical Greece, in: *idem*, Concept of progress 140–155.

22 Burkert, Griechische Religion 371–402.

organization.[23] Oaths were employed much more often than today. Everyone frequently participated in religious activities — probably with all the varying degrees of fervour that can be observed today.

The objects of religious veneration were manifold. Greek religion never officially tried to develop any compulsory strict theology, and this is one of the reasons why traditional views and philosophical concepts about the gods could be held at the same time by one and the same person.[24] Traditional views and forms in Greek religion could easily be given new meanings; and new philosophical concepts about the gods could in turn quickly become conventional and traditional themselves. Traditional religion on the one hand and philosophical religion on the other[25] are fundamentally distinct only from a modern perspective. To the ancient observer, traditional and philosophical religion were rather the extreme positions of a wide spectrum of possible convictions, which admitted of countless gradations. In particular it is hardly possible for the historian to reconstruct in which ways certain individual personalities managed either to make a choice, or eclectically to assimilate disparate concepts and to reconcile them with each other.[26]

The physicians of the fifth and fourth centuries were not theologians; it cannot be ascertained whether they were able to keep the extreme positions strictly apart even theoretically. Furthermore, in their professional situation characterized by a high degree of dependency on their social reputation in their city states, they must have been prudent enough not openly and radically to contradict the public opinion, which traditionally associated disease with curses and demonic influences.[27] The author of a given Hippocratic treatise may have believed both in the traditional, personal gods and, simultaneously, in 'the divine' as postulated by the philosophers. A good example is the writer of the treatise *On Regimen*, books *I–IV*. He has been strongly influenced by philosophy.[28] Parts of book *I* evince even an imitation of a particular philosopher, Heraclitus,

---

[23] Poland, Vereinswesen 5—7, 173—270.

[24] Daniel Babut, La religion des philosophes grecs de Thalès aux stoïciens, Vendôme, 1974, *passim*; Lloyd, Magic 10—58; P. A. Mejer, Philosophers, intellectuals and religion in Hellas, in: H. S. Versnel (ed.), Faith, hope and worship: Aspects of religious mentality in the ancient world, Leiden, 1981, 216—263.

[25] Kudlien, Das Göttliche; Burkert, Griechische Religion 452—495.

[26] Examples of religious beliefs "logically incompatible, but contemporaneously accepted by different individuals or even by the same individual" are given by Dodds, The Greeks 179 (also *ibid.*, ch. V).

[27] On some "general restrictions to the spread of critical inquiry" in Greek *pólis* societies, see Lloyd, Magic 262—264. For the social situation of physicians, see H. W. Pleket, Arts en maatschappij in het oude Griekenland, Tijdschrift voor Geschiedenis 96 (1983), 325—347; Kudlien, Sozialgeschichte des frühgriechischen Arztes.

[28] Joly, Recherches *passim*; Joly (ed.), Hippocrate, Du régime, p. 25—34.

in style and thought.[29] The author says in *I* 2 that it is most important in regimen to know the elements of which man consists.[30] This knowledge enables the physician to recognize if one element abounds, and to administer the appropriate diet, including exercises for the body, provided that he knows also the dietetic properties of the therapeutic measures to be taken. Man and all animals consist of fire and water (ch. 3).[31] The whole of book *II* deals with the corresponding elementary qualities warm/cold and moist/dry of the single foodstuffs and types of exercises. The author's theory is rather logical, and one does not see why any gods should be needed in addition to the elements postulated. Still they occur. They are not mentioned very frequently but are important in the theory of the author, who ends his treatise by using the phrase "with the help of the gods."[32] As far as books *I—III* are concerned, the logical coherence of the theory does not seem to be impaired by the religious component: *I* 11, "The gods have organized the nature of all." ... "What the gods have organized is always right."[33] A little earlier in the same chapter: "The mind of the gods has taught [man] to imitate their [divine] activities."[34] Book *I* 5, "Everything happens through divine necessity."[35] In one passage of book *I* it is intimated that the "divine things" follow the same necessity: *I* 5, "All things divine and human proceed by moving up and down."[36] Perhaps the author wants to suggest that the gods are subject to the very natural laws which they have organized.

An inconsistency in the author's world-picture becomes manifest only in book *IV*, which deals with dreams. Some dreams, he says, are divine (and should be interpreted by diviners), others are signs furnished by the body (and should be interpreted as prognostic signs by the physicians).[37] The latter category, however, must, according to the author, also be divine in some way, because he repeatedly includes prayers in his therapeutical prescriptions. It seems that the patient, not the physician, is advised to execute the prayers (the texts are not absolutely clear as to this point): *IV* 88, "... vomit ..., light food ..., walks ..., sport ..., exercises of the

[29] Diels/Kranz 22 C 1 (vol. 1, p. 182—188).

[30] *Vict. I* 6.468.6—15 Li. = 122.22—124.2 Joly = 4.226 Jones.

[31] 6.472.12—14 Li. = 126.5—6 Joly = 4.230 Jones.

[32] σὺν τοῖσι θεοῖσιν.

[33] 6.486.20—23 Li. = 136.2—4 Joly = 4.248—250 Jones φύσιν δὲ πάντων θεοὶ διεκόσμησαν· ... ὅσα δὲ θεοὶ διέθεσαν αἰεὶ ὀρθῶς ἔχει.

[34] 6.486.14 Li. = 134.22—23 Joly = 4.248 Jones θεῶν γὰρ νοῦς ἐδίδαξε μιμεῖσθαι τὰ ἑωυτῶν.

[35] 6.476.20—478.1 Li. = 128.18—19 Joly = 4.236 Jones πάντα γίνεται δι' ἀνάγκην θείην.

[36] 6.476.12—13 Li. = 128.12 Joly = 4.236 Jones χωρεῖ (χωρεῖ Bernays: χωρὶς θM: complectitur Lat.) δὲ πάντα καὶ θεῖα καὶ ἀνθρώπινα ἄνω καὶ κάτω ἀμειβόμενα. The word θεῖα is not clear.

[37] *IV* 87; see below p. 246.

voice ..., and he should pray to the gods, and the trouble will stop."[38] Particular gods are recommended: in ch. 90, the patient who has dreamed about "terrestrial things" which are abnormal, in particular landscapes, trees, rivers and other waters, is advised to follow certain forms of regimen and to "pray to Gē and Hermes and the heroes."[39] Ch. 89, which deals with dreams about meteorological and astronomical phenomena, even presents the medical indications of prayers to the various deities: "... and praying to the gods; if the dreams are good, to Helios, Zeus Ouranios, Zeus Ktesios, Athena Ktesia, Hermes, and Apollo; otherwise to the ones averting evil and to Gē and the heroes, in order to avoid all evil."[40] If everything relevant in physiology and pathology follows the natural laws of fire and water and of the four elementary qualities, prayer should be useless, even if these laws are divine and instituted by the gods.[41] The

[38] 6.644.3–11 Li. = 220.10–17 Joly = 4.424–426 Jones ...ἔμετον ..., σίτοισι κούφοισι ..., περιπάτοισιν ..., γυμνασίοισιν ..., τοῖσι περιπάτοισι πιέζειν καὶ τοῖσι τῆς φωνῆς πόνοισι χρῆσθαι, καὶ τοῖσι θεοῖσιν εὔχεσθαι, καὶ καταστήσεται ἡ ταραχή. The active form πιέζειν may imply a change of the subject, a grammatical phenomenon customary in recipes.

[39] 6.656.12–658.1 Li. = 228.2 Joly = 4.440 Jones εὔχεσθαι δὲ Γῇ καὶ Ἑρμῇ καὶ ἥρωσιν. The active form ξηραίνειν in the subsequent lines may refer rather to the physician. The dead are mentioned in 658.15–16 Li. = 228.14 Joly = 442 Jones ἀπὸ γὰρ τῶν ἀποθανόντων αἱ τροφαὶ καὶ αὐξήσιες καὶ σπέρματα γίνεται, cf. Joly *ad loc.* and Dodds, Concept of progress 147.

[40] 6.652.19–22 Li. = 224.25–28 Joly = 4.436 Jones καὶ τοῖσι θεοῖσιν εὔχεσθαι, ἐπὶ μὲν τοῖσιν ἀγαθοῖσιν Ἡλίῳ, Διὶ Οὐρανίῳ, Διὶ Κτησίῳ, Ἀθηναίῃ Κτησίῃ, Ἑρμῇ, Ἀπόλλωνι, ἐπὶ δὲ τοῖσιν ἐναντίοισι τοῖσιν ἀποτροπαίοισι, καὶ Γῇ καὶ ἥρωσιν, ἀποτρόπαια τὰ χαλεπὰ εἶναι πάντα.

[41] There was perhaps a discussion among physicians about the usefulness of prayer in medicine. In ch. 46 of the roughly contemporary Hippocratic treatise *On Places in Man* it is said that "chance is sovereign, it cannot be controlled nor can it be summoned through prayer." (*Loc. Hom.* 6.342.9–10 Li. = 76.12–14 Joly ἡ γὰρ τύχη αὐτοκρατὴς καὶ οὐκ ἄρχεται, οὐδ' ἐπ' εὐχῇ ἔστιν αὐτὴν ἐλθεῖν.) The context is not about the divine law immanent in nature: *týkhē* here denotes chance. Yet a religious meaning is referred to. The same applies to the synonymous *tó autómaton* in *On the Art*, ch. 6: "One cannot reasonably make *tó autómaton* responsible for any recoveries that happen without a doctor, because upon examination one finds that *tó autómaton* is nothing: one finds that everything happens through a cause; the cause makes it obvious that *tó autómaton* does not exist as such but only as a word." (*De arte* 6.10.8–12 Li. = 12.26–13.4 Heiberg = 2.198–200 Jones οὐκ ἔστιν ἔτι οὐδενὶ τῶν ἄνευ ἰητροῦ ὑγιαζομένων τὸ αὐτόματον αἰτιήσασθαι ὀρθῷ λόγῳ· τὸ μὲν γὰρ αὐτόματον οὐδὲν φαίνεται ἐὸν ἐλεγχόμενον· πᾶν γὰρ τὸ γινόμενον διά τι εὑρίσκοιτ' ἂν γινόμενον, καὶ ἐν τῷ διά τι τὸ αὐτόματον οὐ φαίνεται οὐσίην ἔχον οὐδεμίην ἀλλ' ἢ οὔνομα.) For *týkhē* see also Hippocrates' (genuine?) tomb-inscription *Anth. Pal. VII* 135 (Annette Stamm, Hippokrates-Epigramme, München [diss.], 1978, 23–40), whose antithesis οὐ τύχᾳ ἀλλὰ τέχνᾳ recalls *De arte*. Around 400 B. C. these and other 'abstract words' (an anachronistic term) came to be widely recognized as deities and to be worshipped (Nilsson, Geschichte der griechischen Religion, vol. 1.812–815; 2.200–210; Burkert, Griechische Religion 286–288). Prayer was, however, becoming problematical if one believed that the world was governed by 'Chance' or 'The Automatism.'

inconsistency is obvious. A professional philosopher around 400 B.C. would perhaps have tried to solve the dilemma by making a decision. For the medical author of *On Regimen*, however, it was certainly easier to live with the inconsistency. He could neither neglect the achievements of contemporary natural speculation without being 'oldfashioned' and jeopardizing his reputation among his colleagues and persons interested in natural philosophy,[42] nor could he shock the less sophisticated citizens by abandoning the religious tradition. Unlike the radical sophist of his time, who attracted a particular clientèle by presenting new fashioned and at times even shocking views, the physician was materially dependent on a public with the broadest possible spectrum of religious and philosophical beliefs, and the less clearly he expressed himself about such matters, the better for him. In the case of the medical amateur-philosopher of *On Regimen*, the result is bizarre because suddenly he recommends traditional prayer after having adopted divine necessity and the elements fire and water as ruling principles.[43]

Prayer or other activities of the popular cult are not recommended elsewhere in the Hippocratic Collection. On the contrary, criticism of certain religious practices is expressed, particularly in the treatise *On the Sacred Disease*. But here, too, the attitude towards the traditional beliefs is as ambivalent as in *On Regimen*.

The 'sacred disease' (epilepsy) seizes people when their phlegm blocks their veins. One of the causes which makes the latent condition manifest is the weather with its changes. Therefore this malady is, according to the author, no more divine than any other disease, and those who first attributed a particularly sacred character to it were magicians, purifiers, charlatans, and quacks, whom he despises. They use purifications and incantations to make their living, he continues, but if this so-called sacred disease could in fact be healed so easily, the action of the god would be disproved. Furthermore, a god can never defile man. On the contrary, the author says, "we ourselves fix boundaries to the sanctuaries and precincts of the gods, so that nobody may cross them unless he be pure; and when we enter, we sprinkle ourselves ... to remove any pollution we may have already contracted. Such is my opinion about purification." (Ch. 1)[44]

---

[42] As Karl Deichgräber's prosopographical research has revealed, the patients of the *Epidemics* belonged in large part to the upper classes of the population, who are likely to have been more interested in philosophical issues (Deichgräber, Patienten, *passim*).

[43] Joly, Recherches 171, summarizes the difficulty met by the historian in this matter: "Il est toujours difficile d'atteindre à travers un texte le sentiment intime de son auteur." A similar case is Herodotus, see, Lloyd, Magic 29–32.

[44] *Morb. Sacr.* 6.352.2–364.8 Li. = 60.2–66.5 Gr. = 2.138–150 Jones; for the aetiology (phlegm) see *passim* in the whole treatise. Generally on *Morb. Sacr.* see Lanata, Medicina magica *passim*; Lloyd, Magic 15–29 *et saepius*.

The use of the same technical vocabulary referring to ritual purity in ch. 1 of *On the Sacred Disease* and in the Koan law inscription quoted shortly above is remarkable. The ambiguity of the author's views becomes particularly apparent in his indiscriminate use of the same terms for the activity of the purifiers and of the physicians ("we"). In fact, all of the rites described (the official purifications in the inscription; the cult in which the physician of *On the Sacred Disease* participated; the business of the magicians and purifiers) belonged to one broad spectrum of religious beliefs. There was no official theology, and there was no authority anxious to fix boundaries against 'heresy.'[45] The individual did not have to make a choice between the various trends in the common cult.

Similarly, no choice was demanded between traditional religion and philosophical opinions. The author of *On the Sacred Disease* held some philosophical beliefs about the gods: ch. 18, "This disease, the so-called sacred one, has the same causes as the other ones, namely matters going into and out of the body, cold, sun, and the ever changing restless winds. *These things are divine.* Therefore, one should not set apart this disease nor regard it as more divine than the others, because all [diseases] are divine and all are human, each has its own nature and power, none is incurable or hopeless ... Someone who knows how to provoke dryness and moisture and coldness and warmth in the patients [lit.: in humans] through diet will be able to cure this disease, too."[46]

The expression "these things are divine" is vague,[47] as is the assertion that all diseases are divine. This physician may have been able to reconcile his philosophical concept of the gods with traditional ideas, but the modern historian cannot know whether, and how, and to what degree he did so. His private theology cannot be reconstructed because his statements are too short and unclear, and because he was probably neither a theologian nor a philosopher. He may have tried eclectically to adopt from traditional religion what was compatible with his philosophical ideas about the divine and with his medical theories and doctrines. The rites of the magicians were incompatible, but participation in the official cult, even where this implied ritual purifications, was (or had to be?) compatible. It is significant that the author of *On the Sacred Disease*, who so violently attacks the "magicians, purifiers, charlatans, and quacks,"[48] does not say a word against priests as such.[49] The very last word of the treatise, used and

---

45 Burkert, Griechische Religion 157–163.

46 6.394.9–396.7 Li. = 88.13–90.27 Gr. = 2.182 Jones ... ταῦτα δ' ἐστὶ θεῖα ὥστε μὴ δεῖν (μὴ δεῖν ci. Wilamowitz: μηδένη θ: μηδὲν M) ἀποκρίνοντα τὸ νόσημα θειότερον τῶν λοιπῶν νομίζειν, ἀλλὰ πάντα θεῖα καὶ πάντα ἀνθρώπινα ...

47 It recalls the (quasi?) divine nature of the air in *On Breaths*, see shortly below p. 244.

48 μάγοι τε καὶ καθαρταὶ καὶ ἀγύρται καὶ ἀλαζόνες.

49 ἱρέες. Parker, Miasma 249.

placed there deliberately as it seems, emphasizes what the author is against: *banausíē*, a substantive which means 'vulgarity,' 'narrow-mindedness,' 'craft of the lower classes.'[50] "I am convinced," he says in ch. 1, "... that if a human body is polluted [this Greek word denotes physical as well as ritual pollution] or suffering something from another cause [a cause other than the gods], it will be purified and cleansed by the god rather than be polluted."[51] No therapeutical prayer is prescribed by the author, but its use would not have contradicted what he intimates about his religious beliefs. "Prayer," says the physician who wrote *On Regimen* (*IV* 87), "is a good thing, certainly; but you must yourself be active while invoking the gods."[52] Perhaps the author of *On the Sacred Disease* could have subscribed to this apophthegm,[53] but this is of course only a more or less plausible conjecture.[54]

---

[50] P. Chantraine, Trois noms grecs de l'artisan, in: Mélanges de philosophie grecque offerts à Mgr. Diès, Paris, 1956, 41–47 (in partic. 43 f.).

[51] 6.362.16–364.2 Li. = 66.92–95 Gr. = 2.148 Jones οὐ μέντοι ἔγωγε ἀξιῶ ὑπὸ θεοῦ ἀνθρώπου σῶμα μιαίνεσθαι, ... ἀλλὰ καὶ ἢν τυγχάνῃ ὑφ' ἑτέρου μεμιασμένον ἤ τι πεπονθός, ὑπὸ τοῦ θεοῦ καθαίρεσθαι ἂν αὐτὸ καὶ ἁγνίζεσθαι μᾶλλον ἢ μιαίνεσθαι.

[52] *Vict. IV* 6.642.8–10 Li. = 218.21–22 Joly = 4.422 Jones καὶ τὸ μὲν εὔχεσθαι ἀγαθόν· δεῖ δὲ καὶ αὐτὸν συλλαμβάνοντα τοὺς θεοὺς ἐπικαλεῖσθαι. The same idea occurs in Euripides (lost earlier version of the *Hippolytos*, frg. 432 Nauck², written before 428 B. C.). It was proverbial. Cf. similar popular formulations collected in Corpus Paroemiographorum Graecorum, I, p. 157 f. (no. 93), 306 (no. 11); II, p. 211 (no. 84), 647 (no. 79), 653 (no. 92), 748 f. (no. 32). See also Joly *ad loc.*

[53] In *Morb. Sacr.* 6.364.3–4 Li. = 66.1 Grensemann = 2.148 Jones, the editions print τὸ θεῖόν ἐστι τὸ καθαῖρον καὶ ἁγνίζον καὶ ῥύμμα γινόμενον ἡμῖν: three words for the same thing; and ῥύμμα is, moreover, a prosaic, if not banal expression. It means 'soap,' 'lye,' 'detergent,' a rather bold metaphor. This is the reading of θ. The mscr. M has ἔρυμα, Reinhold changed ῥύμμα into ῥῦμα, which is synonymous with ἔρυμα, 'protection,' 'defence,' and gives a satisfying sense. If the divine is a 'protection,' prayer is not out of place. – The compiler of *Nat. Mul.* claims in ch. 1 (7.312.2–14 Li. = 70.2–14 Trapp) that with regard to women's diseases μάλιστα μὲν τὸ θεῖον ἐν τοῖσιν ἀνθρώποισιν αἴτιον εἶναι· ἔπειτα αἱ φύσιες τῶν γυναικῶν καὶ χροιαί (and their age), and he recommends: δεῖ δὲ τὸν ὀρθῶς ταῦτα χειρίζοντα πρῶτον μὲν ἐκ τῶν θείων ἄρχεσθαι (by a ritual act such as prayer?). Only subsequently the physician has, according to this author, to examine his patient's constitution (φύσις) and age, the season and the geographic environment. The 'divine' (θεῖον) is obviously not believed here to be identical with any of these latter categories. – The statements on religion found in other Hippocratic treatises (e. g. in *On Airs, Waters, Places* and *Prognostics*) will not be discussed here because they contain still less information about the 'Weltanschauung' of their authors. Cf. Nörenberg, Das Göttliche; Kudlien, Das Göttliche.

[54] Temkin, Falling sickness 14 f. – Theophr. *Hist. pl. IX* 8.5–8 (on herb-diggers, ῥιζοτόμοι) states that "to pray while you are cutting herbs is perhaps not out of place," τὸ δ' ἐπευχόμενον τέμνειν οὐθὲν ἴσως ἄτοπον. The author rejects, however, "what is practised in addition to this," εἴ τι καὶ ἄλλο προστιθέασιν, namely the various superstitious rites performed by the ῥιζοτόμοι (which are in marked contrast to the more 'secular' methods applied by the physicians of the Hippocratic Collection – physicians who *must* have co-operated, at least indirectly, with the ῥιζοτόμοι). On the authenticity of book

Although the available sources are inadequate for reconstructing with any precision the religious convictions of individual medical authors, there is sufficient material to get an overall impression of their religious environment and the range of their possible personal attitudes. Since religion and cult were so important in their society, it is not surprising to note that medical prognosis in the Hippocratic treatises has preserved, besides functional similarities to divinatory practices of the religious cult, also similarities in the form and content of the texts. It is not unlikely that medical prognosis as manifest in the Hippocratic Collection had evolved out of a complex of prognostic activities encompassing, besides augury, such forms of prediction as weather prediction, the forecasting of the year for the farmer or sailor, the determination of favourable and unfavourable days, or the oracular forecast of health and disease. Of course, these activities were distinct from each other, and very early there may have been specialists for each of them; some of the practices formed part of official cults (for the official observation of Sirius on Keos, see above p. 166–168), others did not.

Official as well as private divination was beginning to decline in the fifth century B. C., but still retained much influence; the relationship of the Asklepiads of Kos and Knidos to the Oracle of Delphi (above p. 26) is typical in this respect. Apollo remained the god of divination as well as of medicine.[55] Divination, albeit declining, was still a *tékhnē*, and such also was medicine. Both crafts had to be studied in a long apprenticeship and were passed on in particular families, often of the aristocracy,[56] whose members practised as itinerant specialists.[57] In both crafts similar patterns of thought prevailed, which had originated in popular modes of thought. Both began to produce technical literature in the fifth century. The affinity was always felt. When, in the decades around 400 B. C., it became fashionable for the educated to criticize divination, some physicians thought it advisable to dissociate their methods from those of the diviners. The author of *Prorrhetics II* disqualifies certain medical prognoses as "prophecies" and "divination" (see below, p. 250 f.). Another example is *On Regimen in Acute Diseases*, ch. 3 Li. (= ch. 8 Kw., Jones), an attack by a

---

IX cf. Pauly/Wissowa, Suppl. VII, 1450–1452 s. v. 'Theophrastos 3' (O. Regenbogen). Georg Wöhrle, Theophrasts Methode in seinen botanischen Schriften, Amsterdam, 1985, 42.

[55] *Epist.* 9.342.9–12 Li. = 11.8–10 Putzger. Mark Griffith (ed.), Aeschylus, Prometheus Bound, Cambridge, 1983, p. 173 f. (commentary on 484–490).

[56] Ingrid Löffler, Die Melampodie. Versuch einer Rekonstruktion des Inhalts, Meisenheim, 1963 (Beitr. z. Klass. Philologie, 7), *passim*; Burkert, Griechische Religion 181, with bibliogr.; Parker, Miasma 210; Burkert, Epoche 43 ff.; Kudlien, Sozialgeschichte des frühgriechischen Arztes, with bibliogr.

[57] This applies also to the purifiers; Parker, Miasma 208–211.

physician against certain contradictory methods of contemporary medicine: they are, he complains, just as inconsistent as the methods of contemporary diviners observing birds or intestines, and therefore bring the medical craft into ill repute.[58]

The professional competition which characterized all crafts[59] and in particular Greek medicine[60] affected also medical prognosis, where physicians as in a contest strove to outdo one another.[61] Competition served as a stimulus for developing new modes of prognosis and for refining those that already existed. The Hippocratic Collection presents many examples of this process.[62]

Medicine as a craft (*tékhnē*) in itself manifested specific methods of prediction which had clearly had their origin in medical observation and in professional experience, particularly in the fields of nosology and surgery. In many of the nosological descriptions of specific diseases, information is conveyed about the outcome;[63] also the surgical treatises often indicate the prognosis of wounds and fractures.[64] Yet another method of medical prognosis implied a knowledge of the importance of certain days or periods of days for the development of disease.[65] These latter traditions concerning numbers were based partly on observing the typical course of some diseases such as malaria or pneumonia, and partly on speculation about particular numbers such as that about even and odd.

It was stated earlier that the social function and purpose of divination and prognosis was similar, and that both crafts could insure conformity of opinion. There were also other similarities. One of the aims of divination was to interpret situations of individual or collective impurity (*míasma, akatharsía*) and to indicate methods of purification. Such a *kátharsis* could be effected by a charm or ceremony (*phármakon*). Analogously, one of the aims of prognosis in medicine was to interpret the state of the body. This was done by using the same terms of individual or collective (epidemic) impurity (*akatharsíē*; perhaps also *míasma*), whereupon a treatment was prescribed, which often consisted of purging (*kátharsis*) by means of a

---

[58] *Acut.* 2.240.6–244.1 Li. = 1.112.19–113.12 Kw. = 2.68 Jones. The key words are μαντική, μάντις, and ἱεροσκοπίη.

[59] As early as Hes. *Op.* 23–26.

[60] Edelstein, Περὶ ἀέρων, ch. III.

[61] *Art.* 4.252.14–15 Li. = 2.205.20 Kw. = 3.338 Withington προρρήματα λαμπρὰ καὶ ἀγωνιστικά. *Prorrh. II* 9.8.15 διαγωνίζεσθαι. 10.5 ἀγωνισμάτων.

[62] Relevant examples are *Prognostics; On Airs, Waters, Places; On Regimen.* All of these treatises claim to present better methods of prognosis.

[63] Cf. above p. 55, 60–72.

[64] Mirko D. Grmek, Ancienneté de la chirurgie hippocratique, in: Formes de pensée 285–295. This article, although not directly concerned with prognosis, informs about the relatively high standard of Greek pre-Hippocratic surgery.

[65] Cf. above p. 61–68, 93 ff.

drug (*phármakon*).[66] This technical vocabulary illustrates again that one of the antecedents of medical prognosis was traditional lore such as divination, and that moreover one of the antecedents of medical therapy was ritual purification. "The Hippocratic doctor, in seeing 'impurity' as a cause and symptom of disease, is an heir to the prophet or oracle."[67]

Particularly illustrative of the way in which the religious concept of impurity is manifested in a medical context is the treatise *On Breaths*, whose focus is not that of prognosis but of 'physiology' and 'pathology:' its author[68] aims at explaining health and disease in terms of one major cause, the air. The word *míasma* used in *On Breaths*, ch. 5 and 6 to denote the 'impurity' of the air had a strong ritual connotation. Indeed, this word very rarely signifies a non-ritual contamination.[69] It may, therefore, be safely inferred that the word *míasma* in *On Breaths* serves to extol the air as an (almost?) divine element, whose pollution is, according to the author, not to be explained in terms of infection in a modern sense or of material foulness only,[70] but of ritual impurity. Some statements in *On Breaths* about the air support this religious interpretation. The air is "the greatest ruler over everything in the universe," even the celestial bodies "live" on it: being fiery, they could not live without the air, which guarantees eternal life even to the sun. The earth is the base of the air; the air is the carrier of the earth. (Paraphrase from ch. 3[71])

---

66 Lloyd, Magic 43 f.; Lloyd, Science 131 f.; Parker, Miasma 213 f.; *elatḗrios* (*-on*) had the same double meaning as *phármakon*.

67 Parker, Miasma 2.

68 Menon (pupil of Aristotle), Antiphanes (middle Attic comedy) and Callimachus possibly regarded *On Breaths* as a work of the 'Great' Hippocrates; Langholf, Kallimachos.

69 Parker, Miasma 3 f. The word μίασμα (*Flat.* 6.96.16; 98.11 Li. = 94.4, 20 Heiberg = 2.232 Jones) is used in non-ritual terms by Galen, *Diff. febr.* 7.289 f. K. (on Thuc. *II* 48).

70 The medical terms 'miasma,' '-atic' used until the last century were based on passages in Galen such as 7.289 f. (see note 69); 3.414; 6.58; 9.342; 10.843 K.

71 *Flat.* 6.94.2–22 Li. = 92.21–93.17 Heiberg = 2.230 Jones. In Euripides' *Women of Troy*, Hecuba prays to a deity whom she addresses in almost the same words, "carrier of the earth, having the earth as a base," and whom she equates with Zeus, with the Necessity of Nature, and with the mortals' Mind. (Eur. *Tro.* 884–886 ὦ γῆς ὄχημα κἀπὶ γῆς ἔχων ἕδραν ... Ζεύς, εἴτ' ἀνάγκη φύσεως εἴτε νοῦς βροτῶν ...) This deity closely resembles "the greatest ruler over everything in the universe" of *On Breaths* (Theiler, Teleologische Naturbetrachtung 9, 36, 59). Euripides probably hesitated to have Hecuba equate the deity explicitly with the air after Aristophanes had ridiculed the idea in *Nub.* 220 ff. (provided that the extant comedy scene or a similar one was already contained in the version of 423). That the concept of the air in *On Breaths* was due to a strong influence from the teachings of Diogenes of Apollonia and/or of other pneumatic philosophers is obvious and need not be demonstrated here. Diels/Kranz quote Aristoph. *Nub.*, Hippocr. *Flat.*, Eurip. *Tro.* and other texts under 'Diogenes von Apollonia,' 'C. Nachwirkung' (64 C 1–4, vol. 2.66–69). See also Hans Diller, Die philosophiegeschichtliche Stellung des Diogenes von Apollonia, Hermes 76 (1941), 359–381 (= Kleine

In *On Airs, Waters, Places*, a treatise which, unlike *On Breaths*, is prognostic in content and designed to instruct the itinerant physician on prognostic signs offered by the patients' physical environment, the air is not said to be divine, but it may be impure. Unlike *On Breaths*, impurity is principally material, but still there exists a ritual connotation in so far as the east and the west are specifically associated with purity and impurity respectively. This has a parallel in the Hippocratic Collection. In *On Regimen IV*, ch. 89, where the prognostic meaning of dreams about stars is expounded, it is claimed: "Stars which seem to fall out of their orbit indicate health, if they are pure and bright and move towards the east ... ; but those that are dark and dim and seem to move towards the west ..., indicate diseases."[72] Sources outside of the Hippocratic Collection seem to imply that rites of expiation and purification were performed facing east;[73] the entrances and façades of temples were oriented in the same direction, and when offering sacrifices on the altar in front of a sanctuary, one looked east.[74] The Greeks acknowledged, as Bouché-Leclercq aptly puts it, a "privilège de l'Orient;" the east was "le côté heureux," "la droite du monde."[75] It is, therefore, perhaps not by coincidence that the author of *On Airs, Waters, Places*, ch. 3–6, when describing the healthiness or unhealthiness of cities whose orientation faces one of the four directions, states that the city facing east is the most healthy because "the waters are of necessity clear and fragrant and soft and there is no mist in this city."[76] That "clear" means "pure" here is apparent from the description of the city facing west. Such an opposite site is most unhealthy because "the waters are not clear; the reason is the morning mist mixed with the water and spoiling its limpidity." "The mist is mostly impure and wet there, because it is not thoroughly purified by the northwinds."[77]

Schriften zur antiken Literatur, München, 1971, 162–186), in partic. 369 f., 380 (= 173 f., 185) on the divine nature of the air.

[72] *Vict. IV* 6.650.4–11 Li. = 222.31–224.4 Joly = 4.432 Jones ὅ τι δ' ἂν ἐκ τῆς περιφορῆς ἐκπίπτειν δοκῇ τῶν ἄστρων, ὅσα μὲν καθαρὰ καὶ λαμπρὰ καὶ πρὸς ἠῶ φέρεται, ὑγ⟨ι⟩είην σημαίνει...· ὅ τι δ' ἂν τούτων μέλαν καὶ ἀμυδρὸν καὶ πρὸς ἑσπέρην δοκῇ φέρεσθαι ..., ταῦτα σημαίνει τὰς νούσους.

[73] Parker, Miasma 225 with note 97.

[74] Burkert, Griechische Religion 153.

[75] A. Bouché-Leclercq, Histoire de la divination dans l'antiquité, vol. 1, Paris, 1879 (= repr., Bruxelles, 1963), 137 f., with references; Geoffrey E. R. Lloyd, Right and left in Greek philosophy, Journ. of Hellen. Stud. 82 (1962), 56–66; Lloyd, Polarity and analogy 47; Leo Elders, Aristotle's cosmology: A commentary on the De caelo, Assen, 1966, p. 183–190. Reallex. f. Ant. u. Chr. XV 253–260 (A. Podossinov).

[76] *Aer.* 2.22.21–24 Li. = 1.38.21–24 Kw. = 1.80 Jones τὰ ὕδατα ... πάντα λαμπρά τε εἶναι ἀνάγκη καὶ εὐώδεα καὶ μαλακά, ἠέρα τε μὴ (ἠ. τε μὴ Gad.: ἢ ἐρατεινὰ V) ἐγγίγνεσθαι ἐν ταύτῃ τῇ πόλει.

[77] *Aer.* 2.24.13–26.3 Li. = 1.39.17–40.3 Kw. = 1.82 Jones τὰ ὕδατα οὐ λαμπρά· αἴτιον

Despite the inferable common origin of divination and prognosis, and despite certain similarities between them, these two activities were not considered identical in the decades around 400 B. C. Even the author of *On Regimen IV*, who advocates prognosis from dreams and recommends therapeutic prayer, recognizes this distinction, ch. 87: "As to those dreams which are of divine origin and indicate to the cities or to individuals either bad or good, ... there are people [viz., diviners] to interpret them, and they have their professional technique (*tékhnē*). The soul's premonitions [in dreams] about the affections of the body (such as excessive plethora or evacuation of substances natural to it) are also interpreted by them," sometimes rightly, sometimes wrongly, without their knowing the reasons.[78] The author then seems to plead for a specialization: diviners should confine themselves to non-medical dreams, physicians to the ones with medical importance, and without giving advice in non-medical matters.[79]

Any similarities between oracles and the medical prognoses of the Collection should, therefore, not be interpreted in the sense that these Hippocratic predictions are oracles themselves or have directly arisen out of oracles. On the other hand, these similarities make it difficult to describe the generic difference. The above-mentioned statement of *On Regimen IV* suggests the following social situation: divination is the craft of diviners; medical prognosis is the activity of medical craftsmen. Since for either professional activity specialized craftsmen were available who belonged to specific social groups, the two crafts were considered distinct from each other, even irrespective of their specific methods, which had preserved some similarities. Each of the two crafts had, around 400 B. C., developed its own methods in response to different demands of the public.

How strictly other authors of the Collection kept prognosis and divination apart theoretically we do not know. That they say little about divination does not prove that they all attached little value to it: their

---

δὲ ὅτι ὁ ἀὴρ τὸ ἑωθινὸν ... τῷ ὕδατι ἐγκαταμιγνύμενος τὸ λαμπρὸν ἀφανίζει ...· ... διὰ τὸν ἠέρα, ὅτι ἀκάθαρτος ὡς ἐπὶ τὸ πολὺ αὐτόθι γίγνεται καὶ νοτώδης (νοτ- Lat., Arab.: νοσ- V)· οὔτε γὰρ ὑπὸ τῶν βορείων ἐκκρίνεται σφόδρα. As one cannot detect any reason why the northwind should not be able to reach such a site, one may suspect that this wind has been introduced by the theorist only as an element of superficial rationalization.

[78] *Vict. IV* 6.640.17–642.5 Li. = 218.14–18 Joly = 4.422 Jones.

[79] 6.642.20–644.1 Li. = 220.8–9 Joly = 4.424 Jones περὶ μὲν οὖν τῆς πρήξιος (namely everyday activity of a bad omen) εἴτ' ἀποτρέπειν εἴτε μή, οὐ κρίνω· τὸ δὲ σῶμα θεραπεύεσθαι συμβουλεύω. Further texts of the Hippocratic Collection concerned with prognosis from dreams are quoted in Lloyd, Magic 43. For the Hellenistic period see, P. H. Schrijvers, La classification des rêves selon Hérophile, Mnemosyne, Ser. IV, 30 (1977), 13–27, and the literature quoted there. Of fundamental importance are three articles by Steven M. Oberhelman: The interpretation of prescriptive dreams in ancient Greek medicine, Journ. of the Hist. of Med. 36 (1981), 416–424; Galen, On Diagnosis from Dreams, *ibid.* 38 (1983), 36–47; The diagnostic dream in ancient medical theory and practice, Bull. of the Hist. of Med. 61 (1987), 47–60.

specialized medical subject-matter and the lack of explicitness of their treatises preclude any such *argumentum e silentio*. Obviously many people among the general public did not systematically differentiate between diviners and medical practitioners, and *On the Sacred Disease* exemplifies the situation. The physician had to compete with divining purifiers.[80]

Divination was based essentially on two distinct principles: *(i)* there was 'natural' or 'intuitive' divination, which was effected through divine inspiration, ecstasy, trance, dreams, etc.; *(ii)* 'artificial' divination, which consisted in interpreting signs of all sorts according to certain sets of rules. This latter method is designated 'inductive divination' in modern terminology. Both principles could be combined; for instance, dreams could be interpreted according to rules.

'Natural,' 'intuitive' divination has no counterpart in medical prognosis as described in the Hippocratic Collection; such procedures were, instead, used in the incubation rituals of healing deities such as Asklepios.[81] The interpretation of dreams according to technical rules occurs in *On Regimen IV* (cf. above), for instance ch. 89: "To see the sun and the moon and the heaven and the stars pure ... is good."[82] "If it seems to rain gently in calm weather ..., it is good."[83] ch. 90, "If he seems to swim in a lake or in the sea or in rivers, it is not good ...; but when he has a fever, it is good." An important principle of interpretation was analogy.[84]

By far the largest portion of prognostic texts contained in the Hippocratic Collection corresponds to the 'artificial' or 'inductive' method of divination. In order to illustrate the provenance of medical prognosis from the complex of prognostic activities mentioned above, let us now compare to medical prognostic aphorisms both some oracular texts and some texts

---

80 The general public cannot have failed to compare the *therapeutic success* of the magicians to that of the physicians; such a comparison cannot always have been favourable to the medical practitioners, particularly in the case of epilepsy: Lloyd, Magic 49; cf. Parker, Miasma 238. For details, see Temkin, Falling sickness 65–81.

81 Emma J. Edelstein/Ludwig Edelstein, Asclepius: A collection and interpretation of the testimonies, 2 vols, Baltimore, 1945, *passim*; Burkert, Griechische Religion 186 f., 329, 401.

82 *Vict. IV* 6.644.12–13 Li. = 220.18–19 Joly = 4.426 Jones ἥλιον καὶ σελήνην καὶ οὐρανὸν καὶ ἄστρα καθαρὰ ... ἀγαθά.

83 6.652.11–13 Li. = 224.19–20 Joly = 4.434–436 Jones εἰ δὲ δοκέοι ὕεσθαι ὕδατι μαλακῷ ἐν εὐδίῃ ..., ἀγαθόν.

84 6.658.1–4 Li. = 228.3–5 Joly = 4.440 Jones εἰ δὲ κολυμβῆν ἐν λίμνῃ ἢ ἐν θαλάσσῃ ἢ ἐν ποταμοῖσι δοκεῖ, οὐκ ἀγαθόν ...· πυρέσσοντι δὲ ἀγαθόν. More passages: 642.15 Li. = 220.3 Joly = 424 Jones; 652.8, 10 Li. = 224.16, 18 Joly = 434 Jones; 656.15 Li. = 226.28 Joly = 440 Jones; 658.7, 9, 14, 19 Li. = 228.7, 8, 12, 17 Joly = 442 Jones. For analogy as a principle in the interpretation of dreams and of other presages, see above p. 221 f., note 442, and the literature listed on p. 246, note 79.

of traditional weather lore — all belonging to the 'artificial' or 'inductive' type of prediction.

An unofficial method of divination was the interpretation of signs furnished by the human body.[85] This kind of superstition can be traced back to early times, although most of its attestations are from the Hellenistic and later epochs. In the *Odyssey*, for instance, sneezing is a sign which indicates that a wish uttered shortly before will come true (*XVII* 539—547).[86] People who heard a buzzing in their ears took it as a signal that somebody was thinking or talking about them,[87] or simply as a "voice of the gods."[88] Also itching in various regions of the body was taken to indicate future events, frequently so in Plautus (and probably already in his Hellenistic sources).[89] Other relevant signs were the quiverings in the body: Theocritus 3.37, "My right eye quivers; am I going to see her?"[90] Plautus, *Pseudolus* 104—107, "I hope to get money to help you ... ; my eyebrow quivers like that."[91] According to a note contained in a sixth century A. D. text, the Stoic philosopher Poseidonios wrote on divination effected by interpreting involuntary movements of the human body (palpitations, tics, etc.).[92] Perhaps he did so in his work *On Divination.*[93] The reliability of this evidence can, of course, hardly be assessed; only the hazards of the text transmission, however, seem to be responsible for the fact that the oldest complete work on this mode of divination called palmoscopy dates from late antiquity (fourth to seventh centuries A. D.):

---

85 For a short survey (with bibliography) about the methods of ancient divination see, Der Kleine Pauly III, 968—976 s. v. 'Mantik' (Clemens Zintzen).

86 More material: Arthur S. Pease, The omen of sneezing, Class. Philol. 6 (1911), 429—443; Pease (ed.), Cic., *De div.*, Book II, p. 305 f. (= repr., p. 487 f.).

87 Luc. *Dial. meretr.* 9.2 ἦ που ... ἐβόμβει τὰ ὦτα ὑμῖν; ἀεὶ γὰρ ἐμέμνητο ἡ κεκτημένη. "Didn't your ears keep buzzing? For she always thought of you." Plin. *N. h. XXVIII* 24 (ch. 5), Quin et absentes tinnitu aurium praesentire sermones de se receptum est.

88 Ael. *Var. hist.* 4.17, [Pythagoras said that] ὁ πολλάκις ἐμπίπτων τοῖς ὠσὶν ἦχος φωνὴ τῶν κρειττόνων. Cf. Stat. *Silv. IV* 4.26, Certum est: inde sonus geminas mihi circuit aures.

89 The head, *Bacch.* 1193; the cheeks and teeth, *Poen.* 1315; the teeth, *Amph.* 295; the shoulder-blades, *Pers.* 32; the back, *Mil.* 397.

90 ἄλλεται ὀφθαλμός μευ ὁ δεξιός· ἆρά γ' ἰδησῶ αὐτάν;

91 Spero ... me ... tibi inventurum esse auxilium argentarium ... : ita supercilium salit. Cf. Plaut. *Mil.* 694 on the female diviner "who tells the future from the eyebrow," quae supercilio spicit; Diels, Zuckungsliteratur I, p. 4.

92 Nonnos Abbas (6th c.), Commentary on Greg. Naz. *Or.* 4 (= *Contra Julian.* 1), Migne, Patrol. Graeca 36, 1024; Suda s. v. Οἰωνιστική (οι 163 = vol. 4, p. 627 Adler), and s. v. Ποσειδώνιος (π 2110 = *ibid.* p. 180).

93 Theiler, Poseidonios, vol. 2, p. 307, 415 (following Karl Reinhardt, Kosmos und Sympathie, München, 1926, 234 f.) thinks the testimonies quoted in the preceding note are erroneous. Edelstein/Kidd, Posidonius p. 92 however classify only the work mentioned by Nonnos Abbas as dubious.

Melampous, *On Palpitations.*[94] Its sources must have been considerably older,[95] and the mode of divination as such may be archaic.

A comparison of these so-called prophecies of Melampous (which probably reflect much older texts) with aphoristic medical predictions contained in the Hippocratic Collection reveals that both texts prognosticate future events by reference to somatic signs, or to combinations of such signs; neither contains even traces of any practices involving divine inspiration or magic. The correctness of the predictions in both texts, if put to the test with methods of modern statistics, would possibly prove more or less the same: the prophecies of Melampous must have been applicable to a great number of possible future events, i. e. have often been 'correct' from an ancient user's point of view, because of the vagueness of their wording.[96]

---

[94] Μελάμποδος ἱερογραμματέως περὶ παλμῶν μαντικὴ πρὸς Πτολεμαῖον βασιλέα, edited with its parallel versions by Diels, Zuckungsliteratur I, II. — The codex Athous Iberon 4301 (181) mentioned by Diels I, p. 16, contains on fol. 2r—11v the text of Diels's Melampous (Version A). It is a text source independent of the codices collated by Diels but does not provide considerable text improvements. The name Melampous does not occur in it. Instead, the title reads αἰλιανοῦ περὶ παλμῶν, πρὸς πτολεμαῖον βασιλέα: περὶ παλμῶν μαντικὴ πρὸς βασιλέα πτολεμαῖον (sic). The explicit reads τέλος τῶν παλμῶν δαμαντίνου (sic) σοφιστοῦ πρὸς τὸν πτολεμαῖον βασιλέα. The forms ΑΙΛΙΑΝΟΥ and ΔΑΜΑΝΤΙΝΟΥ (pro ΑΔΑΜΑΝΤΙΟΥ?) may all be majuscule blunders instead of a collateral form of the genitive, ΜΕΛΑΜΠΟΥ, cf. W. Pape/G. Benseler, Wörterbuch der griechischen Eigennamen, Braunschweig, 1911 (= repr. Graz, 1959), s. v., and the classical Οἰδίποδος/Οἰδίπου. — Generally on this kind of divination cf. C. E. Ruelle, La palmomantique, Rev. de Philologie 32 (1908), 137—141.

[95] Diels, Zuckungsliteratur I, p. 8 ff.; II, p. 56 f. Besides the signs furnished by the body through involuntary actions, permanent signs were also interpreted by fortune-tellers (physiognomical features, signs on the hands, birth-marks *et sim.*), Pauly/Wissowa XIV. 1 (27. Halbband), 1287 f. s. v. 'Mantike' (Th. Hopfner). Cf. the ample "Sylloge locorum" of ancient testimonia in Richard Foerster (ed.), Scriptores physiognomonici Graeci et Latini, vol. 2, Leipzig, 1893, 233—352. See also above p. 200 f. (physiognomical signs in the *Epidemics*).

[96] Both the *Koan Prognoses* and the so-called Melampous handbook exhibit a traditional order in describing the phenomena of the body, namely the sequence 'from the head to the heel' (*a capite ad calcem*). In *Coac.*, where also other orders appear, this disposition starts with paragraph 156 (5.617.17 Li.); cf. Littré's translation, also his remark p. 574. The order was in fact traditional. It is found also in the nosological works (Jouanna, Hippocrate, p. 26 f., with a footnote providing bibliography) and in anatomical descriptions (*Loc. Hom., Oss., Anat.*), where perhaps the traditional doctrine about the humours descending from the head and thus causing diseases has prompted this mode of disposition. Also *Prog.* once has the sequence *a capite ad calcem* (*v. supra* p. 160, note 148). Cf., in addition, *Epid. VI* 5.330.2—8, an instruction to start with the head when examining the body. The same order was followed in pre-Greek Egyptian texts, cf. Hermann Grapow, Grundriss der Medizin der alten Ägypter, vol. 1: Anatomie und Physiologie, Berlin, 1954, p. 12. It stayed popular until the Byzantine time and later; see Otmar Schissel—Fleschenberg (Wolfgang Eisner), Eine kosmische Ausdeutung des menschlichen Körpers, Wiener Stud. 61/62 (1943—1947), 88—97.

Here are some isolated medical sentences (aphorisms) exhibiting a rather simple structure, followed by similar predictions of Melampous. *Koan Prognoses* 235: "If the lip is contracted, it indicates a violent bilious bowel-movement."[97] Melampous 39–40: "If the upper lip quivers, it indicates a quarrel with somebody and a victory; for a slave something good, for a virgin a gain. If the lower lip quivers, it indicates something useful or punishment for what one has done."[98] – *Koan Prognoses* 189: "Tinnitus and buzzing in the ears, during acute diseases, is fatal."[99] Melampous 45: "If the right ear quivers or buzzes, this means joy about something; for a slave good luck, for a virgin an acquisition, for a widow something good."[100] – *Koan Prognoses* 8: "Frequent shiverings from the back, which alternate rapidly, indicate a bad condition."[101] Melampous 124–125: "If the right side of the back quivers, it indicates an outrage. The left side indicates profusion in case of a rich person, labour in case of a poor one."[102] – *Koan Prognoses* 292: "Palpitations at the stomach during fever provoke disorders of consciousness."[103] Melampous 113–114: "If the stomach quivers, it indicates good things ... If the right side of the stomach quivers, it indicates a short disease."[104] – *Koan Prognoses* 73: "During fevers, pain in the groin indicates a long disease."[105] Melampous 137–138: "If the right side of the groin quivers, it indicates violence and troubles. If the left side of the groin quivers, it indicates something not good."[106]

The form of the simple medical aphorisms is possibly archaic and rooted in popular lore. The sentences themselves, however, need not be very old (see above, p. 224, note 451, about the nuclei of prognostic aphorisms and their extensions). The author of a rather elaborate Hippocratic treatise on prognosis, *Prorrhetics II*, may have had this simple type

---

97 *Coac.* 5.636.4–5 χεῖλος συσπώμενον σημαίνει κοιλίης χολώδεος κατάρρηξιν (κατάρρηξιν A: καταρραγησομένης IR). The reading of IR would make sense with σημεῖον.

98 χεῖλος τὸ ἄνωθεν ἐὰν ἄλληται, διάκρισιν πρός τινα καὶ νίκην σημαίνει· δούλῳ ἀγαθόν, παρθένῳ κέρδος. χεῖλος τὸ κάτω ἀλλόμενον ὠφέλειαν ἢ ἔργου ζημίαν δηλοῖ.

99 *Coac.* 5.624.18–19 βόμβος ἐν ὀξέσι (β. ἐν ὀ. IR: καὶ β. δὲ A) καὶ ἦχος ἐν ὠσὶ θανάσιμον.

100 ὠτίον δεξιὸν ἀλλόμενον ἢ ἠχοῦν χαρὰν ἐπί τινι σημαίνει· δούλῳ εὐφρασίαν, παρθένῳ ἐπίκτησιν, χήρᾳ ἀγαθόν.

101 *Coac.* 5.588.11–12 αἱ ἐκ νώτου φρῖκαι πυκναὶ καὶ ὀξέως (ὀ. A: ὅπως IR) μεταπίπτουσαι δύσφοροι. Cf. *Prorrh. I* 75 (5.528.12–530.1 Li.).

102 νῶτος δεξιὸς ἀλλόμενος ὕβριν δηλοῖ· ὁ δ' εὐώνυμος πλουσίῳ εὐωχίαν δηλοῖ, πένητι δὲ κάματον.

103 *Coac.* 5.648.16–17 οἱ κατὰ κοιλίην ἐν πυρετῷ παλμοὶ ἐκστάσιας ποιέουσιν. Cf. *Prorrh. I* 144 (5.562.11–564.1 Li.).

104 κοιλία ἀλλομένη ἀγαθὰ σημαίνει ...· κοιλίας δεξιὸν μέρος ἀλλόμενον νόσον ὀλιγοχρόνιον δηλοῖ.

105 *Coac.* 5.600.4–5 ἐν πυρετοῖσι βουβῶνος ἄλγημα νοῦσον χρονίην σημαίνει.

106 βουβὼν δεξιὸς ἀλλόμενος βίας καὶ ταραχὰς δηλοῖ. βουβὼν εὐώνυμος ἀλλόμενος οὐκ ἀγαθὸν σημαίνει.

of prediction in mind[107] when he criticized those physicians who, right upon first entering the room of a patient given up by the other doctors, say: "This man will not die but get blind," or "The man will get well but have a lame arm," or "He will recover, but his toes will get black and putrid and fall off." The author gives other similar examples of allegedly correct "prophesies" (as he calls them) and declares that he does not believe any of these stories about the correctness of such predictions. He adds: "I am not going to practise divination of that sort" [in my book].[108]

Traditional weather lore had for the most part the same structure.[109] It is sufficient to quote a few predictions from Ps.-Theophrastus *On Weather Signs*, a treatise of unknown date which contains peripatetic material also used by *Aratus*:[110] § 30, "If during southwind glued objects make a noise, it indicates a change to northwind. — If the feet swell, there is a change to southwind. — The same indicates storm."[111] § 34, "If the Etesians blow for a long time and the autumn is windy, the winter will be windless. — If the opposite happens, the winter will be opposite."[112] § 41, "If in autumn the sheep or cattle dig holes and sleep keeping their heads close together, it signifies a hard winter ... — Cattle eating more than usual and lying on

---

[107] In *Prorrh. II* 9.20.11—15, the author refers to discussions on prognosis which he had with medical colleagues "and their sons and pupils" (παισί τε καὶ μαθητῇσιν), and to prognostic literature (ξυγγράμματα).

[108] *Prorrh. II* 9.6.3—8.6 ... προφητίζειν καὶ πάντα ἀληθεύειν ...· ἐγὼ δὲ τοιαῦτα μὲν οὐ μαντεύσομαι. In 9.10.21—26, the uncertainty of "human" prognoses is contrasted to spectacular accounts of allegedly "miraculous" predictions (ἀνθρωπίνως/τερατωδεστέρως, cf. ἀνθρωπινωτέρως 8.11); Lloyd, Magic 45, note 195. See also above p. 242f.

[109] Literature with further bibliography: Maximilianus Heeger, De Theophrasti qui fertur ΠΕΡΙ ΣΗΜΕΙΩΝ libro, Leipzig (diss. phil.), 1889; Pauly/Wissowa, Suppl. VII, 1354—1562 s. v. 'Theophrastos 3' (O. Regenbogen), in partic. 1412—1415 (about Περὶ σημείων); Albert Schott (transl.)/Robert Böker (comment.), Aratos, München, 1958 (Das Wort der Antike, VI); Pauly/Wissowa, Suppl. IX, 1609—1692 s. v. 'Wetterzeichen' (R. Böker); Graziano Arrighetti, Problemi di letteratura meteorologica greca, Maia 15 (1963), 399—441; Pauly/Wissowa, Suppl. X, 26—39, and Suppl. XIV, 55 s. v. 'Aratos' (Walther Ludwig); Manfred Erren, Die Phainomena des Aratos von Soloi, Wiesbaden, 1967 (Hermes Einzelschr., 19), 227—300; Der Kleine Pauly, V, 1372f. s. v. 'Wetterzeichen' (F. Lasserre).

[110] Theophrasti Eresii opera, ed. Fridericus Wimmer, Paris, 1866, 389—398; reproduced with English translation in: Theophrastus, ed. Arthur Hort, vol. 2, London, 1916, 390—433.

[111] Ἐὰν δὲ νοτίων ὄντων ψοφῇ τῶν κεκολλημένων, εἰς τὰ †νότια† (τἀναντία scripserim: βόρεια ci. Furlanus) σημαίνει τὴν μεταβολήν. — ἐὰν δὲ πόδες οἰδῶσι, νοτία ἡ μεταβολή. — τὸ δὲ αὐτὸ σημεῖον καὶ ἐκνεφίου. For the prediction of southwind from signs of the body cf. *Hum.* 5.498.7—9 Li. = 4.90 Jones (above, p. 170).

[112] Ἐὰν ἐτησίαι πολὺν χρόνον πνεύσωσι καὶ μετόπωρον γένηται ἀνεμῶδες, ὁ χειμὼν νήνεμος γίνεται. — ἐὰν δ' ἐναντίως, καὶ ὁ χειμὼν ἐναντίος.

their right sides are a sign of storm."[113] § 44, "If the spring and the summer are cold, the late summer and the autumn are hot and windless."[114]

As has been demonstrated in the preceding chapter, most of the prognostic aphorisms of the Collection have a more involved structure, and some of these complex aphorisms might be more recent. As in the case of the medical prescriptions,[115] however, one should be careful not to declare a text recent only because it has a more complex logical form. A fragmentary Ephesian inscription on augury dated from the middle or end of the sixth century B. C. serves as an example. In spite of its early date, it exhibits a rather sophisticated structure:

"If it [the bird] flies from right to left:
 if it disappears, it is good;
 but if it lifts its left wing and if it flies away and if it disappears, it is bad.
But if it flies from left to right:
 if it disappears straight away, it is bad;
 but if it disappears after lifting its right wing and after flying away, it is good."[116]

Similar forms of prognostic aphorisms are contained in the Hippocratic Collection, but rarely:

Epidemics VI 1.13, "Tears in acute diseases, when being in a bad condition:
 if voluntary, good;
 if flowing involuntarily, bad."[117]
Aphorisms VII 37, "Those who vomit blood:
 if without fever, wholesome;
 if with fever, bad."[118]

---

[113] Μετοπώρῳ ἐὰν πρόβατα ἢ βόες ὀρύττωσι καὶ κοιμῶνται ἀθρόοι πρὸς ἀλλήλους ἔχοντες τὰς κεφαλάς, τὸν χειμῶνα χειμέριον σημαίνει ... — βόες μᾶλλον ἐσθίοντες τοῦ εἰωθότος καὶ ἐπὶ τὸ δεξιὸν κατακλινόμενοι χειμέριον.

[114] Ἐὰν τὸ ἔαρ καὶ τὸ θέρος ψυχρὰ γίνηται, ἥ τε ὀπώρα γίνεται καὶ μετόπωρον πνιγηρὸν καὶ οὐκ ἀνεμῶδες.

[115] Cf. above p. 68–72.

[116] [----- ἐγ μὲν δεξι] | [ῆς ἐς τὴν ⁝ ἀριστερὴν ⁝ πετ] | [όμεν]ος ⁝ ἢμ μὲν ⁝ ἀποκρύψε|[ι, δε] ξιός ⁝ ἢν δὲ ⁝ ἐπάρει ⁝ τὴ[ν] | [ε]ὐώνυμον ⁝ πτέρυγα ⁝ κἂν | [ἀπά]ρει ⁝ κἂν ἀποκρύψει ⁝ ε| [ὐώ]νυμος ⁝ ἐγ δὲ ⁝ τῆς ἀριστ | [ερῆ]ς ⁝ ἐς τὴν δεξιὴν ⁝ πετό|[μ]ενος ⁝ ἢμ μὲν ⁝ ἰθὺς ⁝ ἀποκρ | [ύ]ψει ⁝ εὐώνυμος ⁝ ἢν δὲ ⁝ τὴν | [δεξ]ιὴν πτέρυγα ⁝ ἐπάρας | [κἂν ⁝ ἀπάρας ⁝ ἀποκρύψει] | [δεξιός -----------] Quoted after Franciszek Sokolowski, Lois sacrées de l'Asie Mineure, Paris, 1955, no. 30. Wilhelm Dittenberger, Sylloge inscriptionum Graecarum, 3rd ed., Leipzig, 1920 (= repr. Hildesheim, 1960), no. 1167.

[117] *Epid. VI* 5.272.13–14 δάκρυον ἐν τοῖσιν ὀξέσι τῶν φλαύρως ἐχόντων, ἑκόντων μὲν χρηστόν· ἀκόντων δὲ παραρρέον κακόν. Cf., for a similar structure, lines 5 ff.

[118] *Aph.* 4.586.10–588.1 = 4.200 Jones ὁκόσοι (ὁκόσοι M: ὁκόσοισιν C′ V) αἷμα ἐμέουσιν, ἢν μὲν ἄνευ πυρετοῦ, σωτήριον· ἢν δὲ ξὺν πυρετῷ, κακόν. Cf. the preceding aphorism and *Aph. I* 2 (4.458.7–11 Li. = 4.98 Jones).

Koan Prognoses 77, "Those who in a continuous fever lie without voice and blink while their eyes are closed:
if they regain voice and consciousness after nosebleeding and subsequent vomiting, they recover;
if that does not occur, they will have respiratory troubles and die immediately."[119]

Further examples are found even in an early[120] nosological treatise, *On Diseases II*, ch. 22[121] and ch. 57.[122] Both the simple and this more complicated form of prognostic aphorisms may, therefore, be archaic. Even their content may be rather ancient.

That the simple prognostic aphorisms and the phrases which are the nuclei of the expanded type are, as a rule, *affirmative* sentences with the structure "A indicates B,"[123] is a characteristic which these aphorisms have in common with oracular statements like those of Melampous, with weather-lore and the like.[124]

Occasionally, also the apparatus of medical prognosis recalls oracular techniques: One branch of divination in antiquity read the future from observing whether objects thrown into the water floated or went under.[125] The procedure is recommended also in the Hippocratic Collection, *Koan Prognoses* 427: "Patients suffering from *phthísis*, whose purulent expectoration when spat into sea-water sinks to the bottom, will die promptly; but the sea-water must be in a bronze vessel."[126]

A further affinity between divination and prognosis consists in the content of the structure "A indicates B." For "B," the oracular texts have, as standard expressions, "good" and "bad,"[127] just like the prognostic aphorisms, where the same vague expressions abound. For instance, in *Prorrhetics I*, § 39–96, predictions are made by using various synonyms

---

119 *Coac.* 5.600.9–12 ὅσοι ἐν ξυνεχεῖ ἄφωνοι κείμενοι μύοντες καρδαμύσσουσιν (κ- A: σκ- IR), ἢν αἵματος ῥυέντος ἐκ ῥινῶν (post ῥ. add. ῥυῆ AIR) ἐμέσαντες φθέγξωνται καὶ (καὶ A: om. IR) παρ' αὑτοῖσι (παρ' αὑτοῖσι IR: παρὰ τοῖσι A) γένωνται, σῴζονται· μὴ γενομένων δὲ τούτων δύσπνοοι γενόμενοι θνήσκουσι συντόμως. Cf. 616.8–10.

120 See above p. 25, 52 f.

121 *Morb. II* 7.36.14–16 Li. = 156.10–12 Jouanna, quoted above p. 67.

122 *Morb. II* 7.90.2–5 Li. = 197.2–5 Jouanna, quoted above p. 60 f. with note 163.

123 For the structure of the prognostic aphorisms, see above p. 224–226. Rarely the nucleus is a question: above p. 225 f., note 456.

124 Of course, this structure is the most natural and appropriate one anyhow.

125 For instance Paus. *III* 23.8; Zosim. *I* 58, cf. the commentary by François Paschoud (ed.), Zosime I, Paris, 1971, 167 f. Further attestations are listed in Pauly/Wissowa IX.1 (17. Halbband), 84 f. s. v. 'Hydromanteia' (Boehm); XIV.1 (27. Halbband), 1285 s. v. 'Mantike' (Th. Hopfner).

126 *Coac.* 5.680.14–15 Τῶν φθισικῶν οἷσιν ἐπὶ θάλασσαν πτύουσιν ἐς τὸν πυθμένα βαδίζει τὸ πύον, ὀλέθριον συντόμως· ἔστω δὲ ἐν χαλκῷ ἡ θάλασσα.

127 Cf. the augural inscription.

of "bad;" other examples are contained in the prognostic chapters about dreams in *On Regimen IV* quoted above. It seems that medical prognosis, when forecasting simply "bad" or "good," functioned to help in attaining conformity of opinion[128] among physicians, patients, relatives, etc. and in making the decision as to whether treatment should or should not be undertaken. In this context a more detailed prognosis was often not necessary, quite apart from the fact that more details might have entailed the risk of erroneous prediction. Similarly, forecasts in fields other than medicine were often concerned with helping to make a decision rather than with indicating details of the future; divination proper very frequently provided just good omens or bad omens; weather predictions also most often indicated simply "rain," "wind," "cold," "fair weather" in answer to the farmer's or sailor's perennial question as to whether or not one should plow or sail, etc. It is not surprising that in the medical prognostic aphorisms "bad" is more often predicted than "good:" there was less need for the physician to prognosticate a favourable outcome. If the patient recovered, this was not at the practitioner's risk. If, however, the physician failed to predict the death of his patient, he was likely to be held accountable and to risk his professional reputation.

[128] Cf. above p. 232.

Concluding Remarks

With regard to the subject of this book – the application and evolution of medical theories in the fifth and fourth centuries B.C. –, five questions were formulated in the "Introduction." It was stated there that they could not be asked or responded to sequentially. Answers have been proposed in diverse contexts throughout the entire book and remain more or less tentative, given the fragmentary nature of the historical sources.

Question *(i)* was: "What are the medical theories contained in the writings of the Hippocratic Collection?" Since the term 'theory' is anachronistic for the Hippocratic Collection, the present study was not based on a modern definition or concept of 'theory.' The word was, instead, taken in its vague modern colloquial meaning as a heuristic tool, synonymous with 'doctrine.' Textual analysis was concentrated on two groups of sources occupying opposite ends of a chronological continuum: on the relatively early nosological texts of *On Diseases II,* ch. 12–75, which describe the symptoms, treatment, and prognosis of particular diseases (such as *íkteros* or *pleurîtis*); and, on the other hand, more recent texts, especially the *Epidemics* and kindred treatises, which describe symptoms and prognosis rather independently from particular diseases. Other nosological texts besides those of *On Diseases II,* ch. 12–75 were not included systematically, because their relative chronology is unclear. The restricted choice of sources, as well as the impossibility of defining 'theory' account for the fact that the answers given to the first question are inexhaustive, despite the numerous doctrinal details.

In response to questions *(ii)* and *(iii)* – "To what extent do these theories contradict each other?" and "To what extent are they compatible with each other?" – there are no testimonia for the decades around 400 B.C. which prove that the medical centres were opposed to each other and held peculiar, mutually exclusive doctrines: the dichotomy of Kos versus Knidos is unwarranted. In the texts analysed, doctrinal contradictions did not appear to be related to any 'schools,' but to be restricted to marginal features of the doctrines. The theoretical approach of nosology, as represented by the nosological texts *On Diseases II,* ch. 12–75, was based on sensory observation, little aetiological speculation, and a flexibility of application; it was not superseded by that of the *Epidemics* and kindred treatises but remained by and large compatible and was absorbed. Any physician using the *Epidemics* was supposed to have a nosological training.

The answer to questions *(ii)* and *(iii)* implies an affirmative response to question *(iv)*: "Can these theories be grouped as stages of a general historical development of Greek medicine?" Indeed, not only did the relatively ancient nosological works continue to be useful to physicians who adhered to the more recent method of the *Epidemics* and of kindred treatises, but also the new paradigm of the *Epidemics* did not subsequently render the production of new nosological texts superfluous: the evolution of medical theory consisted in a change of interest and viewpoint rather than in the abrogation of doctrines; nosology, though still important, henceforth no longer remained the centre of the Hippocratic physician's attention.

Question *(v)* was bipartite: "On what general outlines did this development take place, and what are the specific steps involved?" The answer to the first part has just been indicated above; as for the second part of the question, the historian can observe that the *Epidemics* presupposed traditional nosology and re-interpreted it in the light of their own new doctrines; but their doctrinal innovations are nowhere set forth systematically in our sources: a characteristic trait of the *Epidemics* and of kindred texts is their lack of explicitness. It is certainly possible to make out single 'steps' such as the evolution of the doctrine of *krísis* (including *pépsis* and *apóstasis*) from rudimentary origins; the growing influence of meteorological doctrines; and the application of prognostic aphorisms to individual cases of disease. Any chronological sequence, however, of these 'steps' cannot be established. It is likewise possible to make inferences about the research methods applied by the authors of the *Epidemics*. Problems discussed in this book were, among others: How did the authors presuppose and use traditional nosology? The answer has just been outlined. – What theoretical questions did they ask, and how did they manage to reconcile their theories with the observed facts? They tended to widen the range of applicability of their doctrines. – How did they collect data? They started from their theories; for certain purposes they used a 'questionnaire.' – What methods of inference did they use? They mentally constructed 'types' and 'groups' of patients and diseases. – How did they verify their findings? Applicability served as a 'proof.' – How sceptical were they? They were cautious with regard to details, but less sceptical with regard to the fundamental assumptions of their own main doctrines, which they never questioned.

Despite the availability of answers concerning single 'steps,' the historical development that led to the *Epidemics* cannot be traced, even though the motives for this development are obvious: physicians reacted to a failure of traditional nosology to describe adequately what they themselves and their patients observed.

The doctrinal system of the *Epidemics* remains in many respects unclear to us. But speculation about what might be concealed behind the veil of inexplicitness did not lie within the scope of this book, since it is not even known how systematic, or coherent, the theories underlying the *Epidemics* were. Instead of 'reconstructing' a 'system' of the Hippocratic doctrines presupposed in these treatises, single doctrinal features and methods were selected for this study. Just as the problem of chronology was averted by selecting text sources from two distant stages (*On Diseases II*, ch. 12–75, and the *Epidemics*), modern systematization was avoided by concentrating on single doctrines and methods of the *Epidemics*. This procedure along with the above-mentioned refusal to define the word 'theory' accounts for the at times fragmentary character of the present book. Its intention has been to contribute details to a reconstruction of Greek intellectual life during an epoch in which medical theories were not the exclusive domain of the professional physician, but were common knowledge at least as far as the principal assumptions were concerned. Often the physician's *tékhnē* served as an intellectual stimulus outside of the medical profession: in Plato, Aristotle, and others, knowledge of medical doctrines is frequently presupposed on the part of the reader, whenever the art of medicine is used as a methodological model for other fields of human activity. On the other hand, medicine mirrored common modes of thought, not only of contemporary philosophy, but also of more traditional provinces such as agriculture, politics, warfare, and religion. To elucidate more comprehensively the rôle of Greek medical theorizing as an integral and influential part of Greek culture in the fifth and fourth centuries B.C. would be a rewarding project for further research.

Bibliography

Works contained in the following selection are referred to by author and/or abridged title. Editions of, and commentaries on, ancient texts are listed under the respective ancient author.

General bibliographies on Hippocrates and the Hippocratic Collection: Bruni Celli, Blas, Bibliografía hipocrática, Caracas, 1984. — Fichtner, Gerhard, Corpus Hippocraticum. Verzeichnis der hippokratischen und pseudohippokratischen Schriften, Tübingen (Institut für Geschichte der Medizin), 1988. — Maloney, Gilles / Savoie, Raymond, Cinq cent ans de bibliographie hippocratique: 1473—1982, St-Jean-Chrysostome (Québec), 1982.

Lexical works: Kühn, Josef-Hans / Fleischer, Ulrich, Index Hippocraticus, Göttingen, 1986—1989. — Maloney, Gilles / Frohn, Winnie, Concordance des œuvres hippocratiques, Montréal, 1984 (= Hildesheim, 1986). — Still a useful tool is the Table alphabétique in Littré, vol. 10, 471—848.

Anonymus Londinensis: Anonymi Londinensis ... eclogae, ed. Diels, Hermann (Supplementum Aristotelicum, III 1), Berlin, 1893.

—: Jones, W. H. S., The medical writings of Anonymus Londinensis, Cambridge, 1947.

[Aristoteles], Problemata physica, übersetzt von Flashar, Hellmut (Aristoteles, Werke in deutscher Übersetzung, 19), 3rd ed., Berlin, 1983.

Bertier, Janine, Mnésithée et Dieuchès (Philosophia antiqua, 20), Leiden, 1972.

Böhme, Joachim, Die Seele und das Ich im homerischen Epos, Leipzig/Berlin, 1929.

Bourgey, Louis, Observation et expérience chez les médecins de la Collection hippocratique, Paris, 1953.

Brunn, L. von, Hippokrates und die meteorologische Medizin (1—3), Gesnerus 3 (1946), 151—173; 4 (1947), 1—18, 65—85.

Burkert, Walter, Griechische Religion der archaischen und klassischen Epoche (Die Religionen der Menschheit, 15), Stuttgart, 1977.

—, Lore and science in ancient Pythagoreanism, Cambridge, Mass., 1972.

—, Die orientalisierende Epoche in der griechischen Religion und Literatur (Sitzungsberichte der Heidelberger Akademie der Wissenschaften, Philosophisch-historische Klasse, 1984, 1), Heidelberg, 1984.

Cicero: Marci Tulli Ciceronis De divinatione libri duo, ed. Pease, Arthur S., Univ. of Illinois Studies in Language and Literature 6 (1920), 161—500, and 8 (1923), 153—474 (books I and II respectively; reprinted in 1 vol., Darmstadt, 1963).

Cohn-Haft, Louis, The public physicians of ancient Greece (Smith College Studies in History, 42), Northampton, Mass., 1956.

La Collection hippocratique et son rôle dans l'histoire de la médecine. Colloque de Strasbourg (23—27 octobre 1972) (Université des Sciences Humaines de Strasbourg, Travaux du Centre de Recherche sur le Proche-Orient et la Grèce Antiques, 2), Leiden, 1975.

"Corpus Hippocraticum." Actes du colloque hippocratique de Mons (22—26 septembre 1975), édités par Joly, Robert (Éditions universitaires de Mons, Série Sciences humaines, IV), Mons, 1977.

Corpus Paroemiographorum Graecorum, edd. von Leutsch, E. L. / Schneidewin, F. G., vols 1—2, Göttingen, 1839, 1851 (= repr. Hildesheim, 1965).

Coulter, Harris L., Divided legacy: A history of the schism in medical thought, vol. 1, Washington, D. C., 1975.
Deichgräber, Karl, Die griechische Empirikerschule, 2nd ed., Berlin, 1965.
—, Die Epidemien und das Corpus Hippocraticum. Voruntersuchungen zu einer Geschichte der koischen Ärzteschule, 2nd ed., Berlin, 1971.
—, Aus der Geschichte der wissenschaftlichen Kritik im Corpus Hippocraticum, Medizinhist. Journ. 6 (1971), 97—112.
—, Zur Milchtherapie der Hippokratiker, in: Medizingeschichte in unserer Zeit. Festgabe für Edith Heischkel und Walter Artelt zum 65. Geburtstag, Stuttgart, 1971, 36—53.
—, Die Patienten des Hippokrates. Historisch-prosopographische Beiträge zu den Epidemien des Corpus Hippocraticum (Akad. d. Wiss. u. d. Lit., Abhandl. d. geistes- u. sozialwiss. Kl. 1982, 9), Mainz/Wiesbaden, 1982.
Di Benedetto, Vincenzo, Cos e Cnido, in: Hippocratica 97—111.
Diels, Hermann, Die Fragmente der Vorsokratiker, hrsg. von Kranz, Walther, vols 1—3, 6th ed., Dublin, 1967 sqq. (repr. of the 6th ed., 1951, 1952).
—, Beiträge zur Zuckungsliteratur des Okzidents und Orients, *I*: Die griechische Zukkungsliteratur (Melampus, Περὶ παλμῶν), Abhandl. der Preuss. Akad. d. Wiss., Philos.-histor. Classe, 1907, no. IV; *II*: Weitere griechische und aussergriechische Literatur und Volksüberlieferung, *ibid.*, 1908, no. IV.
Diller, Hans, Ausdrucksformen des methodischen Bewusstseins in den hippokratischen Epidemien, Archiv f. Begriffsgesch. 9 (1964), 133—150 (= Kleine Schriften zur antiken Medizin 106—123).
—, Ὄψις ἀδήλων τὰ φαινόμενα, Hermes 67 (1932), 14—42 (= Kleine Schriften zur antiken Literatur, München, 1971, 119—143).
—, Kleine Schriften zur antiken Medizin, hrsg. von Baader, Gerhard / Grensemann, Hermann (Ars medica, II 3), Berlin, 1973.
—, Wanderarzt und Aitiologe. Studien zur hippokratischen Schrift Περὶ ἀέρων ὑδάτων τόπων (Philologus Suppl. XXVI 3), Leipzig, 1934.
Dittmer, Hans-L., Konstitutionstypen im Corpus Hippocraticum, Würzburg-Aumühle, 1940 (doctoral thesis).
Dodds, Eric R., The ancient concept of progress, Oxford, 1973.
—, The Greeks and the irrational, Berkeley/Los Angeles, 1968.
Dover, Kenneth J., Ion of Chios: His place in the history of Greek literature, in: Boardman, John / Vaphopoulou-Richardson, C. E. (edd.), Chios: A conference at the Homereion in Chios, Oxford, 1987, 27—37.
Ducatillon, Jeanne, Polémiques dans la Collection hippocratique, Lille/Paris, 1977.
Düring, Ingemar, Aristoteles. Darstellung und Interpretation seines Denkens, Heidelberg, 1966.
Edelstein, Ludwig, Περὶ ἀέρων und die Sammlung der hippokratischen Schriften (Problemata, 4), Berlin, 1931.
—, 'Hippokrates,' in: Pauly/Wissowa, Realencyclopädie, Suppl. VI, 1290—1345.
—, The idea of progress in classical antiquity, Baltimore, 1967.
Edelstein, Ludwig / Kidd, I. G., Posidonius: I. The fragments, Cambridge, 1972.
Emonds, Hilarius, Zweite Auflage im Altertum (Klassisch-philolog. Studien, 14), Leipzig, 1941.
Ermerins, Franciscus Z., De Hippocratis doctrina a prognostice oriunda, Lugduni Batavorum, 1832.
Flashar, Hellmut (ed.), Antike Medizin (Wege der Forschung, CCXXI), Darmstadt, 1971.
—, Melancholie und Melancholiker, Berlin, 1966.
Fleischer, Ulrich, Untersuchungen zu den pseudohippokratischen Schriften Παραγγελίαι, Περὶ ἰητροῦ und Περὶ εὐσχημοσύνης (Neue deutsche Forschungen, Abt. Klassische Philologie, 10), Berlin, 1939.

Formes de pensée dans la Collection hippocratique. Actes du IVe Colloque international hippocratique (Lausanne, 21–26 septembre 1981), édition préparée par Lasserre, François, et Mudry, Philippe (Université de Lausanne, Publications de la Faculté des lettres, 26), Genève, 1983.

Fraser, P. M., Ptolemaic Alexandria, Oxford, 1972.

Fredrich, Carl, Hippokratische Untersuchungen (Philologische Untersuchungen, 15), Berlin, 1899.

Galen: Claudii Galeni opera omnia, ed. Kühn, C. G., vols 1–20, Leipzig, 1821–1833 (= repr. Hildesheim, 1964–1965).

—: Galeni In Hippocratis De natura hominis comm. III, ed. Mewaldt, I.; In Hippocratis De victu acutorum comm. IV, ed. Helmreich, G. (Corpus Medicorum Graecorum, V 9.1), Leipzig, 1914.

—: Galeni In Hippocratis Prorrheticum I comm. III, ed. Diels, H.; De comate secundum Hippocratem, ed. Mewaldt, I.; In Hippocratis Prognosticum comm. III, ed. Heeg, I. (Corpus Medicorum Graecorum, V 9.2), Leipzig, 1915.

—: Galeni In Hippocratis Epidemiarum librum I comm. III, ed. Wenkebach, E.; In Hippocratis Epidemiarum librum II comm. V, in Germanicam linguam transtulit Pfaff, F. (Corpus Medicorum Graecorum, V 10.1), Leipzig, 1934.

—: Galeni In Hippocratis Epidemiarum librum III comm. III, ed. Wenkebach, E. (Corpus Medicorum Graecorum, V 10.2.1), Leipzig, 1936.

—: Galeni In Hippocratis Epidemiarum librum VI comm. I–VI, ed. Wenkebach, E.; comm. VI–VIII, in Germanicam linguam transtulit Pfaff, F. (Corpus Medicorum Graecorum, V 10.2.2), 2nd ed., Berlin, 1956.

Gossen, Hans, 'Hippokrates,' in: Pauly/Wissowa, Realencyclopädie VIII.2 (16. Halbband), 1801–1852.

Grensemann, Hermann, Der Arzt Polybos als Verfasser hippokratischer Schriften (Akad. d. Wiss. u. d. Lit., Abhandl. d. geistes- u. sozialwiss. Kl. 1968, 2), Mainz, 1968.

—, Hippokratische Gynäkologie, Wiesbaden, 1982.

—, Die Krankheit der Tochter des Theodoros. Eine Studie zum siebten hippokratischen Epidemienbuch, Clio Medica 4 (1969), 71–83.

—, Knidische Medizin, Teil I: Die Testimonien zur ältesten knidischen Lehre und Analysen knidischer Schriften im Corpus Hippocraticum (Ars medica, II 4.1), Berlin, 1975.

Grmek, Mirko D., Les maladies à l'aube de la civilisation occidentale, Paris, 1983.

Grmek, Mirko D. / Wittern, Renate, Die Krankheit des attischen Strategen Nikias und die Nierenleiden im Corpus Hippocraticum, Archives internat. d'histoire des sciences 26 (1977), 3–32.

Harris, C. R. S., The heart and the vascular system in ancient Greek medicine, Oxford, 1973.

Heidel, William A., The heroic age of science, Washington, D. C., 1933.

—, Hippocratic medicine: Its spirit and method, New York, 1941.

Herzog, Rudolf, Heilige Gesetze von Kos (Abhandl. d. Preuss. Akad. d. Wiss., Philos.-histor. Klasse, 1928, no. 6), Berlin, 1928.

Hippocrates: Die hippokratische Schrift Prognostikon. Überlieferung und Text, ed. Alexanderson, Bengt (Studia Graeca et Latina Gothoburgensia, XVII), Göteborg, 1963.

—: Hippokratische Gynäkologie. Die gynäkologischen Texte des Autors B, ed. Countouris, Nicolas, Hamburg, 1985 (doctoral thesis).

—: Œuvres choisies d'Hippocrate, traduites par Daremberg, Charles, 2nd ed., Paris, 1855.

—: Hippokrates, Über Entstehung und Aufbau des menschlichen Körpers (Περὶ σαρκῶν), ed. Deichgräber, Karl, Leipzig, 1935.

—: Hippokrates, Über die Umwelt, ed. Diller, Hans (Corpus Medicorum Graecorum, I 1.2), Berlin, 1970.

—: Hippocratis et aliorum medicorum veterum reliquiae, ed. Ermerins, Franciscus Z., vols 1–4, Traiecti ad Rhenum, 1859–1867.

—: Hippocrate, L'ancienne médecine. Introduction, traduction et commentaire, par Festugière, A.-J. (Études et commentaires, 4), Paris, 1948.
—: Hippokrates, Über Achtmonatskinder. Über das Siebenmonatskind (unecht), hrsg., übersetzt und erläutert von Grensemann, Hermann (Corpus Medicorum Graecorum, I 2.1), Berlin, 1968.
—: Die hippokratische Schrift "Über die heilige Krankheit," hrsg., übersetzt und erläutert von Grensemann, Hermann (Ars medica, II 1), Berlin, 1968.
—: Hippocratis opera (Indices librorum, Iusiurandum, Lex, De arte, De medico, De decente habitu, Praeceptiones, De prisca medicina, De aere locis aquis, De alimento, De liquidorum usu, De flatibus), ed. Heiberg, I. L. (Corpus Medicorum Graecorum, I 1), Leipzig, 1927.
—: Hippocrate, Du régime, édité, traduit et commenté par Joly, Robert, avec la collaboration de Byl, Simon (Corpus Medicorum Graecorum, I 2.4), Berlin, 1984.
—: Hippocrate, tome XI (De la génération, De la nature de l'enfant, Des maladies IV, Du foetus de huit mois), ed. Joly, Robert, Paris, 1970.
—: Hippocrate, tome VI, 2e partie (Du régime des maladies aiguës, Appendice, De l'aliment, De l'usage des liquides), ed. Joly, Robert, Paris, 1972.
—: Hippocrate, tome XIII (Des lieux dans l'homme, Du système des glandes, Des fistules, Des hémorrhoïdes, De la vision, Des chairs, De la dentition), ed. Joly, Robert, Paris, 1978.
—: Hippocrates, with an English translation, by Jones, W. H. S. (vols 1, 2, 4) and Withington, E. T. (vol. 3), London/Cambridge, Mass., 1923—1931.
—: Hippocrate, tome X (Maladies II), ed. Jouanna, Jacques, Paris, 1983.
—: Hippocrate, La nature de l'homme, édité, traduit et commenté par Jouanna, Jacques (Corpus Medicorum Graecorum, I 1.3), Berlin, 1975.
—: Hippocratis opera quae feruntur omnia, vols 1—2, ed. Kuehlewein, Hugo, Leipzig, 1894 (vol. 1) and 1902 (vol. 2).
—: Hippokrates, Über Nachempfängnis, Geburtshilfe und Schwangerschaftsleiden, hrsg., übersetzt und erläutert von Lienau, Cay (Corpus Medicorum Graecorum, I 2.2), Berlin, 1973.
—: Œuvres complètes d'Hippocrate, ed. Littré, Émile, vols 1—10, Paris, 1839—1861 (= repr. Amsterdam, 1961—1962).
—: Hippocratic writings, edited with an introduction by Lloyd, Geoffrey E. R. (The Pelican Classics), Harmondsworth, 1978.
—: Ippocrate, Epidemie, Libro sesto. Introduzione, testo critico, commento e traduzione a cura di Manetti, Daniela, e Roselli, Amneris (Biblioteca di studi superiori, 66), Firenze, 1982.
—: Polack, Hilde, Textkritische Untersuchungen zu der hippokratischen Schrift Prorrhetikos I (Hamburger philologische Studien, 44), Hamburg, 1976 [contains a provisional edition of this treatise].
—: Hippokrates, Über die Krankheiten III, hrsg., übersetzt und erläutert von Potter, Paul (Corpus Medicorum Graecorum, I 2.3), Berlin, 1980.
—: Hippocratis quae feruntur epistulae, ed. Putzger, Gualtharius (Wiss. Beilage zum Jahresbericht d. Königl. Gymnasiums in Wurzen), Wurzen, 1914.
—: Ἱπποκράτης, κομιδῇ Reinhold, Carolus H. Th., vols 1—2, Athens, 1864—1867.
—: Die hippokratische Schrift von der Siebenzahl in ihrer vierfachen Überlieferung, hrsg. von Roscher, Wilhelm H. (Studien zur Geschichte u. Kultur des Altertums, VI 3,4), Paderborn, 1913 (= repr. New York, 1967).
—: Die hippokratische Schrift De natura muliebri. Ausgabe und textkritischer Kommentar ... vorgelegt von Trapp, Helga, Hamburg, 1967 (doctoral thesis).
—: Die hippokratische Schrift De morbis I. Ausgabe, Übersetzung und Erläuterungen von Wittern, Renate (Altertumswissenschaftliche Texte und Studien, 3), Hildesheim, 1974.

Hippocratica. Actes du Colloque hippocratique de Paris (4—9 septembre 1978), édition préparée par Grmek, Mirko D. (Colloques internationaux du CNRS, no. 583), Paris, 1980.

Iohannis Alexandrini commentaria in sextum librum Hippocratis Epidemiarum, recogn. Pritchet, C. D., Leiden, 1975.

Jaeger, Werner, Diokles von Karystos, 2nd ed., Berlin, 1963.

Joly, Robert, Le niveau de la science hippocratique. Contribution à la psychologie de l'histoire des sciences, Paris, 1966.

—, La question hippocratique et le témoignage du Phèdre, Rev. Ét. Grecques 74 (1961), 69—92 (German translation with additional comments in: Flashar [ed.], Antike Medizin 52—82).

—, Recherches sur le traité pseudo-hippocratique Du régime, Paris, 1960.

Jouanna, Jacques, Hippocrate. Pour une archéologie de l'école de Cnide, Paris, 1974.

Jurk, Johannes, Ramenta Hippocratea, Berlin, 1900 (doctoral thesis).

Kauder, Egon, Physikalische Modellvorstellung und physiologische Lehre im Corpus Hippocraticum und bei Aristoteles, Hamburg, 1960 (doctoral thesis, unpublished typescript).

Knutzen, Georg H., Technologie in den hippokratischen Schriften περὶ διαίτης ὀξέων, περὶ ἀγμῶν, περὶ ἄρθρων ἐμβολῆς (Akad. d. Wiss. u. d. Lit., Abhandl. d. geistes- u. sozialwiss. Kl. 1963, 14), Mainz, 1964.

Körner, Otto, Die ärztlichen Kenntnisse in Ilias und Odyssee, München, 1929.

Kollesch, Jutta, Die Stellung der knidischen Heilkunde in der wissenschaftlichen Medizin der Griechen, in: "Corpus Hippocraticum" 106—122.

Kudlien, Fridolf, Der griechische Arzt im Zeitalter des Hellenismus (Akad. d. Wiss. u. d. Lit., Abhandl. d. geistes- u. sozialwiss. Kl. 1979, 6), Mainz, 1979.

—, Die Bedeutung des Ungeraden in der hippokratischen Krisenarithmetik, Hermes 108 (1980), 200—205.

—, Der Beginn des medizinischen Denkens bei den Griechen. Von Homer bis Hippokrates, Zürich/Stuttgart, 1967.

—, Bemerkungen zu W. D. Smith's These über die knidische Ärzteschule, in: "Corpus Hippocraticum" 95—103.

—, Das Göttliche und die Natur im hippokratischen Prognostikon, Hermes 105 (1977), 268—274.

—, Early Greek primitive medicine, Clio Medica 3 (1968), 305—336.

—, "Schwärzliche" Organe im frühgriechischen Denken, Medizinhist. Journ. 8 (1973), 53—58.

—, Überlegungen zu einer Sozialgeschichte des frühgriechischen Arztes und seines Berufs, Hermes 114 (1986), 129—146.

Kühn, Josef-Hans, System- und Methodenprobleme im Corpus Hippocraticum (Hermes Einzelschriften, 11), Wiesbaden, 1956.

Kühner, Raphael / Gerth, Bernhard, Ausführliche Grammatik der griechischen Sprache, Zweiter Teil: Satzlehre, vols 1—2, 3rd ed., Hannover, 1898 (vol. 1), 1904 (vol. 2) (= repr. München, 1963).

Kuhn, Thomas S., The structure of scientific revolutions, Chicago/London, 1962.

Kurz, Dietrich, ΑΚΡΙΒΕΙΑ. Das Ideal der Exaktheit bei den Griechen bis Aristoteles (Göppinger Akademische Beiträge, 8), Göppingen, 1970.

Laín Entralgo, Pedro, La historia clínica, 2nd ed., Barcelona/Madrid, 1961.

—, La medicina hipocrática, Madrid, 1970.

Lanata, Giuliana, Medicina magica e religione popolare in Grecia fino all' età di Ippocrate (Filologia e critica, 3), Roma, 1967.

Langholf, Volker, Beobachtungen zur Struktur einiger Traktate des 'Corpus Hippocraticum,' Sudhoffs Archiv 73 (1989), 64—77.

—, Frühe Fälle der "Verwendung" von Analogien in der altgriechischen Medizin, Berichte zur Wissenschaftsgeschichte 12 (1989), 7—18.

–, Generalisationen und Aphorismen in den Epidemienbüchern, in: Die hippokratischen Epidemien. Verhandlungen des Ve Colloque international hippocratique, Berlin 1984, hrsg. von Baader, Gerhard und Winau, Rolf (Sudhoffs Archiv, Beiheft 27), Stuttgart, 1989, 131–143.

–, Kallimachos, Komödie und hippokratische Frage, Medizinhist. Journ. 21 (1986), 3–30.

–, Über die Kompatibilität einiger binärer und quaternärer Theorien im Corpus Hippocraticum, in: Hippocratica 333–346.

–, Symptombeschreibungen in Epidemien I und III und die Struktur des Prognostikon, in: Formes de pensée 109–119.

–, Die parallelen Texte in Epidemien V und VII, in: "Corpus Hippocraticum" 264–274.

–, Syntaktische Untersuchungen zu Hippokrates-Texten. Brachylogische Syntagmen in den individuellen Krankheits-Fallbeschreibungen der hippokratischen Schriftensammlung (Akad. d. Wiss. u. d. Lit., Abhandl. d. geistes- u. sozialwiss. Kl., Einzelveröffentlichung), Mainz/Wiesbaden, 1977.

Lesky, Erna, Die Zeugungs- und Vererbungslehren der Antike und ihr Nachwirken (Akad. d. Wiss. u. d. Lit., Abhandl. d. geistes- u. sozialwiss. Kl. 1950, no. 19), Mainz/Wiesbaden, 1951.

Levine, Edwin B., Hippocrates, New York, 1971.

Lexicon iconographicum mythologiae classicae, vols I.1 ff., Zürich/München, 1981 ff.

Lichtenthaeler, Charles, La médecine hippocratique I: Méthode expérimentale et méthode hippocratique, Lausanne, 1948.

–, La médecine hippocratique II–V, Neuchâtel, 1957.

–, Sur la vocation universitaire de l'histoire de la médecine. (Leçon inaugurale.) Le troisième Épidémique d'Hippocrate vient-il vraiment après le premier? (Sixième étude hippocratique), Genève/Paris, 1960.

–, Quatrième série d'études hippocratiques (VII–X), Genève/Paris, 1963.

–, Der Eid des Hippokrates. Ursprung und Bedeutung (XII. Hippokratische Studie), Köln, 1984.

Liddell, H. G./Scott, R./Jones, H. S., A Greek-English lexicon, Oxford, 1940. Barber, E. A., A supplement, Oxford, 1968.

Lloyd, Geoffrey E. R., Magic, reason, and experience: Studies in the origin and development of Greek science, Cambridge, 1979.

–, Polarity and analogy, Cambridge, 1966.

–, The Hippocratic question, Class. Quart. (N. S.) 25 (1975), 171–192.

–, Science, folklore, and ideology, Cambridge, 1983.

Lonie, Iain M., Cos versus Cnidus and the historians, History of Science 16 (1978), 42–75 (part 1); 77–92 (part 2).

–, Literacy and the development of Hippocratic medicine, in: Formes de pensée 145–161.

–, A structural pattern in Greek dietetics and the early history of Greek medicine, Medical History 21 (1977), 235–260.

–, The Cnidian treatises of the Corpus Hippocraticum, Class. Quart. (N. S.) 15 (1965), 1–30.

–, The Hippocratic treatises "On Generation," "On the Nature of the Child," "Diseases IV" (Ars medica, II 7), Berlin/New York, 1981.

López Férez, Juan Antonio (ed.), Historia de la literatura griega, Madrid, 1988.

Mansfeld, Jaap, Theoretical and empirical attitudes in early Greek scientific medicine, in: Hippocratica 371–391.

Marganne, Marie-Hélène, Sur l'origine hippocratique des concepts de révulsion et de dérivation, Ant. Classique 49 (1980), 115–130.

Müller, Carl Werner, Der Aphorismus 2,1 des sechsten hippokratischen Epidemienbuches, Rhein. Mus. (N. F.) 109 (1966), 120–134.

–, Gleiches zu Gleichem (Klassisch-philologische Studien, 31), Wiesbaden, 1965.

Müri, Walter, Melancholie und schwarze Galle, Mus. Helv. 10 (1953), 21–38 (= repr. in: Flashar [ed.], Antike Medizin 165–191).

Nachmanson, Ernst, Der griechische Buchtitel (Göteborgs Högskolas Årsskrift XLVII 1941: 19), Göteborg, 1941.

Nikitas, Anastasios A., Untersuchungen zu den Epidemienbüchern II IV VI des Corpus Hippocraticum, Hamburg, 1968 (doctoral thesis).

Nilsson, Martin P., Geschichte der griechischen Religion I, II, 3rd ed., München, 1967, 1974.

Nörenberg, Heinz-Werner, Das Göttliche und die Natur in der Schrift Über die Heilige Krankheit, Bonn, 1968.

Onians, Richard B., The origins of European thought about the body, the mind, the soul, the world, time, and fate: New interpretations of Greek, Roman and kindred evidence ..., 2nd ed., Cambridge, 1954.

Oribasius, ed. Raeder, Joannes (Corpus Medicorum Graecorum, VI 1.1–2.2; VI 3), Leipzig, 1926–1933.

Palladii In Hippocratis Epidemiarum librum VI comm. (see in this bibliography under: Scholia in Hippocratem et Galenum, vol. 2, p. 1–204).

Palm, Adolf, Studien zur hippokratischen Schrift Περὶ διαίτης, Tübingen, 1933 (doctoral thesis).

Parker, Robert, Miasma: Pollution and purification in early Greek religion, Oxford, 1983.

Pauly/Wissowa: Paulys Realencyclopädie der classischen Altertumswissenschaft, Neue Bearbeitung ... von Wissowa, Georg, 34 vols (= 68 'Halbbd.'), 15 supplementary vols, 1 index vol., Stuttgart/München, 1893–1980.

Pauly, Der Kleine. Lexikon der Antike, 5 vols, Stuttgart, 1964–1975.

Perazzi, Francesco, Ippocrate. *I.* Valutazione della vita e della personalità. *II.* Le massime prognostiche. Studio del "Prognostico I" e delle "Prognosi di Coo." Torino, 1961.

Pfeiffer, Erwin, Studien zum antiken Sternglauben (ΣΤΟΙΧΕΙΑ, 2), Leipzig/Berlin, 1916.

Phillips, E. D., Aspects of Greek medicine, London, 1973.

Phillips, Joanne H., Early Greek medicine and the poetry of Solon, Clio Medica 15 (1980), 1–4.

–, The Hippocratic physician and ἈΣΤΡΟΝΟΜΊΗ, in: Formes de pensée 427–434.

–, On Varro's *animalia quaedam minuta* and etiology of disease, Transactions and Studies of the College of Physicians of Philadelphia (Ser. 5) 4 (1982), 12–25.

Poeppel, Ottokar, Die hippokratische Schrift Κῳακαὶ προγνώσεις und ihre Überlieferung, Kiel, 1959 (doctoral thesis, unpublished typescript).

Pohlenz, Max, Hippokrates und die Begründung der wissenschaftlichen Medizin, Berlin, 1938.

Poland, Franz, Geschichte des griechischen Vereinswesens (Preisschriften ... der Fürstlich Jablonowskischen Gesellschaft, 38), Leipzig, 1909.

Preiser, Gert, Allgemeine Krankheitsbezeichnungen im Corpus Hippocraticum. Gebrauch und Bedeutung von Nousos und Nosema (Ars medica, II 5), Berlin, 1976.

Realencyclopädie (see in this bibliography under: Pauly/Wissowa).

Regenbogen, Otto, Eine Forschungsmethode antiker Naturwissenschaft, Quellen und Studien zur Geschichte der Mathematik I 2, Berlin, 1930, 131–182 (= Kleine Schriften, München, 1961, 141–194).

Roscher, Wilhelm H., Die enneadischen und hebdomadischen Fristen und Wochen der ältesten Griechen. Ein Beitrag zur vergleichenden Chronologie und Zahlenmystik (Abhandlungen der philol.-histor. Klasse der Königl. Sächsischen Gesellschaft der Wissenschaften, vol. 21, no. 4), Leipzig, 1903.

–, Die Sieben- und Neunzahl im Kultus und Mythus der Griechen (*ibid.* vol. 24, no. 1), Leipzig, 1904.

–, Die Hebdomadenlehren der griechischen Philosophen und Ärzte. Ein Beitrag zur Geschichte der griechischen Philosophie und Medizin (*ibid.* vol. 24, no. 6), Leipzig, 1906.

—, Enneadische Studien. Versuch einer Geschichte der Neunzahl bei den Griechen, mit besonderer Berücksichtigung des älteren Epos, der Philosophen und Ärzte (*ibid.* vol. 26, no. 1), Leipzig, 1907.
—, Über Alter, Ursprung und Bedeutung der hippokratischen Schrift von der Siebenzahl. Ein Beitrag zur Geschichte der ältesten griechischen Philosophie und Prosaliteratur (*ibid.* vol. 28, no. 5), Leipzig, 1911.
—, Die Tessarakontaden und Tessarakontadenlehren der Griechen und anderer Völker. Ein Beitrag zur vergleichenden Religionswissenschaft, Volkskunde und Zahlenmystik sowie zur Geschichte der Medizin und Biologie (Berichte der philol.-histor. Klasse der Königl. Sächsischen Gesellschaft der Wissenschaften zu Leipzig, vol. 61, fasc. 2 [1909]).
—, (ed.), Ausführliches Lexikon der griechischen und römischen Mythologie, 6 vols, Leipzig/ Berlin, 1884—1937.
Scarborough, John, Theoretical assumptions in Hippocratic pharmacology, in: Formes de pensée 307—325.
Schmalzriedt, Egidius, ΠΕΡΙ ΦΥΣΕΩΣ. Zur Frühgeschichte der Buchtitel, München, 1970.
Scholia in Hippocratem et Galenum ed. Dietz, Fridericus R., vols 1—2, Regimontii Prussorum, 1834 (= repr. Amsterdam, 1966).
Schöner, Erich, Das Viererschema in der antiken Humoralpathologie (Sudhoffs Archiv, Beihefte, 4), Wiesbaden, 1964.
Schumacher, Joseph, Antike Medizin. Die naturphilosophischen Grundlagen der Medizin in der griechischen Antike, 2nd ed., Berlin, 1963.
Senfelder, Leopold, Die hippokratische Lehre von den Ausscheidungen und Ablagerungen, Wiener med. Wochenschr. 46 (1896), nos. 21—47; the instalments begin on pp. 925, 983, 1029, 1083, 1125, 1175, 1221, 1269, 1309, 1625, 1655, 1707, 1831, 1873, 1921, 1971, 2015, 2055.
Senn, Gustav, Über Herkunft und Stil der Beschreibungen von Experimenten im Corpus Hippocraticum, Sudhoffs Archiv 22 (1929), 217—289.
Sherwin-White, Susan M., Ancient Cos. An historical study from the Dorian settlement to the imperial period (Hypomnemata, 51), Göttingen, 1978.
Smith, Wesley D., Analytical and catalogue structure in the Corpus Hippocraticum, in: Formes de pensée 277—284.
—, Galen on Coans versus Cnidians, Bull. of the Hist. of Med. 47 (1973), 569—585.
—, Physiology in the Homeric poems, Transact. and Proceed. of the Amer. Philol. Assoc. 97 (1966), 547—556.
—, Implicit fever theory in Epidemics 5 and 7, Medical History, Suppl. 1, 1981, 1—18.
—, The Hippocratic tradition (Cornell Studies in the History of Science), Ithaca, N. Y., 1979.
Snell, Bruno, Die Entdeckung des Geistes, 5th ed., Göttingen, 1980.
Soranus, ed. Ilberg, Ioannes (Corpus Medicorum Graecorum, IV), Leipzig, 1927.
Spaet, Franz, Die geschichtliche Entwickelung der sogenannten hippokratischen Medicin im Lichte der neuesten Forschung, Berlin, 1897.
Steckerl, Fritz, The fragments of Praxagoras of Cos and his school (Philosophia antiqua, 8), Leiden, 1958.
Stückelberger, Alfred, Vestigia Democritea. Die Rezeption der Lehre von den Atomen in der antiken Naturwissenschaft und Medizin (Schweizerische Beiträge zur Altertumswiss., 17), Basel, 1984.
Sudhoff, Karl, Kos und Knidos (Münchener Beiträge zur Geschichte und Literatur der Naturwissenschaften und Medizin, 4/5), München, 1927.
—, Zur Geschichte der Lehre von den kritischen Tagen im Krankheitsverlaufe (1901), Sudhoffs Archiv 21 (1929), 1—22.
Temkin, Owsei, Greek medicine as science and craft, Isis 44 (1953), 213—225 (German transl. in: Flashar [ed.], Antike Medizin 1—28).
—, The falling sickness: A history of epilepsy from the Greeks to the beginnings of modern neurology, 2nd ed., Baltimore/London, 1971.

—, Der systematische Zusammenhang im Corpus Hippocraticum, Leipzig, 1928 (doctoral thesis; repr. from: Kyklos. Jahrbuch des Instituts für Geschichte der Medizin an der Universität Leipzig 1 [1928]).
Theiler, Willy, Zur Geschichte der teleologischen Naturbetrachtung bis auf Aristoteles, 2nd ed., Berlin, 1965.
—, Poseidonios. Die Fragmente, vols 1—2, Berlin/New York, 1982.
Thivel, Antoine, Cnide et Cos? Essai sur les doctrines médicales dans la Collection hippocratique (Publications de la Faculté des lettres et des sciences humaines de Nice, 21), Paris, 1981. — There exists a parallel, almost identical edition with different pagination (reproduction of the typescript): *Idem*, Cnide et Cos? (Thèse présentée devant l'Université de Paris IV le 18 juin 1977), Lille, 1981. Quotations refer to the first-named edition.
Vintró, Eulalia, Hipócrates y la nosología hipocrática (Colección "Convivium," 14), Barcelona, 1972.
Vogel, Claus, Zur Entstehung der hippokratischen Viersäftelehre, Marburg, 1956 (doctoral thesis, unpublished typescript).
Wellmann, Max, Die Fragmente der sikelischen Ärzte Akron, Philistion und des Diokles von Karystos, Berlin, 1901.
Wenskus, Otta, Vergleich und Beweis im hippokratischen Corpus, in: Formes de pensée 393—406.
Wittern, Renate, Zur Krankheitserkennung in der knidischen Schrift "De internis affectionibus," in: Medizinische Diagnostik in Geschichte und Gegenwart. Festschrift für Heinz Goerke, München, 1978, 101—119.
Zink, Norbert, Griechische Ausdrucksweisen für warm und kalt im seelischen Bereich, Heidelberg, 1962 (doctoral thesis, Mainz).

Addendum

It was only after the text of this book was completed that the author obtained the facilities for using the recently published CD ROM, version "C," of the Thesaurus Linguae Graecae (University of California, Irvine). The vast computer-readable and thus lexicographically accessible text corpus stored on this compact disk, which in fact comprises most of ancient Greek literature, could not, therefore, be exploited here except for a few supplementary references. Since the author's equipment was not yet capable of searching the entire disk in a single run, Wesley D. Smith (Philadelphia) very kindly did this on an Ibycus machine for *melágkholos*, an adjective that must have been important in the early history of the concept of black bile (cf. above, p. 46—50). In addition to the abovementioned — intentionally obscure — passage in Sophocles, *Trachiniae* 573, Smith found four references. They all confirm the author's hypothesis about the semantic field of *melágkholos*. Three of them occur in scholia on Aristotle, *Rhet. III* 1408 b 4—10. In an anonymous commentary, which appears to have been compiled in the twelfth century out of "varia variorum scholia," Aristotle's precepts to the orator are interpreted thus: "If your words are harsh, you must pronounce them in a low, not a wild voice, and must show a friendly countenance and look mild. The effect will be that the harsh content of your words is concealed by your low voice and your friendly face, and you do not make the impression of being *melágkholos* and harsh ... If, on the other hand, your words are harsh and you pronounce them in a wild voice, showing a grim face, it becomes only too obvious that you are *melágkholos* and a liar and aggressive with someone whom you are doing injustice." (Εἰ μὲν αἱ λέξεις εἰσὶν ὑβριστικαί, δεῖ σε ταύτας ἐκφέρειν μετὰ φωνῆς ὑφειμένης καὶ μὴ ἀγρίας καὶ πρόσωπον ἔχειν ἱλαρὸν καὶ βλέμμα πρᾶον, ἵνα τὸ τῶν λέξεων τραχὺ συγκαλύπτηται διὰ τῆς ὑφειμένης φωνῆς καὶ τοῦ ἱλαροῦ προσώπου, καὶ μὴ φαίνῃ μελάγχολος καὶ ὑβριστικός ... Εἰ δὲ καὶ αἱ λέξεις εἰσὶ τραχεῖαι καὶ ἐκφέρεις ταύτας μετὰ φωνῆς ἀγρίας καὶ πρόσωπον ἐνδείκνυσαι ἄγριον, φανερὸν γίνεται ὅτι μελάγχολος εἶ καὶ ψευδὴς καὶ ἐπίκεισαί τῳ, ὃν ἀδικεῖς. Anonymi et Stephani In artem rhetoricam commentaria, ed. Hugo Rabe, Berlin, 1896 [= Commentaria in Aristotelem Graeca XXI 2], p. 188. For the date see *ibid.* p. IX f.)

The other compilation of scholia (Ἕτερα σχόλια τοῦ Κυροῦ Στεφάνου), which is equally late Byzantine, has the following interpretation of Aristotle's text: "Above, Aristotle said: 'You should pronounce words, which are harsh against someone, in a friendly manner.' Now somebody might say: 'Well, should I then also pronounce mild and friendly words in the opposite manner,' i. e. in a harsh and angry voice? The philosopher gives the solution: 'No,' he says, 'because you would make the impression of being *melágkholos* and inconsistent.' Thus, he gives the advice not to be harsh even if the words are harsh; but if the words are friendly, you should pronounce them all the more friendly." (Εἶπε γὰρ ἀνώτερον ὅτι "τὰ ὑβριστικὰ κατά τινος ῥήματα ἀπάγγελλε κἂν ἱλαρῶς"· εἶτα εἶπεν ἴσως ἄν τις· "καὶ λοιπὸν ἄρα γε καὶ τὰ μαλακὰ καὶ προσηνῆ ῥήματα ἀπαγγελῶ ἐναντίως", ἤγουν τραχείᾳ καὶ ὀργίλῳ τῇ ἐκφωνήσει; λύει οὖν τὸν λόγον ὁ φιλόσοφος· "οὐχί", φησί, "μελάγχολος γὰρ καὶ ἀνακόλουθος ὀφθήσῃ." παρακαλεῖ οὖν τὸν ἄνθρωπον μὴ εἶναι τραχύν, κἂν καὶ τὰ ὀνόματα ᾖ τραχέα· εἰ δὲ τὰ ὀνόματα ᾖ προσηνῆ, πολλῷ μᾶλλον καὶ προσηνῶς ταῦτα ἐκφωνήσεις. *Ibid.* p. 317. For the date, see p. XIII.)

In these two scholia, which might ultimately be derived from one and the same ancient source, the adjective *melágkholos* has quite obviously nothing to do with any medical humour, but has a semantic field which can be outlined by such words as *harsh, wild, liar, aggressive, unjust, angry, inconsistent* (ὑβριστικός, ἄγριος, ψευδής, ἐπίκειμαι, ἀδικέω, ὀργίλος, ἀνακόλουθος, quoted in the order as they occur in both texts).

The fourth additional occurrence of *melágkholos* is clearly medical. It is from an undated anonymous treatise *On foodstuffs* (*De alimentis,* ed. J. L. Ideler, Physici et medici Graeci minores, vol. 2, Berlin, 1842, p. 278), whose language betrays the Byzantine period, but whose substance is much older. In the chapter *On entrails,* it states: "The liver of all animals has thick humours, is hard to digest, and passes slowly. Better than all other liver is that of pork, except that it has peccant humour and is *melágkholos.* The spleen causes black-biled blood and is harmful. The lung is easier to digest, because it is spongy ..." (Τὸ ἧπαρ ἁπάντων τῶν ζῴων παχύχυμόν τε καὶ δύσπεπτον καὶ βραδύπορον. Κάλλιον δὲ παρὰ πᾶσι τὸ τοῦ χοίρου, πλὴν δὲ κακόχυμον καὶ μελάγχολον. Ὁ δὲ σπλὴν μελαγχολικοῦ γεννητικός ἐστι αἵματος καὶ βλαπτικός. Εὐπεπτότερος δὲ ὁ πνεύμων ὡς χαῦνος ...) Parallel versions of this passage and its context are transmitted in Galen, *De aliment. facult. III* 11 (= p. 343 f. ed. G. Helmreich, CMG V 4.2); Oribas. *Coll. med. II* 39 (= p. 39 f. ed. J. Raeder, CMG VI 1.1); and in Aetius *II* 128 (= p. 199 f. ed. A. Olivieri, CMG VIII 1). Both Oribasius and Aetius claim to be dependent on Galen (cf. the editions by Raeder, p. 28.2, and by Olivieri, p. 196.26). Neither they nor their source, Galen, have the word *melágkholos*. It remains to be investigated whether the anonymous treatise originates in a source independent of, and earlier than, Galen.

The meaning of *melágkholos* is not quite clear in the medical Anonymus. Probably *melágkholos* does not denote the same as *melagkholikós*, an adjective that is terminological and occurs only four words later. While *melagkholikós* here obviously presupposes the medical doctrine about the humour black bile, *melágkholos* may still have preserved a broader meaning even in the medical context of the Anonymus. In any case, the passage exemplifies how *melágkholos* was liable to being reinterpreted in terms of humoral theory.

With regard to the word *mélās* (or *mélaina*; *melag-* in the compounds mentioned above, p. 46–50), the following additional remarks have to be made. Although the adjective is usually, and more or less correctly so, translated as 'black,' a preciser description of its semantic field will prove relevant for reconstructing the early history of black bile, as was pointed out to the author by William Beck, whose article μέλας will appear in the "Lexikon des frühgriechischen Epos."

Any Greek dictionary specifies that *mélās* means also 'dark.' At first sight, this seems to be trivial because 'black' and 'dark' are interchangeable in many contexts and languages. But Greek has a peculiarity. Already in the earliest texts, *mélās* is not infrequently used to denote relatively light hues. Eleanor Irwin (Colour terms in Greek poetry, Toronto, 1974, 111; see her chapters 4 and 5) states, for instance, that men and women, who, to our eyes, do not differ extremely in skin colour are described as "dark" (*mélās*) and "light" (*leukós*) respectively. This 'relational' usage of *mélās* was common still in the fifth and fourth centuries and later. One might, therefore, surmise that not necessarily only deep dark or almost black colours of bodily phenomena were interpreted in terms of a humour 'black bile,' but that also *slightly*, or *relatively* darkish hues of excretions etc., which might even have been rather light in colour, could be called *mélās*. The concept of black bile may thus, at least originally, have been applicable to a large number of phenomena.

Index of Passages

General Index

UNTERSUCHUNGEN ZUR ANTIKEN LITERATUR UND GESCHICHTE

JOACHIM DINGEL

Scholastica materia

Untersuchungen zu den Declamationes minores und der Institutio oratoria Quintilians

Groß-Oktav. XII, 186 Seiten. 1988. Ganzleinen DM 108,– ISBN 3 11 011462 3 (Band 30)

THEO HIRSCHBERG

Senecas Phoenissen

— Einleitung und Kommentar —

Groß-Oktav. VIII, 169 Seiten. 1989. Ganzleinen DM 92,– ISBN 3 11 011630 8 (Band 31)

MICHAEL HILLEN

Studien zur Dichtersprache Senecas: Abundanz — Explikativer Ablativ — Hypallage

Groß-Oktav. XII, 345 Seiten. 1989. Ganzleinen DM 176,– ISBN 3 11 011798 3 (Band 32)

HARTMUT ERBSE

Thukydides — Interpretationen

Groß-Oktav. XIII, 192 Seiten. 1989. Ganzleinen DM 98,– ISBN 3 11 012126 3 (Band 33)

EVELINE KRUMMEN

Pyrsos Hymnon

Festliche Gegenwart und mythisch-rituelle Tradition als Voraussetzung einer Pindarinterpretation (Isthmie 4, Pythie 5, Olympie 1 und 3)

Groß-Oktav. X, 291 Seiten. 1990. Ganzleinen DM 158,– ISBN 3 11 012231 6 (Band 35)

Preisänderungen vorbehalten

Walter de Gruyter · Berlin · New York

Bei Fragen zur Produktsicherheit wenden Sie sich bitte an:
If you have any questions regarding product safety,
please contact:

Walter de Gruyter GmbH
Genthiner Straße 13
10785 Berlin
productsafety@degruyterbrill.com